38.00

D0256954

HORMONAL FUNCTION AND THE KIDNEY

CONTEMPORARY ISSUES
IN NEPHROLOGY
VOL. 4

Series Editors
BARRY M. BRENNER MD
JAY H. STEIN MD

Published 1978
Vol. 1 Sodium and Water Homeostasis
Vol. 2 Acid-Base and Potassium Homeostasis

Published 1979
Vol. 3 Immunologic Mechanisms of Renal Disease
  Curtis B. Wilson MD, Guest Editor

Forthcoming volumes in series

Vol. 5 Nephrolithiasis
  Fredric L. Coe MD, Guest Editor
Vol. 6 Acute Renal Failure

HORMONAL FUNCTION AND THE KIDNEY

Edited by **Barry M. Brenner, M.D.**

Samuel A. Levine Professor of Medicine, Harvard Medical
School; Director, Renal Division and Laboratory of Kidney
and Electrolyte Physiology, Peter Bent Brigham Hospital,
Boston, Massachusetts

and **Jay H. Stein, M.D.**

Professor and Chairman, Department of Medicine and
Director, Division of Renal Diseases, The University of
Texas Health Science Center at San Antonio, San Antonio,
Texas

CHURCHILL LIVINGSTONE
NEW YORK, EDINBURGH AND LONDON 1979

Distributed in the United Kingdom by Churchill Livingstone,
Robert Stevenson House, 1-3 Baxter's Place, Leith Walk,
Edinburgh EH1 3AF and by associated companies, branches
and representatives throughout the world.

First published 1979
Printed in U.S.A.

ISBN 0-443-08039-9

Library of Congress Cataloging in Publication Data

Main entry under title:
Hormonal function and the kidney.
    (Contemporary issues in nephrology; 4)
    Bibliography: p.
    Includes index.
    1. Kidneys. 2. Hormones. 3. Kidneys—Diseases.
I. Brenner, Barry M., 1937–   II.   Stein, Jay H.,
1937–   III. Series. [DNLM: 1. Kidney—Metabolism.
2. Kidney—Drug effects. 3. Metabolism.
W1 C0769MR v. 4 / WJ301 H812]
QP249.H67   612'.463   79–19204
ISBN 0-443-08039-9

Manufactured in the United States of America

Preface

This volume of Contemporary Issues in Nephrology summarizes the recent explosion of knowledge concerning the major hormones that directly or indirectly affect renal function. As with the other volumes in this series, each of the chapters herein is structured to correlate basic physiological and clinical concepts.

In the initial chapter, Schambelan and Stockigt review the various factors known to regulate the renin-angiotensin system and consider the disease entities associated with abnormalities of this important hormonal axis. They also discuss the clinical utility of plasma renin measurements, the effects of various drugs such as diuretics, vasodilators and beta-adrenergic blockers on plasma renin activity, and the usefulness of renin determinations in the diagnosis of hypertension due to renal arterial disease.

In the next chapter, Hollenberg summarizes the current status of the use of angiotensin antagonists in clinical medicine. He describes the pharmacological properties of the beta-adrenergic blocking agents, the converting enzyme inhibitors and the receptor antagonists. He then considers the usefulness of these agents in the treatment of hypertension, in the elucidation of the pathogenesis of various forms of hypertension, and in defining the effects of angiotensin on renal hemodynamics.

The following two chapters review the biochemistry, pharmacology and renal actions of the prostaglandins. Morrison and Needleman provide a lucid review of the biochemistry, metabolism and pharmacology of the renal prostaglandins. Dunn then goes on to explore the possible influences of the various prostaglandins on the regulation of the renin-angiotensin system, and on the control of renal blood flow and sodium and water excretion. He also provides a timely summary of the role of these lipids in the pathogenesis and pathophysiology of hypertension. While each of these areas remains controversial, the reader will find that these chapters provide an objective and balanced summary of our current knowledge in these important areas.

In the fifth chapter, Margolius and Buse describe the renal kallikrein-kinin system. They initially evaluate the biochemical pathways of this important system and then examine the evidence for a role of the kinins in the regulation of renal hemodynamics, sodium excretion, and arterial blood pressure. As with the prostaglandins, the kinin-kallikrein system is an area of renal endocrinology in which major advances have been made in recent years, and the reader is certain to find this chapter both timely and comprehensive.

In Chapter six, Weitzman evaluates the factors regulating the secretion and metabolism of antidiuretic hormone. Since the original observations of Verney, a variety of factors have been found to influence both the release and the metabolism of this important hormone, and these factors are reviewed in lucid fashion. Dr. Weitzman also considers the role of left atrial and carotid sinus baroreceptors as well as the effects of extracellular fluid volume, the renin-angiotensin system, and other stimuli in modulating the secretion and metabolism of vasopressin.

Slatopolsky and his associates then describe the physiologic and metabolic actions of parathyroid hormone. The initial portion of the chapter is concerned with an evaluation of the various factors which govern the synthesis, release and metabolism of this hormone. In the later portions of the chapter the authors consider the effects of PTH on the excretion of calcium, phosphorus, magnesium, bicarbonate and sodium. Lastly, the authors provide a splendid summary of the various disease states associated with an excess or deficiency of parathyroid hormone.

In Chapter eight, Berl and Better evaluate the effects of prolactin, estrogen and progesterone on renal function. The authors examine the controversial evidence in favor of a role for prolactin in renal water excretion. The authors suggest that the antinatriuretic effects of estrogen are due to an intricate hormonal balance involving progesterone and possibly aldosterone. The relationship of this interaction to contraceptive-associated hypertension is also considered.

Levine and Coburn review the biochemistry, mechanism of action and clinical disorders associated with abnormalities of vitamin D metabolism. Here again is an area in which there has been an enormous increase in knowledge in recent years. The authors admirably summarize this new information and describe the factors regulating the production of the active sterol, 1,25 dihydroxycholecalciferol, and consider its actions on bone and kidney.

In the final chapter Dousa reviews the basic features of the renal cyclic nucleotide system and examines the pivotal position played by cyclic nucleotides in the actions of parathyroid hormone, calcitonin, vitamin D, vasopressin, thyroid, and adrenal hormones.

In keeping with the theme of this series, the present volume aims to provide a contemporary and comprehensive overview of the role of various hormones of importance to nephrologists. Emphasis has again been placed on integrating pathogenesis, pathophysiology and practical concepts of diagnosis and management. To this end, the Editors are deeply appreciative of the cooperation and enthusiasm displayed by the authors in preparing the splendid material for this volume.

1979   J.H.S.
                                                                                                                    B.M.B.

Contributors

TOMAS BERL, M.D.
Associate Professor of Medicine, University of Colorado Medical Center, Denver, Colorado

ORI S. BETTER, M.D.
Professor of Medicine, Head, Department of Nephrology, Aba Khoushy School of Medicine, Haifa, Israel

JOHN B. BUSE, A.B.
Student Research Associate, Department of Pharmacology, Medical University of South Carolina, Charleston, South Carolina

JACK W. COBURN, M.D.
Chief, Nephrology Section, Veterans Administration Wadsworth Medical Center; Professor of Medicine, University of California, Los Angeles, School of Medicine, Los Angeles, California

THOMAS P. DOUSA, M.D., Ph.D.
Consultant in Physiology and Medicine, Mayo Clinic and Foundation; Professor of Medicine and Physiology, Mayo Medical School, Department of Physiology and Biophysics, and Department of Medicine (Division of Nephrology), Mayo Clinic and Foundation, Rochester, Minnesota

MICHAEL J. DUNN, M.D.
Hanna Payne Professor of Experimental Medicine, Director, Division of Nephrology, Department of Medicine, University Hospitals, Cleveland, Ohio

JEFFREY FREITAG, M.D.
Post-Doctoral Fellow, National Kidney Foundation, Washington University, School of Medicine, St. Louis, Missouri

NORMAN K. HOLLENBERG, M.D., Ph.D.
Professor of Radiology and Medicine, Departments of Medicine and Radiology, Harvard Medical School, Peter Bent Brigham Hospital, Boston, Massachusetts

KEITH HRUSKA, M.D.
Assistant Professor of Medicine, Washington University, School of Medicine, St. Louis, Missouri

BARTON S. LEVINE, M.D.
Associate Investigator, Veterans Administration Wadsworth Medical Center; Assistant Professor of Medicine, University of California, Los Angeles, School of Medicine, Los Angeles, California

HARRY S. MARGOLIUS, M.D., Ph.D.
Professor of Pharmacology, Associate Professor of Medicine, Departments of Pharmacology and Medicine, Medical University of South Carolina, Charleston, South Carolina

AUBREY R. MORRISON, M.D.
Assistant Professor of Medicine and Pharmacology, Washington University School of Medicine, St. Louis, Missouri

KEITH MARTIN, M.D.
Assistant Professor of Medicine, Washington University School of Medicine, St. Louis, Missouri

PHILIP NEEDLEMAN, Ph.D.
Professor and Chairman, Department of Pharmacology, Washington University School of Medicine, St. Louis, Missouri

EDUARDO SLATOPOLSKY, M.D.
Professor of Medicine, Director, Chromalloy American Kidney Center, Washington University School of Medicine, St. Louis, Missouri

JAN R. STOCKIGT, M.D.
Director, Ewen Downie Metabolic Unit, Alfred Hospital; Honorary Senior Lecturer, Monash University, Department of Medicine, Melbourne, Australia

MORRIS SCHAMBELAN, M.D.
Associate Professor of Medicine, University of California, San Francisco; Assistant Director, Clinical Study Center, San Francisco General Hospital Medical Center, San Francisco, California

RICHARD E. WEITZMAN, M.D.
Assistant Professor of Medicine, University of California, Los Angeles, School of Medicine, Los Angeles, California; Director of Hypertension Services, Division of Nephrology and Hypertension, Harbor-UCLA Medical Center, Torrance, California

Contents

1

Pathophysiology of the renin-angiotensin system

MORRIS SCHAMBELAN
JAN R. STOCKIGT

INTRODUCTION

In 1898 Tigerstedt and Bergman identified and gave the name renin to a component of crude kidney extract that was shown to increase blood pressure, but their finding attracted little interest until 1934, when Goldblatt and his associates reported that an increase in renin secretion and hypertension resulted from renal ischemia in dogs. Since then, studies of this humoral factor have assumed enormous importance in investigations of the pathogenesis of hypertension and of the role of the kidney in the regulation of fluid and electrolyte balance.

Renin, the structure of which is still unknown, is a glycoprotein enzyme that acts on an α_2-globulin substrate in plasma to release angiotensin I. Removal of two C-terminal amino acids from this decapeptide, predominantly in the pulmonary circulation, leads to formation of the octapeptide angiotensin II, which is both a potent pressor substance and a specific stimulus to aldosterone biosynthesis by the adrenal zona glomerulosa. A simplified outline of the renin-angiotensin-aldosterone system is shown in Figure 1.1. Although renin is usually regarded as a hormone, it is probably more correct to regard renin substrate (angiotensinogen) as a prohormone and renin as a specific protease. The main control points in this cycle involve regulation of renin release, alteration of pressor and adrenal sensitivity to angiotensin II, changes in aldosterone secretion and renal sodium reabsorption, and ultimately negative feedback on renin release. These control points identify the components of the system that are most frequently abnormal in disease states, sometimes as primary abnormalities but more often as secondary responses.

Because of the intimate relationships of the renin-angiotensin system with adrenal mineralocorticoid hormones, extracellular fluid volume, and arterial blood pressure, it has become obvious that the functional state of this system can be best evaluated in relation to "effective" blood volume, a term used by physiologists to refer to the relationship between vascular capacity and "fullness" rather than plasma or extracellular fluid volume per se. Because no technique has yet been developed for quantitating effective volume, an estimate for this factor based on clinical assessment is essential in evaluating a particular level of renin.

In clinical settings in which hyperreninemia occurs in association with reduced effective volume, arterial blood pressure is generally within the normal range. When renin secretion is increased or is inappropriately high with a normal effective blood volume, hypertension is a common occurrence. In some patients with renal hypertension, plasma renin levels are in the range usually regarded as normal, but an abnormal relationship between the state of sodium balance and the prevailing level of renin is often invoked to account for the occurrence of hypertension.

When effective blood volume is expanded, as in states of primary mineralocorticoid excess or in association with impaired renal sodium excretion, renin secretion is suppressed. When hypertension occurs in this setting, volume expansion, decreased vascular compliance, and increased vascular sensitivity to angiotensin may each be important. However, because suppression of plasma renin levels in patients with hypertension is an ambiguous finding that may relate to deficient sympathetic function as well as to volume expansion, this finding cannot be considered a specific index of mineralocorticoid excess. Reduced renin secretion can also occur without hypertension as a primary abnor-

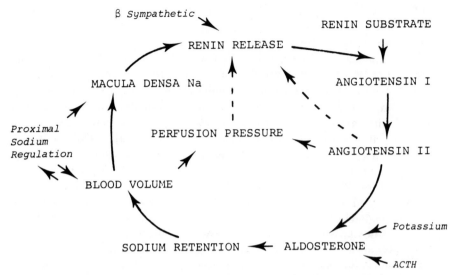

Figure 1.1   Schematic representation of the renin-angiotensin-aldosterone system.

mality of juxtaglomerular cell function with resultant decreased aldosterone secretion. Particularly when associated with chronic renal disease, this abnormality may disturb potassium and acid-base balance.

Thus, it is evident that the pathophysiologic significance of a particular level of plasma renin cannot be interpreted without consideration of its interaction with effective blood volume, autonomic function, steroid hormones, electrolyte balance, and blood pressure. In this chapter we will review certain biochemical features of the renin-angiotensin system, the factors that control the secretion of renin, and the evidence that supports a role for renin in normal physiology as well as in a variety of pathophysiologic states. With this background, we will then consider the role of renin measurements in clinical diagnosis.

COMPONENTS OF THE RENIN-ANGIOTENSIN SYSTEM

It is generally thought that the renin-angiotensin system has five discrete components: renin, renin substrate, angiotensin I, converting enzyme, and angiotensin II. This is probably an oversimplification in view of recent evidence that both renin and its substrate are heterogeneous. Furthermore, it is now apparent than the C-terminal heptapeptide of angiotensin II also has biologic activity. In the following sections, some of these recent advances in our understanding of the components of the renin-angiotensin system will be reviewed briefly. More comprehensive reviews of the biochemistry of this system are available (Oparil and Haber, 1974; Reid, Morris, and Ganong, 1978).

Renin

Renin has been identified in a number of molecular forms. Inagami et al. (1977) have suggested that the large form (MW > 50,000) is the native intrarenal enzyme that is converted by a sulfhydryl-containing enzyme to the circulating form (MW ~ 45,000). A number of investigators have described high molecular weight components in plasma or amniotic fluid that are inactive at physiologic pH but become active after exposure to acid pH or to acid proteases (Day, Leutscher, and Gonzales, 1975; Reid et al., 1978). Acid-activated renin may be related to the cryoactivatable prorenin described by Sealey et al. (1977).

An abnormal inactive form of renin ("big" renin) has been found in the plasma of patients with diabetes mellitus and in association with some renal tumors (Day et al., 1975). In the diabetic patients it has been suggested that failure of renin activation could be a cause of renin deficiency. It is possible that intrarenal modification of renin is a control point in the system, because Derkx et al. (1976) found that stimuli to renin release, such as isoprenaline, upright tilt, or diazoxide, increases active plasma renin and decreases the inactive form. This possibility was supported by Atlas et al. (1977), who found that beta-blockade with propranolol reduces the proportion of enzyme released in active form. The transition from inactive to active forms of renin is reversible in vitro and may be related to dissociation from an inhibitor protein (Skeggs et al., 1977).

Angiotensin-generating activity has been demonstrated in the plasma of anephric subjects, but a large portion of this activity is in the precursor form, suggesting that such renin activity may result from inadvertent activation of prorenin by cold or acid (Sealey et al., 1977). A salivary reninlike enzyme with a molecular weight of 61,000 has been found in anephric subjects (Weinberger et al., 1977), and this may be a source of circulating prorenin.

Without knowledge of its structure, a definition of renin is based mainly on its ability to produce angiotensin, but other acid proteases, such as pepsin or cathepsin D, may easily be misclassified as renin. They may produce angiotensin from natural substrate at an unphysiologic pH (Morris, 1978), or they may show a high affinity for synthetic renin-substrate fragments, while being inactive against the larger more complex natural substrate (Skeggs et al., 1977). This is a major problem when synthetic substrate fragments are used in enzyme purification by affinity chromotography, which has led Haber and Slater (1977) to emphasize that strict specificity for angiotensinogen and lack of general proteolytic activity must be demonstrated before an enzyme can be accepted as genuine renin. Nonspecific acid proteases may also be misclassified because they can convert inactive to active renin (Morris, 1978), thus giving a false impression of intrinsic activity.

There has been extensive interest in the possibility that some extrarenal tissues may contain a discrete renin-angiotensin system, but the problem of exactly which proteolytic enzymes should be called renin remains unresolved.

This dilemma is outside the scope of this chapter, but some extensive recent reviews are available (Ganten et al., 1976; Reid, 1977a).

Renin substrate

Although the amount of active renin in the circulation is clearly the major determinant of angiotensin formation, the amount of substrate is also rate limiting. The normal substrate concentration in human plasma has been estimated as approximately equal to or less than the K_m value (Krakoff, 1973; Skinner et al., 1975). (The K_m value is the substrate level at which the reaction rate is half maximal.) Because substrate levels generally influence a reaction rate until a value at least fivefold in excess of K_m is reached, increases or decreases in substrate are obviously important in determining the rate of angiotensin formation.

Renin substrate is a hepatic glycoprotein of molecular weight 50,000–110,-000, but much smaller fragments, such as the synthetic N-terminal tetradecapeptide, can yield angiotensin I. However, many of the smaller substrates can be split by nonspecific proteases, and the large glycoprotein residue appears to be necessary to avoid nonspecific angiotensin formation. It has been shown that natural renin substrate in plasma is heterogeneous (Lentz et al., 1978), but it is uncertain whether the components are physiologically different or not.

The amount of renin substrate in plasma is increased by glucocorticoid or estrogen excess (Krakoff and Eisenfeld, 1977) and is decreased with glucocorticoid deficiency (Reid et al., 1973). The level increases after nephrectomy, presumably because of diminished utilization, but substrate does not become depleted when renin excess leads to increased utilization. Angiotensin II appears to be the factor that prevents substrate depletion when renin levels are high (Beaty et al., 1976). This effect has been subsequently shown to be abolished by adrenalectomy (Reid, 1977b), confirming the critical role of adrenal steroids in preventing substrate depletion. The clinical significance of these observations has been demonstrated in patients with untreated Addison's disease in whom severe substrate depletion due to glucocorticoid deficiency greatly impaired the effectiveness of circulating renin (Stockigt et al., 1979).

Renin substrate can be measured directly by incubation of diluted plasma with excess renin. The results, expressed in terms of standard angiotensin I formed by complete exhaustion of substrate, give an angiotensin-generating capacity of about 1000 ng/ml in normal subjects (Krakoff, 1973). About one-eighth of this capacity is probably used and replenished each day in active subjects during normal sodium intake.

Angiotensin-converting enzyme

Angiotensin-converting enzyme is a large zinc-containing glycoprotein that is found in the surface membrane of the vascular endothelial cells of the lung, in the brush borders of the proximal renal tubule, in the endothelium of vascular beds, and in plasma (Erdös, 1977). This enzyme removes two C-terminal amino acids from a number of peptide substrates and has been classified as a peptidyl dipeptide hydrolase. Its two most important actions are the inactivation of bradykinin and activation of angiotensin I. However, angiotensin II is resistant to this enzyme and passes through the lung without modification, probably because the enzyme fails to cleave a peptide bond proximate to proline (Erdös, 1977).

The serum level of angiotensin-converting enzyme has been found to be elevated in patients with active sarcoidosis (Lieberman, 1975) and has also been considered as a possible marker of acute lung injury (Barber, Lindauer, and Eger, 1975). The clinical importance of these observations has not been clearly established.

Angiotensin I, II, and III

Numerous direct assays of circulating angiotensin I and II have been described, but the values usually follow renin activity closely and rarely provide additional information. Fragments of angiotensin II lacking up to three N-terminal amino acids are highly reactive in many angiotensin II assays, so that immunologic activity should not be equated with biologic activity. However, it now appears that the heptapeptide, [des-Aspartyl[1]]-angiotensin II (angiotensin III), may have important biologic actions (Freeman et al., 1977). Native angiotensin II and its C-terminal heptapeptide appear to compete for the same receptors in each tissue studied so far, but the receptor may vary in different tissues. Although angiotensin II has more than double the pressor effect of the heptapeptide, the two peptides show approximately equipotent negative effects on renal blood flow and renin release (Freeman, Davis, Lohmeier, 1975a). In contrast to its lower pressor potency, the heptapeptide appears to be more potent in its aldosterone-stimulating effect, and studies with heptapeptide antagonists have shown that adrenal receptors have a higher affinity for des[1] compounds (Freeman et al., 1977) than for angiotensin II. Although circulating levels of the heptapeptide are low, local generation in adrenal tissue was detected (Peach and Chiu, 1974). The view that [des-Aspartyl[1]]-angiotensin II is an important determinant of this system remains speculative, but it is no longer certain that angiotensin II is the sole active principle. The possibility of different angiotensin receptors in various tissues is supported by the divergent effects of sodium depletion on angiotensin responses in vascular and adrenal tissue (Hollenberg et al., 1974; Douglas and Catt, 1976).

REGULATION OF RENIN RELEASE

Renin is synthesized in the juxtaglomerular cells and stored as granules in these specialized myoepithelial cells, which are located in the wall of the afferent renal arteriole. It is released both into the bloodstream and into renal lymphatics in response to numerous stimuli acting on an intrarenal baroreceptor, a sodium sensor at the macula densa, or an intrarenal beta-adrenergic receptor. Many drugs influence renin release via one of these mechanisms, but several humoral agents—including sodium, potassium, and chloride ions; angiotensin II; and prostaglandins—may influence renin release directly.

Major regulatory influences

Baroreceptors
Renin release was initially shown by Skinner, McCubbin, and Page (1964) to be extremely sensitive to small changes in renal perfusion pressure, but in these studies the influence of changes in sympathetic function, macula densa sodium transport, or intrarenal distribution of blood flow was not rigorously controlled. Later studies of the denervated, nonfiltering kidney in adrenalectomized animals (Blaine, Davis, and Prewitt, 1971) clearly demonstrated a discrete vascular receptor, which appeared to respond to changes in transmural pressure gradient or afferent arteriolar wall tension (Davis and Freeman, 1976). Smooth muscle tone appears to be critical for this control mechanism, which can be abolished with papaverine (Witty et al., 1971). Hypotensive hemorrhage and acute renal artery constriction activate this pressure sensor, but it is not clear whether chronically diminished renal perfusion pressure acts by the same mechanism.

Macula densa
The macula densa, that segment of the distal nephron where the distal tubule makes tangential contact with the afferent arteriole just before this vessel enters the glomerulus, may participate in the regulation of renin release in response to variations in tubular fluid composition. However, a precise understanding of the role of the macula densa has been beset with difficulties. Two apparently irreconcilable views have been put forward: (1) that renin release is increased by *decreased* sodium load; and (2) that an *increased* macula densa sodium load activates renin secretion. Results of retrograde micropuncture injections of hypertonic saline into the distal tubule (Thurau et al., 1967) and the renin response to furosemide (Meyer et al., 1968) suggests that increased sodium load activates renin secretion. However, Freeman et al. (1974) found a decrease in renin release with the passage of sodium-rich fluid past the macula densa, which is in accordance with the original hypothesis of Vander and Miller (1964). A renin response to diminished distal tubular sodium load would be appropriate during sodium restriction, but an increase in renin release following excessive or abnormal proximal sodium loss might also be appropriate. Although this type of dual control remains a possibility, the balance of evidence favors the view that decreased sodium movement past, or sodium flux across, the macula densa is the more important stimulus to renin release (Davis and Freeman, 1976).

Autonomic nervous system
There is a wealth of data demonstrating an influence of the autonomic nervous system on renin release, either by humoral catecholamines or via the

renal nerves, an effect that is independent of the macula densa and vascular receptors (Johnson, Davis, and Witty, 1971). This mechanism of renin release is clearly important in the renin secretory response to upright posture, hypoglycemia, cold exposure, exercise, mild volume depletion, and peripheral vasodilatation (Davis and Freeman, 1976). The limitations of the autonomic influence on renin release are demonstrated by the fact that the response to nonhypotensive hemorrhage and mild sodium depletion can be blocked by renal denervation, whereas more extensive sodium depletion causes renin release from denervated kidneys (Gotshall et al., 1973). In humans, beta-blockade with propranolol has been shown to have little influence on the renin response to sodium restriction (Omvik, Enger, and Eide, 1976). Thus, it seems likely that the autonomic nervous system is only one of a number of afferent pathways regulating renin release rather than a final common pathway.

It is not at present clear whether stimulation of renin release involves $beta_1$ or $beta_2$ receptors because the effect of albuterol (salbutamol), a selective $beta_2$ agonist, can be blocked with metoprolol, a selective $beta_1$ blocker (Salvetti et al., 1978), suggesting that the beta receptors that mediate renin release in humans may not correspond to standard beta-subtypes. In contrast to the stimulatory effect of beta-adrenergic activity, an alpha-receptor mechanism appears to inhibit renin release (Pettinger et al., 1976).

The afferent limb of the autonomic pathway appears to involve the vagus nerve, which carries tonic inhibitory impulses from cardiopulmonary receptors. Interruption of vagal afferents by cooling increases renin release, an effect that can be blocked by renal denervation (Mancia, Romero and Shepard, 1975). In further studies of the interaction between cardiopulmonary and carotid baroreceptors, Thames, Jarecki, and Donald (1978) found that cardiopulmonary receptors responded to small decreases in blood volume to which arterial baroreceptors were insensitive. The renin response to vagotomy was smaller when carotid baroreceptors were intact, suggesting a dual tonic inhibitory effect. In contrast to these findings, Schrier et al. (1975) described an effect by which vagotomy during water diuresis decreased renin secretion and increased urine osmolality. Both effects were abolished by hypophysectomy, which led these investigators to suggest that increased vasopressin secretion in response to vagotomy may inhibit renin secretion in some circumstances.

Interaction of control mechanisms

Davis and Freeman (1976) have indicated how these three major control mechanisms might interact in response to varying degrees of hemorrhage or sodium depletion. Minor blood loss, without hypotension, probably increases renin secretion by a beta-adrenergic effect, both neural and humoral, but after blood pressure begins to fall, the renal baroreceptor is activated. They suggested further that with profound hypotension and failure of autoregulation of renal blood flow, the macula densa mechanism becomes increasingly important.

With sodium depletion it seems likely that decreased sodium delivery to the macula densa is the major influence on renin secretion, with an additional stimulus via renal vascular baroreceptors if perfusion pressure falls. With mild sodium depletion the sympathetic nervous component probably plays a relatively minor role, in contrast to its major importance in the response to changes in posture. The importance of central cardiovascular receptors is still difficult to define.

Other regulatory influences

Prostaglandins
Several lines of evidence suggest that renal prostaglandins can influence the release of renin. Direct infusion of PGE_1 into the renal artery has been reported to result in an increase in renal venous renin concentration in anesthetized dogs (Werning et al., 1971) and a similar effect has been seen with direct intrarenal infusion of arachidonic acid, a precursor for prostaglandin synthesis (Larsson, Weber, and Angaard, 1974). In humans intravenous infusion of PGA has been shown to increase both renin and aldosterone secretion (Golub et al., 1976), although it is not certain whether PGA occurs in vivo. That prostaglandins may act directly on the juxtaglomerular cells is suggested by in vitro studies using renal slices or cell suspensions (Weber et al., 1976; Dew and Michelakis, 1974). In these systems arachidonic acid, endoperoxidases, and PGE stimulate and $PGF_{2\alpha}$ inhibit renin secretion. These studies do not exclude a possible role for a hemodynamic mechanism in the mediation of the response of renin secretion to prostaglandins in vivo.

That renal prostaglandins may play a physiologic role in regulating renin secretion has been suggested by studies in which inhibitors of prostaglandin synthesis, such as indomethacin, abolished the renin response to hemorrhage in conscious rabbits (Romero, Dunlop, and Strong, 1976). Infusion of indomethacin in sodium-restricted, anesthetized dogs resulted in a decrease in both renal plasma flow and renin secretion (Yun et al., 1977). In humans administration of indomethacin has been shown to reduce basal renin secretion and to limit the renin secretory response to sodium restriction, upright posture, and administration of pharmacologic agents such as furosemide (Patak et al., 1975). Because it is possible that some action of indomethacin other than inhibition of prostaglandin synthetase could account for the suppression of renin, these studies cannot be taken as conclusive evidence that prostaglandins are normally required for the regulation of renin secretion in response to these physiologic stimuli.

Angiotensin II
Angiotensin II can exert a direct intrarenal "shortloop" negative feedback on renin release without an effect on blood pressure, plasma electrolytes, or sodium excretion (Blair-West et al., 1971). This effect is seen in the isolated perfused kidney (Vandongen, Peart, and Boyd, 1974) and also in the nonfiltering kidney, suggesting a direct intrarenal effect independent of changes in renal blood flow or distal tubular sodium transport (Shade et al., 1973). Studies with competitive angiotensin antagonists show that the effect depends on a

specific intrarenal angiotensin receptor (Ayers et al., 1974). This mechanism may account in part for suppression of renin release from the contralateral kidney in unilateral renal ischemia.

Ionic effects

The concentration of sodium in extracellular fluid can influence renin secretion, and a general inverse relationship between renin and plasma sodium concentration in hypertensive patients has been described (Brown et al., 1965). However, expansion of extracellular fluid volume can clearly exert an overriding influence in the presence of a falling serum sodium level (Newsome and Bartter, 1968). Tuck, Dluhy, and Williams (1974) suggested that the sodium ion has a specific suppressive effect on renin secretion as a result of studies that compared the effects of infusing dextran, glucose, and isotonic saline in sodium-restricted normal subjects. An immediate suppressive effect on renin secretion occurred after infusion of less than 100 ml of isotonic saline, whereas the effect of dextran or glucose infusion was delayed from 4 to 6 hours, indicating that renin release is exquisitely sensitive to intravascular sodium chloride content. Although it was assumed that this suppression was due to the sodium ion, it is now clear that the chloride ion may directly influence renin release, possibly by an effect at the macula densa (Kotchen, Galla, and Luke, 1978). In studies of sodium chloride-deprived rats, renin was inhibited more completely by choline chloride than by sodium chloride, whereas choline bicarbonate and sodium bicarbonate had no effect, thus demonstrating a critical role for the chloride ion in renin suppression. This finding may force a reappraisal of conclusions in studies in which a renin-inhibiting effect was attributed to potassium, administered as potassium chloride (Brunner et al., 1970), or calcium, administered as calcium chloride (Kotchen et al., 1974).

PHYSIOLOGIC AND PATHOPHYSIOLOGIC ROLE OF RENIN

The renin-angiotensin-aldosterone system participates in the normal regulation of blood pressure, sodium balance, and electrolyte and acid-base homeostasis. Renin release increases in response to sodium restriction or depletion, decreased plasma volume, diminished renal perfusion pressure, and upright posture; the consequences of increased renin secretion tend to oppose the circulatory effects of these stimuli. In the following sections, we will review briefly the evidence that supports a role for renin in normal circulatory homeostasis and then consider in more detail the pathophysiology of renin excess or deficiency.

Physiologic role of renin

Response to dietary sodium restriction

Reduction in dietary sodium intake results in a prompt increase in renin secretion that is associated with increased adrenal secretion of aldosterone. The resultant increase in plasma mineralocorticoid activity serves to augment renal sodium reabsorption and represents an important component of the complex mechanisms that permit adaptation to wide variations in sodium intake. The renin-angiotensin system is required for the normal aldosterone secretory response to sodium restriction, demonstrated by the observation that both nephrectomy (Davis, Ayers, and Carpenter, 1961) and administration of angiotensin antagonists (Stephens et al., 1977) block the aldosterone secretory response to salt depletion in dogs.

In humans, simultaneous measurements of components of the renin-angiotensin-aldosterone system have been obtained during induction and rapid correction of sodium deficiency, and the results indicate a close correlation between these parameters under all study conditions (Williams et al., 1977a&b). These studies suggest a strong interdependence between the activity of the renin-angiotensin system and aldosterone secretion during sodium depletion. Yet, factors other than the level of angiotensin II per se may be responsible for stimulation of aldosterone secretion under these conditions. Plasma aldosterone levels for any level of angiotensin II are higher during sodium depletion than during direct infusion of the octapeptide (Boyd et al., 1972), a finding that appears to be due to an increased adrenal sensitivity to angiotensin in this setting (Hollenberg et al., 1974). This effect may be, in turn, due to an increase in the number of specific angiotensin II receptors on the adrenal cell, as has been demonstrated during chronic dietary sodium restriction in the rat (Douglas and Catt, 1976). Even if mediated indirectly, the available evidence suggests that the renin-angiotensin system is normally the major control system for the aldosterone secretory response to sodium depletion or restriction in man.

Response to changes in posture
Assumption of the upright posture is associated with a prompt increase in plasma renin and aldosterone levels. This response, with the associated activation of the sympathetic nervous system, participates in the adaptation of blood pressure to postural changes. In sodium replete subjects, the response of the renin-angiotensin system may be relatively unimportant because administration of an angiotensin-converting enzyme inhibitor did not produce hypotension in response to acute tilting (Haber et al., 1975). In contrast, administration of the converting enzyme inhibitor to subjects on a sodium-restricted intake produced dramatic hypotension (Samuels et al., 1976). These studies suggest that the autonomic response may be inadequate to maintain blood pressure in response to a postural challenge in sodium-depleted states; a normally functioning renin-angiotensin system appears to be required to maintain circulatory homeostasis in this situation.

The close correlation between the changes in renin and aldosterone levels during variations in posture provides additional evidence for the primary role of the renin-angiotensin system in the control of aldosterone secretion (Williams et al., 1972a). It should be noted that, under these experimental conditions, aldosterone levels could increase without a significant change in aldosterone secretory rate, because the metabolic clearance rate of aldosterone, which is closely correlated with hepatic blood flow, may decrease significantly with assumption of the upright posture. Observed decreases in metabolic clearance rate in response to upright tilting (Balikian et al., 1968) could account for a nearly twofold increase in plasma aldosterone concentration without a change in hormone production rate. However, the finding that administration of converting enzyme inhibitor blocks the increases in aldosterone levels with upright tilting in both sodium replete and sodium deplete subjects (Haber et al., 1975; Samuels et al., 1976) supports the view that angiotensin II is a major stimulus to aldosterone secretion under these conditions.

Maintenance of blood pressure

Recent studies with angiotensin antagonists and converting enzyme inhibitor indicate that the renin-angiotensin system does not exert a major influence on normal blood pressure in the sodium replete state. Administration of either an angiotensin antagonist (Noth, Tan, and Mulrow, 1977) or converting enzyme inhibitor (Haber et al., 1975) failed to significantly reduce blood pressure in supine normal subjects maintained on a normal sodium intake. During sodium depletion, however, administration of the converting enzyme inhibitor resulted in hypotension, the degree of which was dependent on the degree of hypovolemia (Samuels et al., 1976). The renin-angiotensin system also appears to play a critical role in the maintenance of blood pressure in response to acute hypovolemia: infusion of an angiotensin antagonist markedly attenuated the circulatory response to acute hemorrhage in dogs (Freeman et al., 1975b). Hence, a physiologic role for the renin-angiotensin system is most apparent when circulatory homeostasis is challenged by salt depletion, hypovolemia, or upright posture.

Renal autoregulation

In addition to the systemic effects attributed to the renin-angiotensin system, several investigators have proposed that intrarenal release of renin and local generation of angiotensin II may contribute to the regulation of renal blood flow and glomerular filtration rate. One line of investigation, principally using micropuncture techniques, has identified an intrarenal mechanism in which alteration of the rate and character of fluid delivery to the distal tubule and/or iron flux across the macula densa can influence the filtration rate of the same nephron (Wright, 1978). That the renin-angiotensin system might serve as the mediator of this feedback regulation has been championed by Thurau (1975), although the available micropuncture data are not entirely in accord with this concept (Wright, 1978).

Studies of whole kidney autoregulation have produced conflicting data with respect to the role of the renin-angiotensin system in the maintenance of renal blood flow during reduction of arterial pressure. Such autoregulation occurs normally in dogs despite both suppression of renin levels by sodium loading and direct intrarenal arterial infusion of angiotensin II (Belleau and Earley,

1967). That the renin-angiotensin system may influence these regulatory processes is suggested by studies in which angiotension antagonists decrease the magnitude of the feedback regulation of the glomerular filtration rate (Stowe and Schnermann, 1974) and prevent the autoregulation of renal artery pressure in conscious dogs with graded renal artery stenosis (Anderson, Johnston, and Korner, 1979). These studies, however, do not indicate whether these antagonists are blocking angiotensin originating in the kidney or from the systemic circulation. Although the available evidence does not permit the conclusion that the renin-angiotensin system is the major intrarenal mediator of autoregulation, it is still possible that this hormonal system, perhaps interacting with other vasoactive substances (e.g., prostaglandins), participates in the control of the glomerular filtration rate and renal blood flow.

Pathophysiologic role of renin in hyperreninemic states associated with hypertension

Experimental models

Prompted by the classic experiments of Goldblatt and his colleagues more than 40 years ago, numerous investigators have continued to study the pathogenesis of hypertension in animal models of renal ischemia. Despite intensive investigation, the role that the renin-angiotensin system plays in the pathogenesis of such experimental renal hypertension remains controversial. In part, much of the difficulty in interpreting the vast literature in this area stems from differences in the animal species used (dog, rat, rabbit, sheep), the experimental model employed (one-kidney and two-kidney Goldblatt hypertension), the stage of the experiment in which hormonal data are obtained (acute versus chronic phase), and the level of dietary sodium intake.

Attempts to implicate the renin-angiotensin system in the pathogenesis of renal hypertension have generally relied upon measurements of renin levels in the course of the experiment and/or an evaluation of the effects of agents that block this system on blood pressure. Administration of antirenin antibodies to dogs with chronic renovascular hypertension was successful in reducing blood pressure (Wakerlin, 1958), but these studies have been criticized because pure preparations of renin were not available for immunization. Similar attempts to block or correct hypertension by immunization with angiotensin II have not been consistently successful (Macdonald et al., 1970). More recently, many investigators have utilized angiotensin II antagonists (e.g., saralasin) or an angiotensin-converting enzyme inhibitor (SQ 20881) for these purposes. The results of these latter studies are reviewed in detail in Chapter 2.

Acute reduction in renal blood flow in the one-kidney Goldblatt model (clamping the solitary renal artery after prior unilateral nephrectomy) results in prompt development of hypertension in association with a marked increase in plasma renin activity (Gutmann et al., 1973). Hypertension persists, however, despite a subsequent decrease in renin levels to control values over the next few days. The reduction in renin levels has been attributed to the positive sodium balance and volume expansion that occurs in this model (Tobian, Coffee, and McCrea, 1969). The transient period of renin hypersecretion may be necessary for the induction of hypertension because both saralasin and SQ 20881 successfully reduce arterial blood pressure in the acute phase of unilateral renal hypertension in the rat (Pals et al., 1971) and dog (Miller et al., 1975). Infusion of SQ 20881 can prevent the occurrence of hypertension in the one-kidney Goldblatt dog, but subsequent injections of the inhibitor become less effective as salt and water retention occur in the chronic stage when plasma renin levels return to normal values (Miller et al., 1975). Similarly, angiotensin antagonists will not reduce elevated blood pressure in the chronic phase of the one-kidney hypertension model in the rat unless the rat has been sodium depleted (Gavras et al., 1973).

A similar pattern may occur in the two-kidney Goldblatt hypertension model (constriction of one renal artery with contralateral kidney intact). In the dog, attempts to produce chronic hypertension in this model have met with varying success, perhaps owing to the rapid development of collateral circulation. This problem has been circumvented to some extent by progressive renal artery plication (Watkins et al., 1976) or a two-stage operative procedure (Masaki et al., 1977) that results in severe unilateral renal ischemia. The renin-angiotensin system is activated in the initial stages (Watkins et al., 1976) but, after 3 to 4 days, tends to return to control levels. Infusion of angiotensin antagonists results in blood pressure reduction in the acute phase but is ineffective in the chronic phase (Masaki et al., 1977) unless the animals are sodium depleted (Watkins et al., 1976). In the rat angiotensin dependence has been demonstrated for as long as 5 weeks after unilateral renal artery constriction, but the response to antagonists may no longer be present when such animals are evaluated several months later (Gavras et al., 1975). The degree to which renin dependency can be demonstrated in the chronic phase appears related to induction of negative sodium balance following severe renal artery constriction (Leenen and de Jong, 1975). Similar variability has been noted in sheep in that a renin mechanism appears to be present only in the most severely hypertensive animals that had the greatest degree of negative sodium balance (Blair-West et al., 1968).

On the whole, then, it appears that hypertension associated with experimental renal ischemia is dependent on increased secretion of renin in the initial stages, but in many models, sodium retention occurs and appears to account for subsequent reduction of renin secretion to control values. Although some investigators have considered the relationship between the state of sodium balance and activity of the renin-angiotensin system to be abnormal in this setting, it has not been possible to demonstrate that hypertension is immediately dependent on angiotensin when such animals are studied in the sodium-replete state. Thus, although there is little doubt that the kidney is of primary importance in the genesis of hypertension in these models, the exact role of the renin-angiotensin system in the maintenance of chronic renal hypertension is still unresolved.

Renovascular and renal parenchymal hypertension

In concert with the development of models of renal hypertension in experimental animals, numerous studies in the past two decades have clearly established that hypertension can result from a variety of renal arterial and parenchymal lesions in man. In addition to stenotic lesions of one or both renal arteries (renovascular hypertension), hypertension may occur in patients with renal infarction, hydronephrosis, solitary cysts, renal tuberculosis, and other parenchymal lesions. In many instances a causal role for such lesions in the pathogenesis of hypertension has been demonstrated by the finding that elevated blood pressure can be reduced to normal or near-normal levels after corrective surgery. Whereas the true prevalence of surgically correctible renal hypertension is not known because almost all large series show some selection bias, it is generally agreed that renal lesions represent the most common cause of surgically reversible hypertension.

Renovascular disease, due either to arteriosclerosis or fibromuscular hyperplasia, is probably the most common and is certainly the best-studied cause of renal hypertension. The role of the renin-angiotensin system in the pathogenesis of renovascular hypertension in man, like that in experimental animals, is uncertain. Plasma renin levels are within normal limits in approximately half of the patients whose hypertension is subsequently benefited by a surgical procedure (Brown et al., 1964; Stockigt et al., 1972). One possible explanation for this finding may be that such levels of renin, although in the normal range, may be "inappropriate" to the pathophysiologic setting. Recent studies with angiotensin II antagonists or angiotensin-converting enzyme inhibitors, reviewed in detail in Chapter 2, indicate that the "angiotensin dependency" of renovascular hypertension can be demonstrated by an acute reduction in blood pressure after administration of these agents (Brunner et al., 1973; Gavras et al., 1974). Nevertheless, these studies have also indicated that the degree of reduction in blood pressure in such patients appears to be strongly dependent on the level of plasma renin activity and on the state of sodium balance at the time of study (Marks, Maxwell, and Kaufman, 1977). Thus, in many patients with chronic renovascular hypertension, the mechanism maintaining elevated blood pressure cannot be shown to be directly due to the prevailing level of renin. An interaction between renin and the state of sodium balance, the exact nature of which is unknown, appears to be responsible for the maintenance of chronic hypertension.

Renin-secreting tumors

One of the rarest, but perhaps most interesting, causes of renal hypertension is that associated with a renin-secreting tumor. The first such report appeared in 1967 (Robertson et al.), and although a number of additional cases have been reported in the subsequent decade, this still appears to be a relatively rare cause of hypertension (Cohn et al., 1972; Schambelan et al., 1973). The majority of patients are young and have severe hypertension that is frequently associated with secondary hyperaldosteronism. In fact, hypokalemia has occasionally been so severe that, prior to the wide availability of renin assays, the initial diagnosis was thought to be primary aldosteronism prompting subtotal adrenalectomy in several cases (Robertson et al., 1967; Schambelan et al., 1973).

The tumors are generally small, well encapsulated, and benign. Histologically, they have been considered to represent hemangiopericytomas. The primary cell component appears to be derived from the granule-containing cells in the wall of the afferent arteriole, which is a modified smooth muscle cell. The characteristics of the granule are similar to those found in the cells of the juxtaglomerular apparatus. However, the tumor also contains tubular components and thus may be a form of hamartoma (Schambelan et al., 1973).

Plasma renin levels have been markedly elevated in patients with renin-secreting tumors. Several lines of evidence support the conclusion that the renal tumor is responsible for the elevated renin levels. Renal vein renin studies showed that the kidney containing the tumor was the predominant source of renin, with selective renin samples further pinpointing the source of renin at the pole containing the tumor (Schambelan et al., 1973). The levels of renin from the contralateral kidney are low, suggesting suppression of renin from that side. The very high renin content of tumor tissue compared with normal kidney tissue and evidence that tumor tissue can secrete renin in tissue culture (Cohn et al., 1972) demonstrate that the tumor is the active site of renin secretion.

In addition to juxtaglomerular cell tumors, several cases of Wilms' tumor have been reported in which the tumor itself appears to be actively secreting renin (Mitchell et al., 1970; Day et al., 1975). The association of hypertension with Wilms' tumor is fairly common, but in many instances it has been thought that these large tumors compromise renal circulation and result in ischemia in the surrounding normal tissue. The presence of a large inactive form of renin in tumor tissue and peripheral plasma suggest the site of origin to be in the tumor rather than normal kidney tissue (Day et al., 1975). Hypertension and hyperreninemia have also been reported to occur in association with a tumor arising in lung (Genest et al., 1975).

Accelerated hypertension
Accelerated hypertension is characterized by marked elevation of blood pressure with evidence of progressive arteriolar necrosis manifested by renal functional impairment and severe retinopathy. Elevated plasma renin activity and associated secondary hyperaldosteronism are often, but not invariably found (McAllister et al. 1971). Increased renin secretion may reflect altered renal hemodynamics that result in renal cortical ischemia (Hollenberg et al. 1969). Hyperreninemia probably contributes to the severity of the hypertension because angiotensin antagonists can reduce blood pressure (Brunner et al., 1973). Nevertheless, the malignant phase of hypertension can occur despite normal plasma renin levels (Johnson et al., 1973).

Normalization of renin and aldosterone levels generally occurs with effective anithypertensive therapy in patients with accelerated hypertension. Hyperaldosteronism may sometimes persist despite normalization of renin levels, suggesting that prolonged stimulation of the adrenal gland can result in "tertiary" hyperaldosteronism (McAllister et al., 1971).

Chronic renal failure

Hypertension occurs commonly in patients with chronic renal disease and tends to increase in frequency and severity with progressive renal failure. In general, two pathogenetic mechanisms have been suggested to account for the hypertension in these patients (Schambelan and Biglieri, 1976). In the majority of patients, elevated blood pressure is associated with increases in plasma volume, extracellular fluid volume, and exchangeable sodium. Administration of diuretic agents or initiation of chronic dialysis to achieve "dry weight" is usually successful in normalizing the blood pressure. Plasma renin levels tend to be within the normal range in this group. In contrast, dialysis fails to control blood pressure adequately in a small subgroup with markedly elevated renin levels. These are patients in whom bilateral nephrectomy may be required to control the severe hypertension.

These two subtypes of hypertensive syndromes have been referred to as "sodium-dependent" and "renin-dependent" hypertension, respectively. It has been suggested that the difference may depend on the extent to which renal damage has affected the renin-secreting capacity of the kidney. In the sodium-dependent form, the renin response to normalization of extracellular fluid volume is limited so that a normal angiotensin-fluid volume relationship occurs after dialysis whereas in the renin-dependent variety, volume reduction leads to an excessive increase in angiotensin resulting in an inappropriate relationship between volume and angiotensin (Schalekamp et al., 1973).

Hypertension following renal transplantation

In the period immediately following renal transplantation, acute rejection is frequently, but not invariably, associated with increases in plasma renin activity (Popovtzer et al., 1973) and hypertension. Subsequently, hypertension can occur despite an otherwise normally functioning renal allograft. The hypertension may be due to stenosis of the transplant renal artery or to redistribution of blood flow with renal cortical ischemia, presumably as a consequence of chronic low grade allograft rejection (Bennett et al., 1974). Evaluation of a possible role for the renin-angiotensin system may be complicated by the presence of the host's kidneys in addition to one or more donor kidneys. In a recent study, administration of an angiotensin II antagonist to patients with posttransplant hypertension indicated that a hypotensive response occurred only after previous sodium restriction and then most commonly in patients who still have their own kidneys (Linas et al., 1978). Determination of the source of increased renin secretion requires venous samples from both host and donor kidneys. If hypertension is not controlled adequately with drug therapy, surgical correction of the renal artery stenosis in the transplanted kidney or removal of the host's kidneys should be considered, depending on the result of selective renin sampling.

Necrotizing vasculitis

Systemic arterial hypertension occurs in approximately 50 percent of patients who have either pathologic or arteriographic evidence of necrotizing vasculitis (periarteritis nodosa). Although the exact pathogenetic mechanisms responsible for the hypertension are not known, a relationship between the renal vasculitis and hypertension might be postulated. We recently studied three patients who had necrotizing vasculitis in association with hepatitis B surface-antigen-positive hepatitis (Topliss, Hewett, and Stockigt, unpublished observations; White and Schambelan, unpublished observations). All three patients presented with severe hypertension and hypokalemia with renal potassium wasting due to hyperreninemic hyperaldosteronism. Renal vein renin studies showed bilateral renal ischemia. Renal vasculitis with microaneurysms was noted on arteriography. The pathophysiologic role of angiotensin was shown in one patient by a hypotensive response to acute administration of saralasin and in a second by normalization of blood pressure and reversal of secondary hyperaldosteronism with chronic administration of the orally active angiotensin-converting enzyme inhibitor, SQ 14225. These results suggest that renin excess, probably due to patchy renal ischemia, may be an important factor in the pathogenesis of hypertension in patients with necrotizing vasculitis.

Estrogen therapy

The occurrence of hypertension in patients receiving estrogen-containing compounds has been recognized for more than a decade (Laragh et al., 1967). Components of the renin-angiotensin system are altered during treatment with estrogens and the possible pathogenetic role of these changes has been investigated in detail. Characteristically, increased levels of renin substrate and plasma renin activity (Laragh et al., 1967; Skinner, Lumbers, and Symonds, 1969) as well as angiotensin II (Cain, Walters, and Catt, 1971) occur during estrogen treatment. The levels of the renin enzyme per se appear to be suppressed, indicated by decreased levels of plasma renin concentration when determined in an assay in which exogenous substrate is added to the reaction mixture (Beckerhoff et al., 1972). However, the relationship between these hormonal changes and the occurrence of hypertension is not clear because estrogen treatment increases renin substrate and plasma renin activity in normotensive as well as hypertensive women. The suggestion that hypertension may be related to a failure of normal suppression of renin release in response to the increased levels of substrate and angiotensin II (Skinner et al., 1969) is not supported by the measurements of plasma renin concentration, which are equally reduced in normotensive and hypertensive women who are taking oral contraceptives (Beckerhoff et al., 1972). Thus, hypertension can occur despite normal feedback suppression of renin release.

Coarctation of the aorta

Coarctation of the thoracic aorta is frequently associated with arterial hypertension proximal to the site of stenosis and decreased blood pressure and pulse wave distal to the stenosis. That the kidney might be involved in the pathogenesis of prestenotic hypertension has been suggested by experiments in which renal autotransplantation to a site proximal to the stenosis resulted in a significant decrease in blood pressure (Scott and Bahnson, 1951). However, attempts to document increased activity of the renin-angiotensin system in patients with coarctation have been disappointing. Levels of plasma renin activity in both peripheral and renal venous blood have generally been within normal limits (Amsterdam et al., 1969). The significance of these "normal" levels of plasma renin activity should probably be reassessed in light of our current understanding of the relationship between sodium balance and the renin-angiotensin system. Administration of an angiotensin antagonist to two patients with coarctation resulted in a significant decrease in both systolic and diastolic blood pressures during the infusion. Both patients had been treated with a diuretic before the study and had elevated levels of plasma renin activity under these study conditions (Ribeiro and Krakoff, 1976). Thus, a hyperresponsive renin-angiotensin system may be present in such patients (Van Way et al., 1976) and thereby contribute to chronic hypertension.

Hyperreninemic states without hypertension

Hyperreninemia and secondary hyperaldosteronism are characteristic findings in several syndromes associated with a reduced effective blood volume, in which increased activity of the renin-angiotensin system is a direct response to the abnormal circulatory state. Hypertension is absent, in contrast to the syndromes previously discussed in which hyperreninemia was "inappropriate" to the state of the effective volume. These syndromes, which have recently been reviewed in detail (Stockigt, 1979), are mentioned here only briefly to distinguish their characteristic pathophysiologic abnormalities from other syndromes of secondary hyperaldosteronism.

Extrarenal and renal sodium loss
Sodium loss of sufficient magnitude to cause even modest degrees of contraction of extracellular fluid volume characteristically results in a marked stimulation of the renin-angiotensin system. When the route of sodium depletion is extrarenal (vomiting, diarrhea, sweating), increased aldosterone is responsible in part for renal sodium conservation. Depletion of the extracellular fluid volume can also occur when sodium loss is primarily of renal origin, from administration of diuretic agents, or from impairment of the normal mechanisms of sodium conservation. The latter can occur as a consequence of deficient production of mineralocorticoid hormones (Addison's disease, adrenal enzymatic defects) or when renal tubular resistance to mineralocorticoid hormone action is present (pseudohypoaldosteronism, salt-wasting nephritis).

Edema is characteristically absent in these syndromes. Administration of saline and correction of the underlying disorder usually results in a prompt return of renin and aldosterone levels to normal values. Determination of renin levels may provide a means of adjusting mineralocorticoid therapy and/or salt intake to optimal levels in such patients (Oelkers and L'age, 1976).

Edematous states

Increased levels of plasma renin activity and secondary hyperaldosteronism are frequent findings in patients with decompensated hepatic cirrhosis, congestive heart failure, and nephrotic syndrome. In patients with cirrhosis, increased renin secretion probably results from altered renal hemodynamics (Tristani and Cohn, 1967), but impaired hepatic inactivation of renin may also contribute (Barnardo, Strong, and Baldus, 1969). Similar abnormalities occur in patients with congestive heart failure, in whom hyperreninemia and secondary hyperaldosteronism may represent an important initial compensatory mechanism to maintain blood pressure. In dogs with experimental congestive heart failure, administration of converting enzyme inhibitor resulted in a significant fall in blood pressure in the early phase when renin levels were elevated (Watkins et al., 1975). As weight gain and edema occurred, renin and aldosterone returned to control levels and the administration of converting enzyme inhibitor no longer resulted in hypotension. Normal renin levels have been reported in most patients with untreated chronic congestive heart failure (Sanders and Melby, 1964).

Secondary hyperaldosteronism undoubtedly contributes to, but is not entirely responsible for, edema formation in these conditions (Chonko et al., 1977). Enhanced proximal tubule sodium reabsorption, increased perfusion of juxtamedullary nephrons, decreased delivery of filtrate to the diluting segment, and increased secretion of antidiuretic hormone all contribute to increased sodium and water reabsorption by the kidney (Humes, Gottlieb, and Brenner, 1978). Aldosterone antagonists such as spironolactone may limit sodium reabsorption to some degree but are relatively ineffective when severe hemodynamic abnormalities are present. Administration of all diuretics should be cautious, particularly in patients with severe hepatic decompensation, and therapy should aim, wherever possible, to correct the underlying disorder.

Bartter's syndrome

The so-called Bartter's syndrome is characterized by the presence of hypokalemic alkalosis, hyperreninemia, secondary hyperaldosteronism, and resistance to the pressor effects of infused angiotensin II (Bartter et al., 1962). Edema is characteristically absent. A detailed consideration of the pathophysiology of this interesting disorder has appeared in an earlier volume in this series (Bardgette and Stein, 1978). Vascular insensitivity to the pressor effects of angiotensin II, impaired renal sodium or chloride reabsorption, and increased renal production of prostaglandin E have been proposed to account for the findings in this syndrome. Alternatively, a primary renal defect resulting in renal potassium wasting could account for many of the features. This latter possibility is attractive because it is consistent with the observation that no form of therapy, including bilateral adrenalectomy, has been shown to fully ameliorate hypokalemia.

Hyporeninemic states

Hyporeninemia in syndromes of primary mineralocorticoid excess is commonly associated with hypertension. Renin is also low in a subgroup of patients with essential hypertension and in some normotensive patients with chronic renal disease. The interpretation of hyporeninemia, therefore, is always dependent on the associated clinical findings.

Syndromes of mineralocorticoid excess

Exogenous administration or primary adrenal hypersecretion of mineralocorticoid hormones results in sodium retention, expansion of extracellular fluid volume and renal potassium wasting. The expansion of extracellular fluid volume initiates responses that result in the eventual escape from the sodium-retaining effects of the hormone and achievement of a new steady state (Relman and Schwartz, 1952). The hypertension that occurs frequently in clinical states of primary mineralocorticoid excess appears to be initiated by sodium retention and to be sustained by an increase in peripheral vascular resistance (Wenting et al., 1977), perhaps mediated by a change in ionic composition of vascular smooth muscle (Berecek and Bohr, 1977). Plasma renin levels are characteristically suppressed (Conn, Cohen, and Rovner, 1964), presumably as a consequence of the expanded extracellular fluid volume.

The various clinical states of mineralocorticoid excess have been reviewed in a previous volume in this series (Schambelan, Sebastian, and Hulter, 1978). Primary aldosteronism owing to adrenal adenoma, hyperplasia, or carcinoma is the most frequently recognized of these syndromes (Biglieri, Stockigt, and Schambelan, 1972). In addition to aldosterone, increased adrenal production of other mineralocorticoid hormones can result in similar pathophysiologic features. Increased production of deoxycorticosterone accounts for hypertension and hypokalemia in patients with 11β- and 17α-hydroxylase deficiency and in certain patients with Cushing's syndrome, particularly when the underlying cause is an adrenal malignancy or ectopic ACTH production. Rarely, ingestion of large quantities of licorice or the drug carbenoxolone may result in a syndrome of mineralocorticoid excess.

Low renin essential hypertension

The finding of a suppressed plasma renin level in a hypertensive patient cannot be taken as conclusive evidence of the presence of mineralocorticoid excess because approximately 25 percent of patients with essential hypertension have this finding (Dunn and Tanner, 1974). Unlike the classic syndromes of mineralocorticoid excess, patients with low renin essential hypertension do not have hypokalemia, and total body sodium content is generally not increased (Lebel et al., 1974). The possible role of a mineralocorticoid hormone in such patients is suggested by the finding that inhibitors of adrenal biosynthesis (Woods et al., 1969) or of mineralocorticoid action (Spark and Melby, 1971) ameliorate hypertension in these patients but not in those with normal plasma renin levels. When assayed in adrenalectomized rats, urine extracts from patients with low renin essential hypertension have been reported to contain more mineralocorticoid activity than can be accounted for by the known steroids in the extracts (Sennett et al., 1975). In contrast to these findings, no evidence of an increased level of mineralocorticoid hormones was found in plasma of patients with low renin essential hypertension when assayed using a rat kidney receptor system (Baxter et al., 1976).

The presence of normal aldosterone levels in many patients with low renin essential hypertension is puzzling because in other hyporeninemic states (anephric patients, hyporeninemic hypoaldosteronism) aldosterone levels are generally below the normal range. The recent observation that the aldosterone secretory response to infusion of angiotensin II may be enhanced in patients with low renin essential hypertension suggests the possibility that increased adrenal sensitivity to angiotensin may be characteristic of this condition (Wisgerhof and Brown, 1978).

Hyporeninemic hypoaldosteronism

Impaired adrenal production of aldosterone in the presence of normal glucocorticoid production has been recognized with increasing frequency in the past six years (Schambelan, Stockigt, and Biglieri, 1972; Weidmann et al., 1973). In the majority of patients, the defect in aldosterone production appears to result from impaired renal secretion of renin rather than from an intrinsic defect in the adrenal gland. Several pathophysiologic mechanisms may account for the defect in renin secretion (Schambelan and Sebastian, 1978). In diabetic patients, who appear particularly prone to this disorder, hyalinization of the afferent arteriole and arteriolar sclerosis may result in destruction of the juxtaglomerular cells. Diabetics are also prone to develop autonomic neuropathy, which can result in reduced renin secretion. Some patients have increases in extracellular fluid volume and total exchangeable sodium that could result in suppression of renin secretion, a mechanism that may account for the frequent occurrence of hypertension in such patients. Finally, the observation of increased levels of "big renin" in some patients suggests that the hyporeninemia could result from impaired conversion of an inactive renin precursor to the normal active form of renin (Day et al., 1975).

CLINICAL USE OF RENIN MEASUREMENTS

Principles of renin measurement

Because no direct mass unit of purified renin is available, most assays measure either angiotensin I or II formed during incubation of plasma, with results expressed as mass, per volume, per incubation time. Assay details vary so widely for pH, duration, ionic milieu, and enzyme inhibitors that direct comparison of results between laboratories is often impossible. Replacement of bioassay by radioimmunoassay has greatly improved the quantitation of angiotensin, but the incubation conditions remain a major source of variation. Incubation at the pH optimum of the renin-human substrate reaction (pH

5.5–5.7)—without dilution and in the presence of antibacterial agents as well as inhibitors of angiotensin I degradation—has been shown to give a higher rate of angiotensin I formation than is found with many commercial kits (Sealey and Laragh, 1973), thus making the measurement of low renin levels more reliable.

The term plasma renin *activity* describes the result of incubating plasma with its own content of substrate; such methods are influenced both by the amount of renin and the amount of substrate. The term plasma renin *concentration* indicates the amount of angiotensin generated when a large excess of heterologous substrate is added to ensure zero-order kinetics. A third term, plasma renin *reactivity*, has been introduced to describe the amount of angiotensin generated in vitro in response to a standard amount of added renin. This last technique indicates the presence of any accelerator or inhibitor of the renin reaction and has shown that plasma from normal subjects, but not from patients with uremia or renovascular hypertension, contains a neutral lipid that inhibits the renin reaction (Kotchen et al., 1976). Although measurements of plasma renin activity are generally satisfactory for clinical purposes, assessment of renin concentration or renin reactivity becomes essential if substrate abnormalities or accelerators or inhibitors are to be assessed.

Because angiotensin I and II are both degraded during incubation of plasma, it is necessary to add angiotensinase inhibitors to ensure a stable end product of the renin reaction. Because it is virtually impossible to inhibit angiotensinases without also inhibiting plasma-converting enzyme, angiotensin II assays are unsuitable for renin measurement; angiotensin I has proved to be a much more convenient end product. However, conversion of angiotensin I must be completely inhibited because any angiotensin II formed will not be detected by antibodies to the C-terminal portion of angiotensin I. For this reason, the demonstration of quantitative recovery of added angiotensin I through the incubation procedure should be an essential step in assay validation.

Methods that involve preparation of samples by acid dialysis at pH < 4 can activate prorenin and often give a higher value than assays performed without acid pretreatment. The difference can be used to estimate prorenin (Derkx et al., 1976). The demonstration that prorenin can also be activated by cold temperatures means that storage or slow processing of samples between −5° C and +5° C should be avoided. Prolonged storage at room temperature in the presence of EDTA is unsatisfactory because this allows slow generation of angiotensin, which can falsify the final result. Therefore, speed in the handling of samples followed by freezing below −20° C is recommended.

Effects of drugs on the renin-angiotensin system

Numerous drugs may alter the level of plasma renin activity (Table 1.1), resulting in effects that are important in several ways: (1) interactions between various drug effects have been used to investigate the physiology of renin release; (2) the changes in renin have suggested possible modes of action of some antihypertensive drugs; (3) drugs can be used therapeutically in an attempt to

Table 1.1 Drug effects on plasma renin activity

Increase	Decrease
Diuretics	Beta blockers
Vasodilators	Alpha agonists
Hydralazine	Clonidine
Minoxidil	Reserpine
Diazoxide	Alpha methyldopa
Nitroprusside	Prazosin
Bupicomide	Labetalol
Beta agonists	Ganglion blockers
Theophylline	Prostaglandin inhibitors
Caffeine	Indomethacin
Alpha blockers	Ibuprofen
Chlorpromazine	Aspirin
Converting enzyme inhibitors	Carbenoxolone
Mineralocorticoid antagonists	Vasopressin
Glucagon	Somatostatin
Anesthetics	Saralasin[a]
Saralasin[a]	
Estrogen[b]	
Glucocorticoids[b]	

[a] Effect depends on renin level and sodium status.
[b] Effect by increasing renin substrate.

diminish renin secretion; (4) drug effects may be used to accentuate diagnostically important findings, such as lateralization of renin secretion in renal hypertension; and (5) the effects may create diagnostic confusion when the clinical significance of renin measurement is assessed.

As the therapy of hypertension becomes more clearly based on modification of normal physiology, distortions of normal hormonal levels will become more marked. Hence, it is important to perform critical diagnostic investigations before introducing agents that modify the levels of potassium, renin, angiotensin, and aldosterone. Therapeutically induced artifacts can usually be reversed by cessation of treatment, but a major difficulty arises if the hypertension is so severe that treatment cannot be safely stopped when diagnostic investigations are indicated. Guanethidine has been advocated as a drug that has only minor effects on renin levels (Lowder and Liddle, 1975, and it may be useful in such investigations. However, cautious drug withdrawal during hospitalization, perhaps with moderate dietary sodium restriction, may sometimes be the only safe procedure.

Diuretic agents

The renin-stimulating effect of diuretics is largely related to their effect in producing salt and water loss, but furosemide has been shown to increase renin even if volume depletion is prevented (Meyer et al., 1968), an effect that is only partially inhibited by beta blockade (Osborn, Hook, and Bailie, 1977). Determinations of renin response to various diuretics has been advocated for detection of patients with suppressed plasma renin levels. Prolonged therapy with diuretics may reverse extreme degrees of renin suppression (Woods et al., 1976), an effect that may create diagnostic confusion. If spironolactone is used before definitive investigation, the potential for misclassification is great because its renin-stimulating effect can persist for several months (Lowder and Liddle, 1974).

Vasodilators

Vasodilators have generally been found to increase plasma renin levels, an effect that is partly the result of a reactive increase in beta-adrenergic activity. O'Malley et al. (1975) examined the effect of propranolol on the minoxidil-induced increase in renin in patients with severe essential hypertension. Propranolol, 160–640 mg daily, only partly abolished the renin response to minoxidil, suggesting that a nonadrenergic mechanism was at least partly involved in the renin response. Pettinger and Keeton (1975) reported studies of rats in which the renin response to both hydralazine and minoxidil was impaired by beta blockade and was associated with potentiation of the hypotensive response to vasodilators. Because beta blockade did not enhance the hypotensive response to vasodilators in rats previously treated with saralasin, they concluded that impairment of renin release is an important factor in the interaction between vasodilators and beta blockers.

Prazosin, a quinazoline derivative that blocks the constrictor action of catecholamines and that had been initially classified as a vasodilator, has been shown to decrease plasma renin levels (Bolli, Wood, and Simpson, 1976), an effect that may be related to its direct catechol antagonism.

Beta blockers

Beta blockers generally decrease renin, and this inhibition has been suggested as an important factor in their antihypertensive action. Hollifield et al. (1976) showed that low-to-moderate doses of propranolol reduced blood pressure in patients with normal and high renin hypertension but not in patients with low renin hypertension. However, higher doses of propranolol (160–960 mg daily) effected a favorable blood pressure response irrespective of renin status, suggesting that the hypotensive effect on this beta blocker is only partly mediated by its renin-lowering effect. The intrinsic beta-agonist activity of drugs such as prindolol may be associated with an increase in renin, but this does not preclude a hypotensive effect (Weber, Stokes, and Gain, 1974).

Labetalol, which has both alpha- and beta-blocking activity, reduces plasma renin despite its effects of postural hypotension and markedly increased urinary excretion of epinephrine (Weidmann et al., 1978). When this drug was used in combination with chlorthalidone, plasma renin doubled and blood pressure decreased further, suggesting a hypotensive action independent of its effect on renin (Weidmann et al., 1978).

Drugs that act on the central nervous system

Clonidine has been shown in animals to decrease renin by a centrally mediated decrease in renal sympathetic activity (Nolan and Reid, 1978). Although the mechanism of its renin-lowering effect in man is less clear, depression of renin and aldosterone secretion may be important in its hypotensive action (Weber et al., 1976). Methyldopa has also been shown to decrease renin levels in man, although the effect is of minor significance in normal subjects and is most marked in patients with severe hypertension when renal function is impaired or when renin levels are high (Weidmann et al., 1974).

Renal vein renin measurement

Numerous studies have clearly established the usefulness of renal vein renin measurements in the evaluation of patients with suspected unilateral renal hypertension (Bourgoignie et al., 1970; Stockigt et al., 1972). Comparison of renin levels in the renal veins can indicate asymmetry in renin secretion and thereby suggest the presence of unilateral renal ischemia. In view of the low morbidity of this procedure and the nearly 90 percent accuracy in predicting which patients are likely to benefit from surgery, renal vein renin measurements are mandatory in any patient in whom corrective surgery for presumed renin-mediated hypertension is contemplated.

The renal vein renin ratio

An increased concentration of renin in the venous effluent from an ischemic kidney reflects an increase in renin secretion rate as well as a decrease in ipsilateral renal blood flow (Woods and Michelakis, 1968). The ratio of renin levels between the affected and contralateral kidneys is usually a more reliable index of renal ischemia than the absolute level of renin in the renal veins. In our experience a ratio of 1.5 or greater correlates well with postoperative improvement in blood pressure following technically successful surgery (Stockigt et al., 1972). The level of 1.5 was selected in part on the basis of considerations of assay precision, and it is probably advisable for each laboratory to determine independently the ratio of diagnostic significance.

If a renal vein renin ratio greater than 1.5 is to be regarded as suggestive of surgically curable hypertension, such a ratio should be uncommon in essential hypertension. Although Stockigt et al. (1972) found a ratio less than 1.3 in all but one of 13 patients with radiologically normal kidneys, others have found a greater frequency of false-positive studies. Stone, Talner, and Coel (1977) reported a renal vein renin ratio greater than 1.5 in 20 percent of patients with normal arteriograms, a disturbing incidence of false-positive findings. Multiple sampling to assure proper catheter placement and repetition of sampling after an acute stimulus may obviate the problem of false-positive results in many cases.

Additional information with respect to the possible pathophysiologic significance of a renal lesion can be obtained by comparison of the renin level from the unaffected kidney to that in the peripheral circulation (Stockigt et al., 1972). Suppression of contralateral renin release is demonstrated when renin levels are similar in contralateral renal venous effluent and in peripheral blood. Regardless of renal blood flow in the contralateral kidney, net secretion of renin is then zero. Under these circumstances one can conclude that all of the renin is being secreted by the affected kidney, a finding that is highly predictive of a good response to surgery.

Conditions of study

Careful attention must be given to the conditions under which renal vein renin specimens are collected. The patient should be studied after a period of recumbency to assure that basal conditions of renin secretion are present. Recent upright posture can result in transient stimulation of renin release with subsequent cessation of secretion and loss of a diagnostic ratio (Michelakis et al., 1969). For similar reasons, drugs known to effect release of renin should also be avoided before the study. Although it has not been clearly demonstrated that drugs that suppress renin secretion can result in a false-negative study, it is preferable to avoid such agents before renal vein catheterization; patients should be observed closely during this interval to avoid dangerous increases in blood pressure.

In our usual protocol patients are admitted on the evening before the study and are kept flat overnight and during transfer to the radiology department. Plasma samples are obtained from the renal venous effluent and caudal inferior vena cava by retrograde catheterization of the femoral vein. Small volumes of radiopaque material can be used to verify the sampling site. Insofar as possible, the time period between collection of the two renal vein samples should be minimal to avoid the influence of any fluctuations in renin secretion. It is unlikely that significant fluctuations occur during collections of base-line samples, but this may become a more important problem when renin secretion is acutely stimulated. In general, we have preferred to obtain renin samples both before and after acute stimulation of renin secretion, because the latter will occasionally identify renal ischemia when unstimulated samples do not yield a diagnostic ratio or may demonstrate symmetric secretion when a false-positive ratio is present in the unstimulated samples. Upright tilting (Michelakis et al., 1969), vasodilators such as diazoxide (Stockigt et al., 1976), and angiotensin-converting enzyme inhibitor (Re et al., 1978) have been used as stimuli. After such acute stimuli, renin levels from the affected kidney often increase twofold to threefold above control values within 10 to 30 minutes, and the ratio of renin between the renal veins may be greater than that in the basal period. Contralateral suppression of renin secretion is confirmed if the effluent from the unaffected kidney remains the same as the peripheral level.

A recent modification of the venous sampling technique has enhanced detection of localized areas of renal ischemia in patients with renal artery branch stenosis, segmental infarction, and renin-secreting tumors (Schambelan et al., 1974; Korobkin, Glickman, and Schambelan, 1976). Determination of renin levels in the main renal veins in such patients may fail to indicate the presence of an area of renin hypersecretion, presumably because of dilution by blood draining normal areas of the affected kidney. Comparison of the renin levels draining the affected segment with those from the contralateral kidney may yield a ratio that is considerably greater than that from the main renal veins.

For optimal results multiple samples should be obtained by selective catheterization of various segments of the affected kidney under fluoroscopic control. Venograms should be obtained at the time of sampling to verify the sampling site and allow more accurate interpretation.

Relationship to arteriography

Renal arteriography and renal vein renin sampling are commonly performed as two closely related studies. Although Whelton et al. (1977) and Stone et al. (1977) failed to find any consistent change in renal vein renin activity after injection of intra-arterial contrast material, certain individual patients had large changes that could not be accounted for in that study (Stone et al., 1977). In an experimental canine model, intra-arterial injection of contrast material resulted in an immediate decrease and subsequent increase in renal vein renin activity that persisted for up to 20 minutes (Katzberg et al., 1977). In view of the possible alteration of renin secretion by contrast material, it would seem preferable to perform renal vein renin sampling before arteriography if both studies are to be performed as a single procedure. This approach has the inherent disadvantage of sampling with incomplete knowledge of arterial and intrarenal pathology so that it may be preferable to obtain renal vein renin samples as a separate procedure after the results of arteriography are known. On occasion, we have obtained renal vein samples in a "blind" fashion in patients with no apparent lesion on the intravenous pyelogram or midstream aortogram and detected lesions that cause hypertension (Schambelan et al., 1974). This approach will probably be most productive in patients with unexplained elevated peripheral levels of renin.

Peripheral renin measurements

The possibility that a single peripheral blood measurement can be used to categorize a disorder as diverse in etiology as hypertension has been pursued with great enthusiasm. It has been claimed that measurement of renin can screen for renal hypertension, suggest the presence of mineralocorticoid excess, provide a guide to optimal therapy, and indicate the prognosis of hypertensive disorders. However, each of these claims, after an initial vogue, has met increasing resistance. The diversity of opinion stems not only from fundamental differences of interpretation of experimental results but also from differences in the populations studied, the measurement techniques employed, and conditions under which samples were obtained. A priori, it seems unlikely that a physiologically labile enzyme with a short plasma half-life, which circulates in active and inactive forms and which must be incubated with a variable rate-limiting amount of substrate under conditions that arrest this reaction at an intermediate stage, will prove to be a satisfactory screening test. Furthermore, the effects of age, race, sex, drug therapy, sodium intake, and posture make it difficult to define "normality" for renin levels.

Despite these limitations, measurement of renin in a peripheral blood sample is crucial in the investigation of hypertensive patients with hypokalemia because it clearly distinguishes between primary and secondary hyperaldosteronism, except in the rare case of accelerated hypertension owing to primary aldosteronism (McAllister et al., 1971). The degree of suppression of renin is also useful in distinguishing between the adenomatous and hyperplastic forms of primary hyperaldosteronism (Biglieri et al., 1972). Demonstration of subnormal renin levels can readily distinguish patients with isolated hypoaldosteronism due to hyporeninemia from those with generalized adrenal insufficiency (Addison's disease) in which there is usually gross renin excess (Schambelan et al., 1972). In contrast to these conditions in which peripheral renin measurement is the key to correct diagnosis, there are many disorders, such as hepatic cirrhosis with ascites, nephrotic syndrome, or cardiac failure, in which renin excess is an expected finding and thus documentation of the abnormality adds little of diagnostic or therapeutic value.

Swales (1976) has advocated peripheral renin measurement as a screening test for renal hypertension because radiologic screening is too expensive and time consuming for studies of large populations. However, a quarter to one-half of cases of renal artery stenosis, treated successfully by surgery, may have normal peripheral renin levels (Stockigt et al., 1972; Laragh et al., 1975). Furthermore, peripheral renin levels are usually within normal limits in patients with the various forms of parenchymal renal disease (Vaughan et al., 1975), which together may make up almost one-third of surgically correctable cases (Stockigt et al., 1972). Renin is also usually within normal limits in patients with bilateral renal artery stenosis or with stenosis of the artery to a single kidney (Kurtzman et al., 1974). The possibility that renin measurement after a suppressive maneuver might better identify patients with renal hypertension appears unlikely from the findings reported by Grim et al. (1977). Peripheral renin levels after infusion of 2 liters of isotonic saline in 4 hours were similar in patients with renal hypertension compared with those with high renin essential hypertension. Hence, the diagnosis of renal hypertension is better sought by radiologic means and by renal vein renin sampling rather than by measurement of peripheral renin levels.

The present status of peripheral renin measurement in the assessment and treatment of patients with essential hypertension remains uncertain. Laragh (1973) has suggested that therapy can be chosen more rationally after classification of patients into low, normal, and high renin groups, using a categorization based on the relationship between plasma renin activity and 24-hour urinary excretion of sodium during mild dietary sodium restriction. Initial studies by Bühler et al. (1973) have shown that propranolol is most effective in high renin and least effective in low renin hypertensives, whereas other studies (Vaughan et al., 1973) have indicated that low and normal renin subjects tend to respond better than the high renin group to either spironolactone or chlorthalidone. However, several recent studies indicate that the response to a diuretic or beta blocker is not closely related to the plasma renin levels. Woods et al. (1976) showed that fixed dosages of propranolol (3.5 mg/kg/day) or chlorthalidone (100 mg daily) have a comparable hypotensive effect in low and normal renin hypertensive patients, whereas Hollifield et al. (1976) found that propranolol, at doses up to 160 mg daily, effects a similar hypotensive response in normal and high renin hypertensive patients.

Assumptions with respect to pathogenetic mechanisms in hypertensive patients that are based on renin measurements should be made cautiously, because quite different types of hypertensive patients may fall into the same renin group. For example, high renin hypertensive patients may represent either young subjects with mild hypertension of neurogenic origin or persons with severe or accelerated disease in whom renal function may be impaired (Esler et al., 1977). Similarly, low renin hypertension may result from mineralocorticoid excess, suppression of sympathetic nervous function, diminished renal mass, the effects of advanced age, or long-standing hypertension (Esler et al., 1976).

Assessment of peripheral renin levels is complicated further by the multitude of sampling conditions used by different investigators. Although renin measurement after stimulation of secretion magnifies the difference between low and high values, such conditions differ widely from the individual's day-to-day environment and therefore may be of doubtful significance. It may, in fact, be more appropriate to make this assessment after a suppressive maneuver, if abnormal persistence of renin secretion is important in the pathogenesis of hypertension as suggested by Tuck et al. (1976). Renin classification after stimulation can vary widely when the same subject is retested by a different procedure or even by the same procedure (Modlinger and Gutkin, 1975; Woods et al., 1976), and different ways of plotting the same data may alter the classification (Woods et al., 1976). Dietary sodium restriction plus upright posture probably gives the most satisfactory assessment, but routine use of this procedure is difficult to supervise. Administration of chlorthalidone for 5 days has been shown to correlate well with sodium restriction (Drayer, Kloppenborg, and Benraad, 1975) although longer use of this drug (6 weeks) may reverse even extreme degrees of renin suppression (Woods et al., 1976). Shorter tests, using oral or parenteral forms of furosemide, are less satisfactory because they tend to correlate poorly with the effects of sodium restriction and may fail to influence renin in hypertensive patients with normal basal levels (Padfield et al., 1975).

Even if it is accepted that renin classification provides a useful guide to optimal therapy, it is not necessarily appropriate to assess the renin status of patients with mild benign essential hypertension who have a satisfactory response to empirical first-line therapy (Woods et al., 1976; Gavras and Brunner, 1976). It seems likely that peripheral renin measurement will continue to be most important when there are features suggestive of secondary hypertension or when the response to usual drug therapy is poor (Williams, 1976; Noth, 1978).

REFERENCES

Amsterdam, E. A., Albers, W. H., Christlieb, A. R., Morgan, C. L., Nadas, A. S. & Hickler, R. B. (1969). Plasma renin activity in children with coarctation of the aorta. *American Journal of Cardiology*, **23**, 396–399.

Anderson, W. P., Johnston, C. I. & Corner, P. I. (in press). Acute renal haemodynamic and renin-angiotensin system responses to graded renal artery stenosis in the dog. *Journal of Physiology (London)*.

Atlas, S. A., Sealey, J. E., Laragh, J. H. & Moon, C. (1977). Plasma renin and "prorenin" in essential hypertension during sodium depletion, beta-blockade, and reduced arterial pressure. *Lancet*, II, 785–788.

Ayers, C. R., Vaughan, E. D., Yancy, M. R., Bing, K. T., Johnson, C. C. & Morton, C. (1974). Effect of 1-sarcosine-8-alanine angiotensin II and converting enzyme inhibitor on renin release in dog acute renovascular hypertension. *Circulation Research*, 34–35 (suppl. I), I-27–I-33.

Balikian, H. M., Brodie, A. H., Dale, S. L., Melby, J. C. & Tait, J. F. (1968). Effect of posture on the metabolic clearance rate, plasma concentration and blood production rate of aldosterone in man. *Journal of Clinical Endocrinology and Metabolism*, 28, 1630–1640.

Barber, R. E., Lindauer, J. M. & Eger, E. I, II. (1975). A serum enzyme test to detect pulmonary capillary injury. *Critical Care Medicine* 3, 31–35.

Bardgette, J. J. & Stein, J. H. (1978). Pathophysiology of Bartter's syndrome. In *Contemporary Issues in Nephrology*, ed. Brenner, B. M. & Stein, J. H. Vol. 2, New York: Churchill Livingstone.

Barnardo, D. F., Strong, C. G. & Baldus, W. P. (1969). Elevated hepatic venous renin activity in cirrhosis: Evidence for impaired hepatic inactivation and portal venous origin. *Annals of Internal Medicine*, 70, 1065.

Bartter, F. C., Pronove, P., Gill, J. R., Jr., & MacCardle, R. C. (1962). Hyperplasia of the juxtaglomerular complex with hyperaldosteronism and hypokalemic alkalosis: A new syndrome. *American Journal of Medicine*, 33, 821–828.

Baxter, J. D., Schambelan, M., Matulich, D. T., Spindler, B. J., Taylor, A. A. & Bartter, F. C. (1976). Aldosterone receptors and the evaluation of plasma mineralocorticoid activity in normal and hypertensive states. *Journal of Clinical Investigation*, 58, 579–589.

Beaty, O., III, Sloop, C. H., Schmid, H. E., Jr., & Buckalew, V. M., Jr. (1976). Renin response and angiotensinogen control during graded hemorrhage and shock in the dog. *American Journal of Physiology*, 231, 1300–1307.

Beckerhoff, R., Luetscher, J. A., Wilkinson, R., Gonzales, C. & Nokes, G. W. (1972). Plasma renin concentration, activity, and substrate in hypertension induced by oral contraceptives. *Journal of Clinical Endocrinology and Metabolism*, 34, 1067–1073.

Belleau, L. J. & Earley, L. (1967). Autoregulation of renal blood flow in the presence of angiotensin infusion. *American Journal of Physiology*, 213, 1590–1595.

Bennett, W. M., McDonald, W. J., Lawson, R. K. & Porter, G. A. (1974). Posttransplant hypertension: Studies of cortical blood flow and the renal pressor system. *Kidney International*, 6, 99–108.

Berecek, K. H. & Bohr, D. F. (1977). Structural and functional changes in vascular resistance and reactivity in the deoxycorticosterone acetate (DOCA)—hypertensive pig. *Circulation Research* 40 (suppl. I), I-146–I-152.

Biglieri, E. G., Stockigt, J. R. & Schambelan, M. (1972). Adrenal mineralocorticoids causing hypertension. *American Journal of Medicine*, 52, 623–632.

Blaine, E. H., Davis, J. O. & Prewitt, R. L. (1971). Evidence for a renal vascular receptor in control of renin secretion. *American Journal of Physiology*, 220, 1593–1597.

Blair-West, J. R., Coghlan, J. P., Denton, D. A., Funder, J. W., Scoggins, B. A. & Wright, R. D. (1971). Inhibition of renin secretion by systemic and intrarenal angiotensin infusion. *American Journal of Physiology*, 220, 1309–1315.

Blair-West, J. R., Coghlan, J. P., Denton, D. A., Orchard, E., Scoggins, B. A. & Wright, R. D. (1968). Renin-angiotensin-aldosterone system and sodium balance in experimental renal hypertension. *Endocrinology*, 83, 1199–1209.

Bolli, P., Wood, A. J. & Simpson, F. O. (1976). Effects of prazosin in patients with hypertension. *Clinical Pharmacology and Therapeutics*, 20, 138–141.

Bourgoignie, J., Kurz, S., Catanzaro, F. J., Serirat, P. & Perry, H. M., Jr., (1970). Renal venous renin in hypertension. *American Journal of Medicine*, 48, 332–342.

Boyd, G. W., Adamson, A. R., Arnold, M., James, V. H. T. & Peart, W. S. (1972). The role of angiotensin II in the control of aldosterone in man. *Clinical Science*, 42, 91–104.

Brown, J. J., Davies, D. L., Lever, A. F. & Robertson, J. I. S. (1964). Variations in plasma renin concentration in several physiological and pathological states. *Canadian Medical Association Journal*, 90, 201–206.

Brown, J. J., Davies, D. L., Lever, A. F. & Robertson, J. I. S. (1965). Plasma renin concentration in human hypertension. I: Relationship between renin, sodium and potassium. *British Medical Journal,* **2,** 144–148.

Brunner, H. R., Baer, L., Sealey, J. E., Ledingham, J. G. G. & Laragh, J. H. (1970). The influence of potassium administration and of potassium deprivation on plasma renin in normal and hypertensive subjects. *Journal of Clinical Investigation,* **49,** 2128–2138.

Brunner, H. R., Gavras, H., Laragh, J. H. & Keenan, R. (1973). Angiotensin-II blockade in man by sar-ala⁸-angiotensin II for understanding and treatment of high blood-pressure. *Lancet,* II, 1045–1048.

Bühler, F. R., Laragh, J. H., Vaughan, E. D., Brunner, H. R., Gavras, H. & Baer, L. (1973). The antihypertensive action of propranolol. *American Journal of Cardiology,* **32,** 511–522.

Cain, M. D., Walters, M. A. & Catt, K. J. (1971). Effects of oral contraceptive therapy on the renin-angiotensin system. *Journal of Clinical Endocrinology and Metabolism,* **33,** 671–676.

Chonko, A. M., Bay, W. H., Stein, J. H. & Ferris, T. F. (1977). The role of renin and aldosterone in the salt retention of edema. *American Journal of Medicine,* **63,** 881–889.

Cohn, J. W., Cohen, E. L., Lucas, C. P., McDonald, W. J., Mayor, G. H., Blough, W. M., Jr., Eveland, W. C., Bookstein, J. J. & Lapides, J. (1972). Primary reninism. *Archives of Internal Medicine,* **130,** 682–696.

Conn, J. W., Cohen, E. L. & Rovner, D. R. (1964). Suppression of plasma renin activity in primary aldosteronism. *Journal of the American Medical Association,* **190,** 213–221.

Davis, J. O., Ayers, C. R. & Carpenter, C. C. J. (1961). Renal origin of an aldosterone-stimulating hormone in dogs with thoracic caval constriction and in sodium-depleted dogs. *Journal of Clinical Investigation,* **40,** 1466–1474.

Davis, J. O. & Freeman, R. H. (1976). Mechanisms regulating renin release. *Physiological Reviews,* **56,** 1–56.

Day, R. P., Luetscher, J. A. & Gonzales, C. M. (1975). Occurrence of big renin in human plasma, amniotic fluid and kidney extracts. *Journal of Clinical Endocrinology and Metabolism,* **40,** 1078–1084.

Derkx, F. H. M., Gool, J. M. G. V., Wenting, G. J., Verhoeven, R. P., Man in't Veld, A. J. & Schalekamp, M. A. D. H. (1976). Inactive renin in human plasma. *Lancet,* II, 496–498.

Dew, M. E. & Michelakis, A. M. (1974). Effect of prostaglandins on renin release *in vitro. Pharmacologist,* **15,** 198A.

Douglas, J. & Catt, K. J. (1976). Regulation of angiotensin II receptors in the rat adrenal cortex by dietary electrolytes. *Journal of Clinical Investigation,* **58,** 834–843.

Drayer, J. I. M., Kloppenborg, P. W. C. & Benraad, T. J. (1975). Detection of low-renin hypertension; evaluation of out-patient renin-stimulating methods. *Clinical Science and Molecular Medicine,* **48,** 91–96.

Dunn, M. J. & Tanner, R. L. (1974). Low-renin hypertension, *Kidney International,* **5,** 317–325.

Erdös, E. G. (1977). The angiotensin I converting enzyme. *Federation Proceedings, Federation of American Societies for Experimental Biology,* **36,** 1760–1765.

Esler, M., Julius, S., Zweifler, A., Randall, O., Harburg, E., Gardiner, H. & De Quattro, V. (1977). Mild high-renin essential hypertension. Neurogenic human hypertension? *New England Journal of Medicine,* **296,** 405–411.

Esler, M., Zweifler, A., Randall, O., Julius, S., Bennett, J., Rydelek, P., Cohen, E. & De Quattro, V. (1976). Suppression of sympathetic nervous function in low-renin essential hypertension. *Lancet,* II, 115–118.

Freeman, R. H., Davis, J. O., Gotshall, R. W., Johnson, J. A. & Spielman, W. S. (1974). The signal perceived by the macula densa during changes in renin release. *Circulation Research,* **35,** 307–315.

Freeman, R. H., Davis, J. O. & Lohmeier, T. E. (1975a). Des-asp¹ angiotensin II: possible intrarenal role in homeostasis in the dog. *Circulation Research,* **37,** 30–34.

Freeman, R. H., Davis, J. O., Johnson, J. A., Spielman, W. S. & Zatzman, M. L. (1975b). Arterial pressure regulation during hemorrhage: Homeostatic role of angiotensin II (38735). *Proceedings of the Society for Experimental Biology and Medicine,* **149,** 19–22.

Freeman, R. H., Davis, J. O., Lohmeier, T. E. & Spielman, W. S. (1977). (Des-asp¹) angiotensin II; mediator of the renin-angiotensin system? *Federation Proceedings, Federation of American Societies for Experimental Biology and Medicine,* **36,** 1766–1770.

Ganten, D., Schelling, P., Vecsei, P. & Ganten, U. (1976). Iso-renin of extrarenal origin: "The tissue angiotensinase systems." *American Journal of Medicine,* **60,** 760–772.

Gavras, H. & Brunner, H. R. (1976). Renin profiling in hypertension. *New England Journal of Medicine*, **295**, 734.

Gavras, H., Brunner, H. R., Laragh, J. H., Sealey, J. E., Gavras, I. & Vukovich, R. A. (1974). An angiotensin converting-enzyme inhibitor to identify and treat vasoconstrictor and volume factors in hypertensive patients. *New England Journal of Medicine*, **291**, 817–821.

Gavras, H., Brunner, H. R., Thurston, H. & Laragh, J. H. (1975). Reciprocation of renin dependency with sodium volume dependency in renal hypertension. *Science*, **188**, 1316–1317.

Gavras, H., Brunner, U. R., Vaughn, E. D., Jr., & Laragh, J. H. (1973). Angiotensin-sodium interaction in blood pressure maintenance of renal hypertensive and normotensive rats. *Science*, **180**, 1369–1371.

Genest, J., Rojo-Ortega, J. M., Kuchel, O., Boucher, R., Nowaczynski, W., Lefebvre, R., Chrétien, M., Cantin, J. & Granger, P. (1975). Malignant hypertension with hypokalemia in a patient with renin-producing pulmonary carcinoma. *Transactions of the Association of American Physicians*, **88**, 192–201.

Goldblatt, H., Lynch, J., Hanzal, R. F. & Summerville, W. W. (1934). Studies on experimental hypertension. I. The production of persistent elevation of systolic blood pressure by means of renal ischemia. *Journal of Experimental Medicine*, **59**, 347–379.

Golub, M. S., Speckart, P. F., Zia, P. K. & Horton, R. (1976). The effect of prostaglandin A_1 on renin and aldosterone in man. *Circulation Research*, **39**, 574–579.

Gotshall, R. W., Davis, J. O., Shade, R. E., Spielman, W., Johnson, J. A. & Braverman, B. (1973). Effects of renal denervation on renin release in sodium-depleted dogs. *American Journal of Physiology*, **225**, 344–349.

Grim, C. E., Weinberger, M. H., Higgins, J. T. & Kramer, N. J. (1977). Diagnosis of secondary forms of hypertension: A comprehensive protocol. *Journal of the American Medical Association*, **237**, 1331–1335.

Gutmann, F. D., Tagawa, H., Haber, E. & Barger, A. C. (1973). Renal arterial pressure, renin secretion, and blood pressure control in trained dogs. *American Journal of Physiology*, **224**, 66–72.

Haber, E., Sancho, J., Re, R., Burton, J. & Barger, A. C. (1975). The role of the renin-angiotensin-aldosterone system in cardiovascular homeostasis in normal men. *Clinical Science and Molecular Medicine*, **48**, 49s–52s.

Haber, E. & Slater, E. E. (1977). Purification of renin: A review. *Circulation Research* 40 (suppl. I), I-36–I-40.

Hollenberg, N. K., Chenitz, W. R., Adams, D. F. & Williams, G. H. (1974). Reciprocal influence of salt intake on adrenal glomerulosa and renal vascular responses to angiotensin II in normal man. *Journal of Clinical Investigation*, **54**, 34–42.

Hollenberg, N. K., Epstein, M., Basch, R. I., Couch, N. P., Hickler, R. B. & Merrill, J. P. (1969). Renin secretion in essential and accelerated hypertension. *American Journal of Medicine*, **47**, 855.

Hollifield, J. W., Sherman, K., Vander Zwagg, R. & Shand, D. G. (1976). Proposed mechanisms of propranolol's antihypertensive effect in essential hypertension. *New England Journal of Medicine*, **295**, 68–73.

Humes, H. D., Gottlieb, M. N. & Brenner, B. M. (1978). The kidney in congestive heart failure. In *Contemporary Issues in Nephrology*, ed. Brenner, B. M. & Stein, J. H., Vol. 1. New York: Churchill Livingstone.

Inagami, T., Hirose, S., Murakami, K. & Matoba, F. (1977). Native form of renin in the kidney. *Journal of Biological Chemistry*, **252**, 7733–7737.

Johnson, J. A., Davis, J. O. & Witty, R. T. (1971). Effects of catecholamines and renal nerve stimulation on renin release in the nonfiltering kidney. *Circulation Research*, **29**, 646–653.

Johnson, J. G., Lee, S., Acchiardo, S., Cuestas, C., Share, L. & Hatch, F. E. (1973). Normal plasma-renin activity in malignant hypertension. *Journal of Clinical Investigation*, **52**, 43a–44a.

Katzberg, R. W., Morris, T. W., Burgener, F. A., Kamm, D. E. & Fischer, H. W. (1977). Renal renin and hemodynamic responses to selective renal artery catheterization and angiography. *Investigative Radiology*, **12**, 381–388.

Korobkin, M., Glickman, M. G. & Schambelan, M. (1976). Segmental renal vein sampling for renin. *Radiology*, **118**, 307–313.

Kotchen, T. A., Galla, J. H. & Luke, R. G. (1978). Contribution of chloride to the inhibition of plasma renin by sodium chloride in the rat. *Kidney International*, **13**, 201–207.

Kotchen, T. A., Maull, K. I., Luke, R., Rees, D., & Flamenbaum, W. (1974). Effect of acute and chronic calcium administration on plasma renin. *Journal of Clinical Investigation*, **54**, 1279–1286.

Kotchen, T. A., Talwalker, R. T., Miller, M. C. & Welsh, J. C. (1976). Modification of renin reactivity by lipids extracted from normal, hypertensive and uremic plasma. *Journal of Clinical Endocrinology and Metabolism*, **43**, 971–981.

Krakoff, L. R. (1973). Measurement of plasma renin substrate by radioimmunoassay of angiotensin I: Concentration in syndromes associated with steroid excess. *Journal of Clinical Endocrinology and Metabolism*, **37**, 110–117.

Krakoff, L. R. & Eisenfeld, A. J. (1977). Hormonal control of plasma renin substrate. *Circulation Research*, **41** (suppl. II), II-43–II-46.

Kurtzman, N. A., Pillay, V. K. G., Rogers, P. W. & Nash, D. (1974). Renal vascular hypertension and low plasma renin activity. *Archives of Internal Medicine*, **133**, 195–199.

Laragh, J. H. (1973). Vasoconstriction-volume analysis for understanding and treating hypertension: The use of renin and aldosterone profiles. *American Journal of Medicine*, **55**, 261–274.

Laragh, J. H., Sealey, J. E., Bühler, F. R., Vaughan, E. D., Brunner, H. R., Gavras, H. & Baer, L. (1975). The renin axis and vasoconstriction volume analysis for understanding and treating renovascular and renal hypertension. *American Journal of Medicine*, **58**, 4–13.

Laragh, J. H., Sealey, J. E., Ledingham, J. G. C. & Newton, M. A. (1967). Oral contraceptives. Renin, aldosterone, and high blood pressure. *Journal of the American Medical Association*, **201**, 918.

Larsson, C., Weber, P. & Anggard, E. (1974). Arachidonic acid increases and indomethacin decreases plasma renin activity in the rabbit. *European Journal of Pharmacology*, **28**, 391–394.

Lebel, M., Schalekamp, M. A., Beevers, D. G., Brown, J. J., Davies, D. L., Fraser, R., Kremer, D., Lever, A. F., Morton, J. J., Robertson, J. I. S., Tree, M. & Wilson, A. (1974). Sodium and the renin-angiotensin system in essential hypertension and mineralocorticoid excess. *Lancet*, **II**, 308–309.

Leenen, F. H. H. & de Jong, W. (1975). Plasma renin and sodium balance during development of moderate and severe renal hypertension in rats. *Circulation Research*, **36** and **37** (suppl. I), I-179–I-186.

Lentz, K. E., Dorer, F. E., Kahn, J. R., Levine, M. & Skeggs, L. T. (1978). Multiple forms of renin substrate in human plasma. *Clinica Chimica Acta*, **83**, 249–257.

Lieberman, J. (1975). Elevation of serum angiotensin-converting-enzyme (ACE) level in sarcoidosis. *American Journal of Medicine*, **59**, 365–372.

Linas, S. L., Miller, P. D., McDonald, K. M., Stables, D. P., Katz, F., Weil, R., & Schrier, R. W. (1978). Role of the renin-angiotensin system in post-transplantation hypertension in patients with multiple kidneys. *New England Journal of Medicine*, **298**, 1440–1444.

Lowder, S. C. & Liddle, G. W. (1975). Effects of guanethidine and methyldopa on a standardized test for renin responsiveness. *Annals of Internal Medicine*, **82**, 757–760.

Lowder, S. C. & Liddle, G. W. (1974). Prolonged alteration of renin responsiveness after spironolactone therapy. *New England Journal of Medicine*, **291**, 1243–1244.

Macdonald, G. J., Louis, W. J., Renzini, W., Boyd, G. W. & Peart, W. S. (1970). Renal-clip hypertension in rabbits immunized against angiotensin II. *Circulation Research*, **27**, 197–211.

Mancia, G., Romero, J. C. & Shepard, J. T. (1975). Continuous inhibition of renin release in dogs by vagally innervated receptors in the cardiopulmonary region. *Circulation Research*, **36**, 529–535.

Marks, L. S., Maxwell, M. H. & Kaufman, J. J. (1977). Renin, sodium, and vasodepressor response to saralasin in renovascular and essential hypertension. *Annals of Internal Medicine*, **87**, 176–182.

Masaki, Z., Ferrario, C. M., Bumpus, F. M., Bravo, E. L. & Khosla, M. C. (1977). The course of arterial pressure and the effect of Sar^1-Thr^8-angiotensin II in a new model of two-kidney hypertension in conscious dogs. *Clinical Science and Molecular Medicine*, **52**, 163–170.

McAllister, R. G., Jr., Van Way, C. W., III, Dayani, K., Anderson, W. J., Temple, E., Michelakis, A. M., Coppage, W. S., Jr., & Oates, J. A. (1971). Malignant hypertension: Effect of therapy on renin and aldosterone. *Circulation Research*, **28** and **29** (suppl. II), II-160–II-173.

Meyer, P., Menard, J., Papanicolaou, N., Alexandre, J. M., Devaux, C. & Milliez, P. (1968). Mechanism of renin release following furosemide diuresis in rabbits. *American Journal of Physiology*, **215**, 908–915.

Michelakis, A. M., Woods, J. W., Liddle, G. W. & Klatte, E. C. (1969). A predictable error in use of renal vein renin in diagnosing hypertension. *Archives of Internal Medicine*, **123**, 359–361.

Miller, E. D., Jr., Samuels, A. I., Haber, E. & Barger, A. C. (1975). Inhibition of angiotensin conversion and prevention of renal hypertension. *American Journal of Physiology*, **228**, 448–453.

Mitchell, J. D., Baxter, T. J., Blair-West, J. R. & McCredie, D. A. (1970). Renin levels in nephroblastoma (Wilms' tumour): Report of a renin secreting tumour. *Archives of Disease in Childhood*, **45**, 376–384.

Modlinger, R. S. & Gutkin, M. (1975). Normal plasma renin activity in low renin hypertension. *Journal of Clinical Endocrinology and Metabolism*, **40**, 380–382.

Morris, B. J. (1978). Activation of human inactive ("Pro-") renin by cathepsin D and pepsin. *Journal of Clinical Endocrinology and Metabolism*, **46**, 153–157.

Newsome, H. H. & Bartter, F. C. (1968). Plasma renin activity in relation to serum sodium concentration and body fluid balance. *Journal of Clinical Endocrinology and Metabolism*, **28**, 1704–1711.

Nolan, P. L. & Reid, I. A. (1978). Mechanism of suppression of renin secretion by clonidine in the dog. *Circulation Research*, **42**, 206–211.

Noth, R. L. (1978). Interpretation of plasma renin activity. *Archives of Internal Medicine*, **138**, 528–529.

Noth, R. H., Tan, S. Y. & Mulrow, P. J. (1977). Effects of angiotensin II blockade by saralasin in normal man. *Journal of Clinical Endocrinology and Metabolism*, **45**, 10–15.

Oelkers, W. & L'age, M. (1976). Control of mineralocorticoid substitution in Addison's disease by plasma renin measurement. *Klinische Wochenschrift*, **54**, 607–612.

O'Malley, K., Velasco, M., Wells, J. & McNay, J. L. (1975). Control plasma renin activity and changes in sympathetic tone as determinants of minoxidil-induced increase in plasma renin activity. *Journal of Clinical Investigation*, **55**, 230–235.

Omvik, P., Enger, E. & Eide, I. (1976). Effect of sodium depletion on plasma renin concentration before and during adrenergic β-receptor blockade with propranolol in normotensive man. *American Journal of Medicine*, **61**, 608–614.

Oparil, S. & Haber, E. (1974). The renin-angiotensin system. *New England Journal of Medicine*, **291**, 389–401, 446–457.

Osborn, J. L., Hook, J. B. & Bailie, M. D. (1977). Control of renin release. Effects of D-propranolol and renal denervation on furosemide-induced renin release in the dog. *Circulation Research*, **41**, 481–486.

Padfield, P. L., Allison, M. E. M., Brown, J. J., Lever, A. F., Luke, R. G., Robertson, C. C., Robertson, J. I. S. & Tree, M. (1975). Effect of intravenous furosemide on plasma renin concentration: Suppression of response in hypertension. *Clinical Science and Molecular Medicine*, **49**, 353–358.

Pals, D. T., Masucci, F. D., Denning, G. S., Jr., Sipos, F. & Fessler, D. C. (1971). Role of the pressor action of angiotensin II in experimental hypertension. *Circulation Research*, **29**, 673–681.

Patak, R. V., Mookerjee, B. K., Bentzel, C. J., Hysert, P. E., Babej, M. & Lee, J. B. (1975). Antagonism of the effects of furosemide by indomethacin in normal and hypertensive man. *Prostaglandins*, **10**, 649–659.

Peach, M. J. & Chiu, A. J. (1974). Stimulation and inhibition of aldosterone biosynthesis in vitro by angiotensin II and analogs. *Circulation Research*, **34** and **35** (Suppl. I), I-7–I-13.

Pettinger, W. A., & Keeton, K. (1975). Altered renin release and propranolol potentiation of vasodilatory drug hypotension. *Journal of Clinical Investigation*, **55**, 236–243.

Pettinger, W. A., Keeton, T. K., Campbell, W. B. & Harper, D. C. (1976). Evidence for a renal alpha-adrenergic receptor inhibiting renin release. *Circulation Research*, **38**, 338–346.

Popovtzer, M. M., Pinnggera, W., Katz, F. H., Corman, J. L., Robinette, J., Lanois, B., Halgrimson, C. G. & Starzl, T. E. (1973). Variations in arterial blood pressure after kidney transplantation. *Circulation*, **47**, 1297–1305.

Re, R., Novelline, R., Escourrou, M.-T., Athanasoulis, C., Burton, J. & Haber, E. (1978). Inhibition of angiotensin-converting enzyme for diagnosis of renal-artery stenosis. *New England Journal of Medicine*, **298**, 582–586.

Reid, I. A. (1977a). Is there a brain renin-angiotensin system? *Circulation Research*, **41**, 147–153.

Reid, I. A. (1977b). Effect of angiotensin II and glucocorticoids on plasma angiotensinogen concentration in the dog. *American Journal of Physiology*, **232**, E234–E236.

Reid, I. A., Morris, B. J. & Ganong, W. F. (1978). The renin-angiotensin system. *Annual Review of Physiology*, **40**, 377–410.

Reid, I. A., Tu, W. H., Otsuka, K., Assaykeen, T. A. & Ganong, W. F. (1973). Studies concerning the regulation and importance of plasma angiotensinogen concentration in the dog. *Endocrinology*, **93**, 107–114.

Relman, A. S. & Schwartz, W. B. (1952). The effect of DOCA on electrolyte balance in normal man and its relation to sodium chloride intake. *Yale Journal of Biology and Medicine*, **24**, 540–558.

Ribeiro, A. B. & Krakoff, L. R. (1976). Angiotensin blockade in coarctation of the aorta. *New England Journal of Medicine*, **295**, 148–150.

Robertson, P. W., Klidjian, A., Harding, L. K. Walters, G., Lee, M. R. & Robb-Smith, A. H. T. (1967). Hypertension due to a renin-secreting renal tumour. *American Journal of Medicine*, **43**, 963–976.

Romero, J. C. Dunlap, C. L. & Strong, C. G. (1976). The effect of indomethacin and other anti-inflammatory drugs on the renin-angiotensin system. *Journal of Clinical Investigation*, **58**, 282–288.

Salvetti, A., Poli, L., Arzilli, F., Sassono, L., Pedrinelli, R. & Motolese, M. (1978). Effects of salbutamol and metoprolol on plasma renin activity and plasma potassium of normal subjects and of hypertensive patients. *Journal of Endocrinological Investigation*, **1**, 1–8.

Samuels, A. I., Miller, E. D., Jr., Fray, J. C. S., Haber, E. & Barger, A. C. (1976). Renin-angiotensin antagonists and the regulation of blood pressure. *Federation Proceedings, Federation of American Societies for Experimental Biology*, **35**, 2512–2520.

Sanders, L. L., & Melby, J. C. (1964). Aldosterone and the edema of congestive heart failure. *Archives of Internal Medicine*, **113**, 331–341.

Schalekamp, M. A., Beevers, D. G., Briggs, J. D., Brown, J. J., Davies, D. L., Fraser, R., Lebel, M., Lever, A. F., Medina, A., Morton, J. J., Robertson, J. I. S. & Tree, M. (1973). Hypertension in chronic renal failure: an abnormal relation between sodium and the renin-angiotensin system. *American Journal of Medicine*, **55**, 379–390.

Schambelan, M. & Biglieri, E. G. (1976). Hypertension and the role of the renin-angiotensin-aldosterone system in renal failure. In *The Kidney*, ed. Brenner, B. M. & Rector, F. C., Jr. Philadelphia: W. B. Saunders.

Schambelan, M., Glickman, M., Stockigt, J. R. & Biglieri, E. G. (1974). Selective renal-vein renin sampling in hypertensive patients with segmental renal lesions. *New England Journal of Medicine*, **290**, 1153–1157.

Schambelan, M., Howes, E. L., Jr., Stockigt, J. R., Noakes, C. A. & Biglieri, E. G. (1973). Role of renin and aldosterone in hypertension due to a renin-secreting tumor. *American Journal of Medicine*, **55**, 86–92.

Schambelan, M. & Sebastian, A. (1978). Hyporeninemic hypoaldosteronism. *Advances in Internal Medicine*, **24**, 385–405.

Schambelan, M., Sebastian, A. & Hulter, H. N. (1978). Mineralocorticoid excess and deficiency syndromes. In *Contemporary Issues in Nephrology*, ed. Brenner, B. M. & Stein, J. H. Vol. 2, New York: Churchill Livingstone.

Schambelan, M., Stockigt, J. R. & Biglieri, E. G. (1972). Isolated hypoaldosteronism in adults. A renin-deficiency syndrome. *New England Journal of Medicine*, **287**, 573–578.

Schrier, R. W., Reid, I. A., Berl, T. & Earley, L. E. (1975). Parasympathetic pathways, renin secretion and vasopressin release. *Clinical Science and Molecular Medicine*, **48**, 83–89.

Scott, W. H., Jr. & Bahnson, H. T. (1951). Evidence for a renal factor in the hypertension of experimental coarctation of the aorta. *Surgery*, **30**, 206–217.

Sealey, J. E. & Laragh, J. H. (1973). Searching out low renin patients: limitations of some commonly used methods. *American Journal of Medicine*, **55**, 303–314.

Sealey, J. E., Moon, C., Laragh, J. H. & Atlas, S. A. (1977). Plasma prorenin in normal, hypertensive and anephric subjects and its effect on renin measurements. *Circulation Research*, **40** (suppl. I), I-41–I-45.

Sennett, J. A., Brown, R. D., Island, D. P., Yarbro, L. R., Watson, J. T., Slaton, P. E., Hollifield, J. W. & Liddle, G. W. (1975). Evidence for a new mineralocorticoid in patients with low-renin essential hypertension. *Circulation Research*, **36** and **37** (suppl. I), I-2–I-9.

Shade, R. E., Davis, J. O., Johnson, J. A., Gotshall, R. W. & Spielman, W. S. (1973). Mechanism of action of angiotensin II and antidiuretic hormone on renin secretion. *American Journal of Physiology*, **224**, 926–929.

Skeggs, L. T., Levine, M., Lentz, K. E., Kahn, J. R. & Dorer, F. E. (1977). New developments in our knowledge of the chemistry of renin. *Federation Proceedings, Federation of American Societies for Experimental Biology and Medicine*, **36**, 1755–1759.

Skinner, S. L., Dunn, J. R., Mazzetti, J., Campbell, D. J. & Fidge, N. H. (1975). Purification, properties and kinetics of sheep and human renin substrates. *Australian Journal of Experimental Biology and Medical Science*, **53**, 77–88.

Skinner, S. L., Lumbers, E. R. & Symonds, E. M. (1969). Alteration by oral contraceptives of normal menstrual changes in plasma renin activity, concentration and substrate. *Clinical Science*, **36**, 67–76.

Skinner, S. L., McCubbin, J. W. & Page, I. H. (1964). Control of renin secretion. *Circulation Research*, **15**, 64–76.

Spark, R. F. & Melby, J. C. (1971). Hypertension and low plasma renin activity: Presumptive evidence for mineralocorticoid excess. *Annals of Internal Medicine*, **75**, 831–836.

Stephens, G. A., Davis, J. O., Freeman, R. H., Watkins, B. E. & Khosla, M. C. (1977). The effects of angiotensin II blockade in conscious sodium-depleted dogs. *Endocrinology*, **101**, 378–388.

Stockigt, J. R. (in press). Mineralocorticoid excess. In *The Adrenal Gland*, ed. James, V. H. T. & Martini, L. New York: Raven Press.

Stockigt, J. R., Collins, R. D., Noakes, C. A., Schambelan, M., & Biglieri, E. G. (1972). Renal-vein renin in various forms of renal hypertension. *Lancet*, I, 1194–1198.

Stockigt, J. R., Hewett, M. J., Topliss, D. J., Higgs, E. J. & Taft, P. (in press). Renin and renin substrate in primary adrenal insufficiency: Contrasting effects of glucocorticoid and mineralocorticoid deficiency. *American Journal of Medicine*.

Stockigt, J. R., Higgs, E. S. & Sacharias, N. (1976). Diazoxide-induced stimulation of renin release in renal vein renin sampling. *Clinical Science and Molecular Medicine*, **51**, 235S–237S.

Stone, R. A., Talner, L. B. & Coel, M. N. (1977). Renal vein renin activity in primary hypertension: Variability and influence of contrast material. *Investigative Radiology*, **12**, 455–461.

Stowe, N. T. & Schnermann, J. (1974). Renin-angiotensin mediation of tubuloglomerular feedback control of filtration rate. *Federation Proceedings, Federation of American Societies for Experimental Biology*, **33**, 347.

Swales, J. D. (1976). The hunt for renal hypertension. *Lancet*, I, 577–579.

Thames, M. D., Jarecki, M. & Donald, D. E. (1978). Neural control of renin secretion in anesthetized dogs. Interaction of cardiopulmonary and carotid baroreceptors. *Circulation Research*, **42**, 237–245.

Thurau, K. (1975). Modification of angiotensin-mediated tubuloglomerular feedback by extracellular volume. *Kidney International*, **8**, S-202–S-207.

Thurau, K., Schnermann, J., Nagel, W., Horster, M. & Wohl, M. (1967). Composition of tubular fluid in the macula densa segment as a factor regulating the function of the juxtaglomerular apparatus. *Circulation Research*, **20** and **21** (suppl. II), II-79–II-90.

Tigerstedt, R. & Bergman, P. G. (1898). Niere und Kreislauf. *Skandinavisches Archiv für Physiologie*, **8**, 223–271.

Tobian, L., Coffee, K. & McCrea, P. (1969). Contrasting exchangeable sodium in rats with different types of Goldblatt hypertension. *American Journal of Physiology*, **217**, 458–460.

Tristani, F. E. & Cohn, J. N. (1967). Systemic and renal hemodynamics in oliguric hepatic failure: Effect of volume expansion. *Journal of Clinical Investigation*, **46**, 1894–1906.

Tuck, M. L., Dluhy, R. G. & Williams, G. H. (1974). A specific role for saline or the sodium ion in the regulation of renin and aldosterone secretion. *Journal of Clinical Investigation*, **53**, 988–995.

Tuck, M. L., Williams, G. H., Dluhy, R. G., Greenfield, M. & Moore, T. J. (1976). A delayed suppression of the renin-aldosterone axis following saline infusion in human hypertension. *Circulation Research*, **39**, 711–716.

Vander, A. J. & Miller, R. (1964). Control of renin secretion in the dog. *American Journal of Physiology*, **207**, 537–545.

Vandongen, R., Peart, W. S. & Boyd, G. W. (1974). Effect of angiotensin II and its nonpressor derivatives on renin secretion. *American Journal of Physiology*, **226**, 277–282.

Van Way, C. W., III, Michelakis, A. M., Anderson, W. J., Manlove, A. & Oates, J. A. (1976). Studies of plasma renin activity in coarctation of the aorta. *Annals of Surgery*, **183**, 229–238.

Vaughan, E. D., Buhler, F. R., Laragh, J. H., Sealey, J. A., Gavras, H. & Baer, L. (1975). Hypertension and unilateral parenchymal renal disease. *Journal of the American Medical Association*, **233**, 1177–1183.

Vaughan, E. D., Laragh, J. H., Gavras, H., Bühler, F. R., Guras, H., Brunner, H. R. & Baer, L. (1973). Volume factor in low and normal renin essential hypertension: Treatment with either spironolactone or chlorthalidone, *American Journal of Cardiology*, **32**, 523–532.

Wakerlin, G. E. (1958). Antibodies to renin as proof of the pathogenesis of sustained renal hypertension. *Circulation*, **17**, 653–657.

Watkins, B. E., Davis, J. O., Hanson R. C., Lohmeier, T. E. & Freeman, R. H. (1976). Incidence and pathophysiological changes in chronic two-kidney hypertension in the dog. *American Journal of Physiology*, **231**, 954–960.

Watkins, L., Burton, J. A., Haber, E. & Barger, A. C. (1975). Renin in the pathogenesis of congestive failure. *Federation Proceedings, Federation of American Societies for Experimental Biology*, **34**, 367.

Weber, M. A., Case, D. B., Baer, L., Sealey, J. E., Drayer, J. I. M., Lopez-Ovejero, J. A. & Laragh, J. H. (1976). Renin and aldosterone suppression in the antihypertensive action of clonidine. *American Journal of Cardiology*, **38**, 825–830.

Weber, M. A., Stokes, G. S. & Gain, J. M. (1974). Comparison of the effects on renin release of beta-adrenergic antagonists with differing properties. *Journal of Clinical Investigations*, **54**, 1413–1419.

Weber, P. C., Larsson, C., Anggard, E., Hamberg, M., Corey, E. J., Nicolaou, K. C. & Samuelsson, B. (1976). Stimulation of renin release from rabbit renal cortex by arachidonic acid and prostaglandin endoperoxides. *Circulation Research*, **39**, 868–874.

Weidmann, P., De Chatel, R., Ziegler, W. H., Flammer, J. & Reubi, F. (1978). Alpha- and beta-adrenergic blockade with orally administered labetalol in hypertension. *American Journal of Cardiology*, **41**, 570–576.

Weidmann, P., Hirsch, D., Maxwell, M. H., Okun, R. & Schroth, P. (1974). Plasma renin and blood pressure during treatment with methyldopa. *American Journal of Cardiology*, **34**, 671–676.

Weidmann, P., Reinhart, R., Maxwell, M. H., Rowe, P., Coburn, J. W. & Massry, S. G. (1973). Syndrome of hyporeninemic hypoaldosteronism and hyperkalemia in renal disease. *Journal of Clinical Endocrinology and Metabolism*, **36**, 965–977.

Weinberger, M. H., Wade, M. B., Aoi, W., Usa, T., Dentino, M., Luft, F. & Grim, C. E. (1977). An extrarenal source of "renin-like" activity in anephric man. *Circulation Research*, **40** (suppl. I), I-1–I-4.

Wenting, G. J., Man in't Veld, A. J., Verhoeven, R. P., Derkx, F. H. M. & Schalekamp, M. A. D. H. (1977). Volume-pressure relationships during development of mineralocorticoid hypertension in man. *Circulation Research*, **40** (suppl. I), I-163–I-170.

Werning, C., Vetter, W., Weidmann, P., Schweikert, H. U., Stiel, D. & Siegenthaler, W. (1971). Effect of prostaglandin E₁ on renin in the dog. *American Journal of Physiology*, **220**, 852–856.

Whelton, P. K., Harrington, D. P., Russell, R. P., White, R. I. & Walker, W. G. (1977). Renal vein renin activity: A prospective study of sampling techniques and methods of interpretation. *Johns Hopkins Medical Journal*, **141**, 112–118.

Williams, G. H. (1976). Measurement of renin activity—when is it useful? *New England Journal of Medicine*, **294**, 1176–1177.

Williams, G. H., Cain, J. P., Dluhy, R. G. & Underwood, R. H. (1972a). Studies of the control of plasma aldosterone concentration in normal man. I. Response to posture, acute and chronic volume depletion, and sodium loading. *Journal of Clinical Investigation*, **51**, 1731–1742.

Williams, G. H., Tuck, M. L., Rose, L. I., Dluhy, R. G. & Underwood, R. H. (1972b). Studies of the control of plasma aldosterone concentration in normal man. III. Response to sodium chloride infusion. *Journal of Clinical Investigation*, **51**, 2645–2652.

Wisgerhof, M. & Brown, R. D. (1978) Increased adrenal sensitivity to angiotensin II in low-renin essential hypertension. *Journal of Clinical Investigation*, **61**, 1456–1462.

Witty, R. T., Davis, J. O., Johnson, J. A. & Prewitt, R. L. (1971). Effects of papaverine and hemorrhage on renin secretion in the non-filtering kidney. *American Journal of Physiology*, **221**, 1666–1671.

Woods, J. W., Liddle, G. W., Stant, E. G., Jr., Michelakis, A. M. & Brill, A. B. (1969). Effect of an adrenal inhibitor in hypertensive patients with suppressed renin. *Archives of Internal Medicine*, **123**, 366–370.

Woods, J. W. & Michelakis, A. M. (1968) Renal vein renin in renovascular hypertension. *Archives of Internal Medicine*, **122**, 392–393.

Woods, J. W., Pittman, A. W., Pulliam, C. C., Werk, E. D., Waider, W. & Allen, C. A. (1976). Renin profiling in hypertension and its use in treatment with propranolol and chlorthalidone. *New England Journal of Medicine*, **294**, 1137–1143.

Wright, F. S. (1978). Regulation of glomerular filtration rate and renal salt excretion by a single-nephron feedback pathway. *Cardiovascular Medicine*, **3**, 731–753.

Yun, J., Kelly, G., Bartter, F. C. & Smith, H. (1977). Role of prostaglandins in the control of renin secretion in the dog. *Circulation Research*, **40**, 459–464.

2

Angiotensin antagonists in clinical medicine: Implications for diagnosis, treatment, and understanding the pathophysiology of hypertension

NORMAN K. HOLLENBERG

INTRODUCTION

Rarely has the development of pharmacologic agents been applied with such speed to such a wide variety of questions ranging from fundamental physiology through pathophysiology in animal models to applied clinical questions. In the 9 years since the first reports of these agents, the literature has grown so rapidly that it is now unlikely that any one individual has read critically and digested every published report; like obtaining a census in China, the number changes during the attempt. The reasons for this explosive application are several. First, and perhaps most important, the agents were developed in a setting in which there was already long-standing and widespread interest in the possible role of the renin-angiotensin system in a variety of areas. Second, they have come to play a logical role as replacements for surgical ablation in providing evidence that this system is important in pathogenesis: Removal of the source of a hormone has played a key role in proving that a specific organ and its secretory products were important in the body economy. Thus, for example, adrenalectomy, followed by replacement with adrenal extracts, made it clear that the adrenal secreted a substance or substances responsible for certain bodily functions. In the case of the renin-angiotensin system, where the kidney is both the source of the hormone and the major responding organ, this experiment was impossible. Pharmacologic interruption has been employed in place of surgical ablation to assess angiotensin's contribution to a specific function.

The goal of this review will be to assess the insights that we have gained from the clinical application of the agents. In the diagnosis of renovascular hypertension, angiotensin analogues that act as antagonists at the receptor site are already showing promise in identifying patients likely to benefit from surgery. In their application to therapy, the agents that block conversion of angiotensin I to angiotensin II are showing promise in the treatment of essential and secondary hypertension, largely because a nonpeptide analogue of the original peptide antagonist has been developed. Because of the absence of a systematic clinical implication at present (and because of necessary editorial constraint), we will not review here the evidence that shows how the appropriate employment of agents now being developed will improve renal perfusion and function in a number of states in which the renin-angiotensin system is activated and the renal function is distorted with a reduction in glomerular filtration rate and sodium retention. This subject has been reviewed in detail elsewhere (Hollenberg, 1978). Where the agents have implications for the kidney in hypertension, however, their actions will be explored.

To achieve our goals it will be necessary to review the relevant pharmacology of the agents, with special emphasis on their specificity and sensitivity rather than their pharmacokinetics, structure-action relationships, and metabolic fate. The latter aspects have been reviewed in detail recently (Regoli, Park, and Rioux, 1974; Marshall, 1976; Bumpus, 1977; Hollenberg, 1978) and will be raised only when the information is immediately germane to the primary goals of this review.

PHARMACOLOGIC PROPERTIES OF THE AGENTS

The renin-angiotensin enzyme cascade offers a series of sites that have been exploited for more or less selective inhibition (Table 2.1). Because renin release from the kidney is mediated, at least in part, by sympathetic activity acting on the beta receptors, beta-adrenergic blocking agents have been effective in reducing renin release (Haber, 1976). More recently, evidence has accumulated that some agents, such as clonidine, reduce renin release via an action on a presynaptic alpha-adrenergic receptor (Pettinger et al., 1976).

Among many others, two actions of the beta-adrenergic blocking agents are clearly established. They lower an elevated blood pressure; they diminish the

Table 2.1 Pharmacologic interruption of the renin-angiotensin system

Mechanism	Product	Pharmacologic blockade
Renin release	Renin	(1) Beta-adrenergic blocking agents[a]
		(2) Alpha-adrenergic agonists[a]
Renin's action on substrate	A I	(1) Substrate analogues
		(2) Pepstatin
		(3) Antibody to renin
A I conversion to A II	A II	(1) Peptide inhibitors of peptidyl dipeptide hydrolase[a]
		(2) Nonpeptide inhibitors of peptidyl dipeptide hydrolase[a]
A II & A III action on receptor	Response—BP	(1) Peptide analogues of angiotensin II[a]
	adrenal & kidney	(2) Peptide analogues of angiotensin III[a]

[a] Agents that have been employed in man.

release of renin from the kidney. It was tempting, therefore, to suggest a causal relationship between these two effects, an hypothesis originally made by Bühler and coworkers in 1972. As several recent reviews indicate, it is unlikely that these agents have the specificity required to support this concept; indeed, the available evidence suggests they do not (Gross, 1977; Holland and Kaplan, 1976). For example, all known beta-adrenergic blocking agents, independent of whether they have intrinsic sympathetic activity, or are relatively cardioselective, reduce elevated blood pressure when given in appropriate dosage, but their suppressant effect on the renin-angiotensin system is clearly more variable (Gross, 1977). The time course and dose relationships do not parallel the blood pressure response. Thus, for example, intravenously administered propranolol will reduce plasma renin activity with a time course measured in minutes, without modifying blood pressure (Sullivan et al., 1976). Conversely, the plasma renin response is generally complete with chronic oral therapy within days, whereas the blood pressure response often evolves over a much longer time period, measured in weeks. Moreover, relatively cardioselective agents such as oxprenolol, alprenolol, and pindolol are considerably less effective in inhibiting renin release than propranolol or timolol although they induce an equivalent fall in blood pressure (Gross, 1977). Pindolol, the beta-adrenergic blocking agent with the most marked intrinsic sympathetic activity, may even increase plasma renin activity. It is of some interest that Bühler, who originated the attractive hypothesis linking suppression of plasma renin activity and reduction of arterial blood pressure, has recently presented evidence that patients who respond to propranolol show a parallel reduction in circulating plasma catecholamines, whereas nonresponders do not, raising the interesting possibility that propranolol acts at least in part via a central nervous system effect (Bühler et al., 1977). This would be consistent with the absence of orthostatic hypotension when they are used for treatment. Because of the lack of specificity of these agents, the following review on pharmacologic interruption of the renin-angiotensin system and renin's role in hypertension will not include a detailed discussion of beta-adrenergic blockade. It will be useful, however, to examine the renal response to beta-adrenergic blockers in the section on the renin-angiotensin system and the kidney.

Following release, renin acts upon a substrate synthesized by the liver to release the decapeptide, angiotensin I, which is considerably less active on smooth muscle and on the adrenal than angiotensin II. Renin's action on substrate was antagonized initially by antibody to renin and by nonspecific proteases such as pepstatin (Haber, 1976). More recently, a specific blockade has been demonstrated in animal models by structural analogues of the substrate on which renin acts (Marshall, 1976). Because this action not only reduces angiotensin I formation but also generates a modified angiotensin I and II that act as converting enzyme inhibitors and angiotensin antagonists, respectively, this approach may ultimately produce the most complete, effective pharmacologic interruption of the system.

Angiotensin I is hydrolyzed in lung and peripheral tissues by an enzyme that cleaves the carboxyterminal dipeptide leaving the active octapeptide, angiotensin II. The enzyme responsible for this action is known in this system as "converting enzyme," although it lacks the specificity implicit in that name. The same enzyme is also responsible for the degradation of bradykinin (where it is known as "kininase II") and for the hydrolysis of the beta chain of insulin (Erdös, 1975). This enzyme has been blocked by a number of agents, including a series of peptides that were initially shown to potentiate bradykinin by inhibiting its degradation and were thus initially termed bradykinin-potentiating-factor (BPF). The most widely studied peptide in this series is a nonapeptide (Table 2.1) which was distributed as SQ 20881 (Ondetti et al., 1971). Decapeptide analogues have also been shown to compete with angiotensin I for converting enzyme (Marshall, 1976). We will use the term "converting enzyme" in the context of this review, but it is important to keep in mind that the best term for this enzyme is dipeptidyl-peptide hydrolase.

The recent synthesis of a novel, nonpeptide blocker of this enzyme is likely to have an important impact in this field (Ondetti et al., 1977). The achievement was remarkable because the agent was designed on the basis of a working model of the receptor site on the enzyme. The model in turn was based on the peptide structure-action relationships and on what is known of the structure of carboxypeptidase A. The advantages of a nonpeptide obviously include activity when the agent is taken by mouth and relatively inexpensive synthesis. Work in this field has often been delayed until recently by the relative unavailability of the peptide analogues. Never has serendipity in research been more striking. The goal of the investigation was to design and synthesize a nonpeptide with affinity for the site on the enzyme responsible for hydrolysis of angiotensin I, with the ultimate objective of using this action for therapy in hypertension. The serendipity lies not in the creation of the agent, which was carefully planned, but rather in its remarkable effectiveness even in cases of hypertension that are resistant to current medical therapy. This effectiveness probably reflects an action or actions unrelated to the renin-angiotensin system, as reviewed below.

Octapeptide analogues of angiotensin II and its 1-des asp analogue (angiotensin III) act as antagonists by competing with angiotensin at its receptor site in vascular smooth muscle, the adrenal cortex, the kidney, and the nervous system (Regoli et al., 1974; Marshall, 1976; Bumpus, 1977; Hollenberg, 1978). There is some evidence that the heptapeptide analogue has a preferential action on the adrenal (Peach and Chiu, 1974) and the kidney (Taub, Caldicott and Hollenberg, 1977) but, especially for the former, the evidence is mixed. With only a rare exception, an analogue of angiotensin II in which the tyrosine residue in position 4 was substituted, all of the angiotensin antagonists synthesized to date have been modified in position 8 (Marshall, 1976). The first agents synthesized in this class, in which 8-alanine or tyrosine were introduced in the 8 position, were effective in vitro but lacked potency. The former was even thought to be inactive in vivo (Regoli et al., 1974). The closer the resemblance of the C-terminal side chain to phenylalanine in size the more potent both the antagonist and, unfortunately, the agonist properties of the agent.

The N-terminal aspartyl residue in the 1-position has also been subject to considerable investigation. Because a major route of degradation involves aminopeptidase attack on the N-terminal amino acid, Pals et al. (1971) synthesized 1-sar-8-ala-angiotensin II (P-113; saralasin acetate) and demonstrated a striking increase in the inhibitory effect, especially in vivo. While the initial goal of removal of the carbamyl group of aspartic acid was to protect the molecule from degradation, this substitution has also been shown to have an additional influence: The resultant agent is considerably less polar and thus potentially reaches the receptor site more easily. Perhaps more important is the interesting evidence that the binding affinity of the analogue for the receptor site is also enhanced by the substitution.

One of the major difficulties in this field is that the structure-action studies have not defined true competitive antagonists, but rather partial agonists: All of the agents retain significant angiotensinlike agonist properties, which have often been missed because of the insensitive assay systems employed, such as rabbit aorta and blood pressure in the rat. When sensitivity to angiotensin is enhanced, as for example in patients with low-renin hypertension, the agent's angiotensinlike properties become dominant. Not only is this a practical limitation, but it has had significant implications for interpretation of data.

Information is available on the metabolic fate of the most widely used angiotensin analogue, saralasin (Pettinger et al., 1975). The half-life of angiotensin II, which is about 20 seconds, has been extended by substitution of sarcosine in the 1-position to about 3 minutes in the rat and in humans. Consistent with that observation, pharmacokinetic equilibrium of the influence of the agent on blood pressure is generally reached within 10 to 20 minutes when the agent is infused continuously.

The toxicity of these agents has largely been related to their primary action.

In animals and in patients with an extracellular or plasma volume deficit, they induce hypotension, which may be severe (Schroeder et al., 1976). This factor limits their utility in attempts to reverse the renal actions of angiotensin. It is for this reason that attempts have been made to develop relatively selective agents for the renal vascular angiotensin receptor, with initial partial success (Taub et al., 1977). Hypotension has also been reported in a single patient who received SQ 20881, while also receiving a thiazide, triamterene, hydralazine, and guanethidine (Duhme et al., 1974). Perhaps the hypotension in this complex setting was not surprising. Severe hypotension has also been reported in one patient during saralasin infusion; the patient had received neither vasodilator nor autonomic blocking drugs, but rather aggressive diuretic therapy had led to a 440 mEq sodium deficit (Beckerhoff et al., 1976). Neither patient suffered long-term ill effects, but these factors must be considered when employing these agents. At the other end of the spectrum, the partial agonist properties of saralasin and 1-sar-8-ile-angiotensin II has induced striking pressor responses in patients with low renin hypertension or primary aldosteronism (Ogihara, Yamamoto, and Kumahara, 1974; Anderson, Streeten, and Dalakos, 1977). To date no important pathology has resulted from this action, but the observations suggest that caution should be employed in their use, especially if bolus administration is employed (Marks, Maxwell, and Kaufman, 1977). The agonist properties of these agents are also probably responsible for the sharp reduction in renal blood flow which occurs when they are administered in the usual dosage (Hollenberg et al., 1976). Again, no untoward effect on the kidney has been documented from the relatively short periods of administration that have been employed, but in states in which renal vasoconstriction already exists, this influence could potentiate the damage.

About 10 percent of patients receiving SQ 14225 (captopril), generally in very high dosage ranging from 600 to 1,000 mg/day, have suffered a reversible, pruritic rash. This is likely to be dose-related rather than idiosyncratic because in some patients reduction of the dosage has reversed the rash. A transient rise in blood urea nitrogen and serum creatinine associated with normalization of blood pressure occurred in a patient with previously uncontrolled hypertension (Gavras et al., 1978). The influence on renal function reversed when the agent was withdrawn. This action, well-known with other antihypertensive agents, probably reflects a nonspecific effect of blood pressure reduction rather than a specific renal action of the agent.

HYPERTENSION

It is not surprising that major emphasis has been given to assessing angiotensin's contribution to the pathogenesis of hypertension in animal models and in humans. The blockers have already provided important insights into the contribution of angiotensin to the pathogenesis of hypertension with renal artery stenosis; the angiotensin antagonists especially appear to provide some hope in predicting the patient's response to surgery. The agents have been applied to assessing angiotensin's contribution to the pathogenesis of hypertension in renal parenchymal disease as well, but information is surprisingly meager on the subject. There is a substantial literature already available on the use of the agents to assess angiotensin's contribution to the pathogenesis of essential hypertension, and a major and growing controversy exists because the available agents provide a different message. The oral converting enzyme inhibitor is showing outstanding promise for the therapy of hypertension, perhaps as indicated earlier by virtue of some action unrelated to its influence on the renin-angiotension system in many patients. It is the prognostic potential of the angiotensin antagonists and therapeutic potential of the converting enzyme inhibitors that justify an essay today on these agents in "clinical medicine."

Renal artery stenosis

In this, perhaps the simplest model of "renal hypertension," considerable unanimity has been achieved concerning angiotensin's role during the early period following unilateral renal artery stenosis in animals, but with more prolonged hypertension—even in this simple model—debate continues concerning angiotensin's contribution (Davis, 1977). All of this debate, of course, has immediate clinical relevance.

In the rat, rabbit, or dog in which a unilateral renal artery stenosis is induced in the presence of a healthy contralateral kidney, a highly programmed, reproducible response occurs. Within hours and for the first few days, plasma renin activity rises strikingly and the blood pressure elevation is rapidly reversed with either angiotensin antagonists or converting enzyme inhibitors (Davis, 1977). During the following week a second phase occurs. Plasma renin activity tends to drift back toward normal and, in parallel, the responsiveness of the elevated blood pressure to pharmacologic interruption is reversed. In several weeks plasma renin has returned to control, and blood pressure is unresponsive to the antagonists.

It is important not to confuse this sequence with an alternative three-phase sequence following renal artery stenosis in which initially (in a period measured in many weeks) the hypertension is reversed in toto by removing the clamp inducing the stenosis or by nephrectomy. In a second phase the hypertension is reversed only in part, and in the third phase—many months after the stenosis was induced—the hypertension is not cured. No evidence suggests that this sequence involves the renin-angiotensin system or sodium homeostasis whereas in the case of the three phases described above, strong evidence suggests that the fall in plasma renin activity with time following renal artery stenosis is due to sodium retention and a reactive suppression of the system. If animals with a unilateral lesion are brought into balance on a low sodium intake prior to drug infusion, as shown in Figure 2.1, their response returns (Gavras et al., 1973). Moreover, if animals are maintained on a restricted sodium intake following renal artery stenosis, as is evident in Figure 2.2, plasma renin activity remains elevated well into the interval in which plasma renin

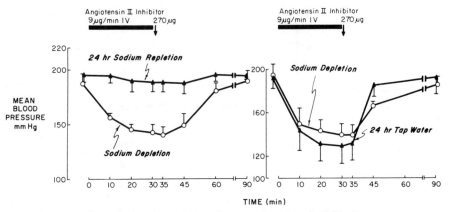

Figure 2.1 In sodium-depleted, one-kidney hypertensive animals (left), the angiotensin antagonist, saralasin, produced a striking fall in blood pressure; whereas 24 hours after sodium repletion, decrements in blood pressure were insignificant. In similar animals (right), the inhibitor produced a marked fall in blood pressure during the first phase of the experiment, and again 24 hours later if sodium was not administered. (From Gavras et al., 1973; reproduced by permission of the author and publisher).

activity generally falls. Moreover, the hypertension remains responsive to pharmacologic interruption (Rocchini and Barger, 1979).

Bilateral renal artery stenosis or unilateral renal artery stenosis, accompanied by contralateral nephrectomy, appears to differ fundamentally in pathogenesis. Plasma renin activity is typically suppressed; the hypertension is not responsive to pharmacologic interruption unless vigorous sodium depletion is employed; and, from studies in animals and in humans, evidence suggests that in this setting sodium retention and plasma volume expansion play a major role in the genesis of the hypertension (Brunner et al., 1971). All of the functioning renal parenchymal mass lies distal to the stenosis, in this case blunting the adjustment of total body sodium with hypertension. Again, these observations have immediate clinical relevance.

In summary, there is uniform agreement that, in the hours to several days following acute renal artery stenosis, activation of the renin-angiotensin system with a direct vascular action of angiotensin is responsible for the hypertension. There is growing evidence that the fall in the plasma renin activity and resistance to pharmacologic interruption of the renin-angiotensin system in the following days reflects sodium retention, consequent volume expansion, and a reactive suppression of the renin-angiotensin system that is prevented or reversed by restriction of sodium intake. These studies in general have not extended beyond 30 days. In the late stages of renal artery stenosis—which in animal models generally extends beyond 6 months—it is not yet clear, when nephrectomy or reversal of the stenosis does not cure the hypertension, whether or not the influence of the renin-angiotensin system has dissipated. No report of such extended studies has as yet appeared.

A number of reports indicate that patients with unilateral renal artery stenosis of undetermined duration (but presumably much longer than the animal

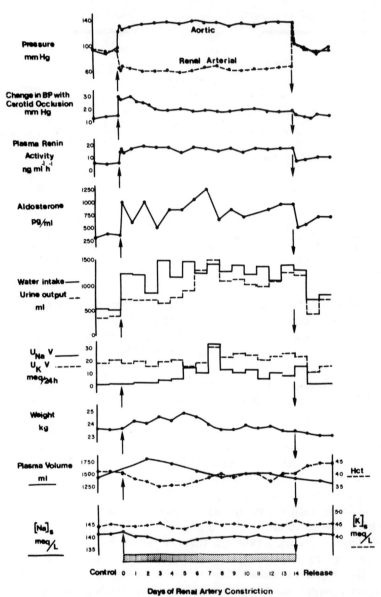

Figure 2.2 Hypertension occurs after renal artery stenosis in the dog, despite a sodium intake reduced to a level which prevented positive sodium balance. This maneuver also prevented the typical progressive fall in plasma renin activity and reduction in responsiveness to angiotensin antagonists that occurs in the dog when free access is provided to sodium and water. Much of the reduction in plasma renin activity and responsiveness which typically occurs in the weeks following renal artery stenosis, therefore reflect the impact of sodium retention. (From Rocchini and Barger, 1979; reproduced by permission of the authors and publishers.)

studies) also show a dramatic response to angiotensin antagonists (Marks et al., 1977; Hollenberg et al., 1979; Wilson et al., 1977; Beckerhoff et al., 1976; Baer et al., 1977). Why has this subject received the attention it has? First, the studies in animal models of the implications of duration raised important questions concerning whether in humans the renin-angiotensin system could be implicated in the hypertension of chronic renal artery stenosis. Second, review of the results of the Cooperative Study on Renovascular Hypertension reveals that significant clinical problems remain. Both of the commonly employed screening procedures, the intravenous pyelogram and the radiohippuran renogram, suffer from a significant false-positive and false-negative rate (Maxwell, 1975). In the case of the IVP, the combination of a reduction in renal size of at least 1.5 cm, delay in the appearance of contrast agent in the involved kidney in early films, and late hyperconcentration of contrast on the involved side had excellent specificity because there were no false positives, but only 22 percent of renovascular hypertensives had the triad. Sensitivity was low. The presence of any single abnormality was identified in 78 percent of renovascular hypertensives, but with a sharp reduction in specificity, since 11 percent of essential hypertensives had at least one manifestation, most commonly a significant difference in the renal size. In the same study, the renogram identified about 85 percent of renovascular hypertensives, with a false-positive rate that was larger—24 percent. For this reason, an alternative screening test for renovascular hypertension would be useful. Moreover, because all arterial lesions are not hemodynamically significant, additional tests—especially the measurement of renal vein renin activity—have become widely employed to assess the functional significance of the lesion. When the test is lateralizing, that is, when the test reveals a plasma renin activity in the renal vein draining the involved side that exceeds the contralateral renal venous concentration by at least 50 percent, 93 percent of patients will have an excellent surgical result (Maxwell, 1975). The false-negative rate is only 7 percent. Here, too, an ancillary test would be useful. Finally, the Cooperative Study has also provided a clear picture of the results of surgery. Whereas surgery for fibromuscular disease was gratifying, with a cure rate that exceeded 90 percent and a mortality of no more than 3 percent, the story was different in patients with atherosclerotic disease. Here the failure rate exceeded 25 percent, with a mortality that was slightly over 9 percent (Maxwell, 1975). For these reasons a test that would predict the presence of renal vascular hypertension and a surgically reversible lesion would have both pathophysiologic and diagnostic implications.

To assess the blood pressure response to angiotensin antagonists, it is necessary to place that assessment in the context of the response in normal persons and patients with essential hypertension. In a normal person, when the renin-angiotensin system is suppressed by recumbency and there is a liberal intake of sodium and potassium, neither angiotensin analogues nor converting enzyme inhibitors reduce arterial blood pressure (Haber, 1976). Despite modest activation of the renin-angiotensin system induced by standing in subjects ingesting a liberal salt intake, the contribution of angiotensin to blood pressure maintenance remains minimal. Neither class of agent reduces blood pressure under these circumstances. When the system is activated further by restriction of sodium intake, however, both classes of agents induce a reproducible reduction in arterial blood pressure despite recumbency (Hollenberg et al., 1978; Haber, 1976). In this setting the response is modest. In our study of 50 normal subjects in balance on a 10 mEq sodium intake, for example, the average fall of diastolic blood pressure with saralasin was only 5 mmHg, with a maximum fall of 10 mmHg computed from the 95 percent confidence limits. Sitting or standing, however, potentiates the response to the antagonists (Haber, 1976). It is important that increasing degrees of negative sodium balance will result in an increasing role for angiotensin in maintaining arterial pressure. Indeed, aggressive sodium depletion induced by restricted sodium intake plus diuretic administration will even make the "low renin hypertensive" dependent on angiotensin for blood pressure maintenance (Gavras et al., 1976). The relation between the state of sodium balance and angiotensin's contribution to normal pressure maintenance is probably best conceived as a continuum.

A potentiated response to saralasin occurs in about 10 percent of patients with essential hypertension, when large series have been studied (Hollenberg et al., 1979). In patients with renovascular hypertension, proved by arteriography and a 6-month followup after surgery which revealed striking improvement or cure, over 80 percent responded to saralasin with a significant hypotensive response (Hollenberg et al., 1979). With a 10 mmHg fall in diastolic pressure as the criterion, 86 percent (31 of 36) of renovascular hypertensives responded whereas only 8.5 percent of several hundred patients with essential hypertension did so (Fig. 2.3). Thus the specificity and sensitivity of this procedure compares favorably with the intravenous pyelogram and radiohippuran renogram. When one considers that the data described for the former identified an arteriographic lesion rather than surgical cure, the comparison is even more favorable.

As indicated above, both false-positive and false-negative responses occur. Not all lesions demonstrated by angiography, as indicated above, are hemodynamically significant. It is not surprising, therefore, that some patients with essential hypertension will carry a high plasma renin activity and also have a functionally insignificant renal artery stenosis. Presumably this accounts for the false-positive result that has been reported (Fagard, 1978).

Some insight has been gained into the pathogenesis of the false-negative reaction (Hollenberg et al., 1979). Among the five patients in whom a fall in blood pressure with saralasin did not occur, and yet who showed an excellent response to vascular reconstructive surgery, three had bilateral renal artery stenosis. As indicated above, the pathogenesis of this syndrome differs significantly from that in typical, unilateral renal arterial disease: Sodium retention is probably more important than the direct vascular action of angiotensin in its pathogenesis (Brunner et al., 1971). On this basis a negative response, or even a pressor response to angiotensin antagonists, would be anticipated. Unfortunately, it is precisely under these circumstances that the alternative tests, the

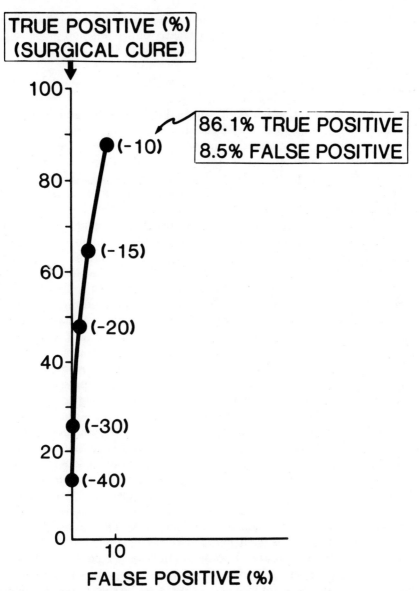

Figure 2.3 Receiver operating characteristic curve that relates the prevalence of depressor responses of a given magnitude (indicated in the brackets) in patients with renovascular hypertension who were strikingly improved or cured 6 months following surgery ("true-positive") and in patients with proven essential hypertension ("false-positive"). Note that a fall in diastolic pressure of 10 mmHg identifies 86 percent of the renovascular hypertensives with a false-positive rate of *about* 8.5 percent—a ratio that compares favorably with the intravenous pyelogram and radiohippuran renogram. (Data from Hollenberg et al., 1979, with permission of the publisher.)

intravenous pyelogram and radiohippuran renogram, are also weakest. Because in both cases they are tests for asymmetry of delivery and processing of the tracer, bilateral disease may be missed (Maxwell, 1975).

Renal parenchymal disease

Given the attention that has been paid to the state of the renin-angiotensin system in renal parenchymal disease and the obvious importance of hypertension in this setting, the amount of information available on the response of blood pressure to pharmacologic interruption in such patients is disappointing.

An inverse correlation has been reported between the level of plasma renin activity and glomerular filtration rates in patients with renal parenchymal disease: As glomerular filtration rate falls, plasma renin activity rises (Schalekamp et al., 1974). There is also a weak but statistically significant correlation between the height of diastolic blood pressure and plasma renin activity. These data are compatible with a role for renin in the chronic latent phase of renal parenchymal disease well before terminal uremic stage. Schalekamp and coworkers have recently reviewed evidence that suggests how an interaction between a variable expansion of total body sodium, measured directly, and an inappropriately elevated plasma renin activity could play a role in the pathogenesis. They demonstrated a modest abnormality in patients with chronic renal parenchymal disease and mild hypertension. Much greater distortion of the relationship was evident in patients with uncontrollable hypertension. It is likely, although not clearly stated, that the latter group represent primarily patients who have end-stage renal disease and are developing accelerated hypertension, patients in whom the responsible mechanisms are grossly distorted and therefore becoming clearer. In patients with early parenchymal disease, where a more modest physiological abnormality might be anticipated, Schalekamp et al. suggest that a modest elevation of plasma renin activity, which is still well within the normal range, is inappropriately high relative to total body sodium. If the hypertension was angiotensin mediated in this stage, it would be reasonable to expect that the elevated blood pressure in such patients would be responsive to angiotensin antagonists. This has been denied in chronic glomerulonephritis (Hollenberg et al., 1978; Brod et al., 1978).

An example of the depressor response to saralasin in a patient with typical chronic glomerulonephritis in its early chronic stage is shown in Figure 2.4. Only scattered data are as yet available on responses in such patients and those data are published only in abstract form (Brod et al., 1978), but the response in our patient is apparently typical. In chronic pyelonephritis we found a significant hypotensive response in only 4 of 12, in each case associated with an unequivocal increase in plasma renin activity and substantial hypertension, and evidence of hydronephrosis on the IVP. None of the patients with a plasma renin activity in the normal range and relatively modest hypertension responded. The failure of the angiotensin antagonist to reduce blood pressure in this setting is clearly not in accord with the evolving concept of an inappro-

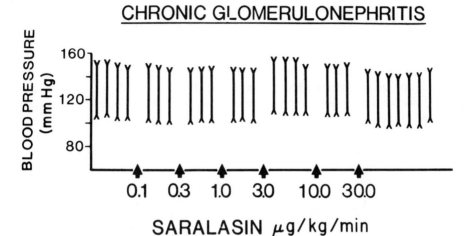

CHRONIC GLOMERULONEPHRITIS

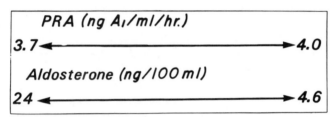

Figure 2.4 Failure of a patient with chronic glomerulonephritis and moderately advanced hypertension to respond to the angiotensin antagonist, saralasin, which was infused in graded dosage over the range effective in identifying angiotensin's contribution to renovascular hypertension. Current hypotheses which suggest that hypertension in this setting reflects a subtle abnormality in the relationship between total body sodium and renin—both of which are mildly to moderately abnormal—are not consistent with this observation. Note that plasma renin activity (PRA) was normal and that plasma aldosterone concentration—which was elevated by restriction of sodium intake—fell strikingly.

priate elevation of plasma renin activity, relative to total body sodium. Whereas the angiotensinlike agonist activity that is still retained by currently available angiotensin analogues may have been responsible for an underestimate of angiotensin's role—as has been claimed (Case et al., 1977)—this does not appear to be a problem, for example, in identifying critical renal stenosis, as reviewed above.

In the terminal stage, when accelerated hypertension supervenes, pharmacologic interruption has often produced dramatic falls in arterial blood pressure (Gavras et al., 1973), results that are consistent with the current hypothesis that this syndrome, too, is renin mediated.

Renin and the pathogenesis of essential hypertension

The application of pharmacologic interruption to the assessment of angiotensin's contribution to the pathogenesis of essential hypertension has created a dilemma. As pointed out above, significant hypotensive responses to saralasin which exceed the normal occur only in a small fraction of patients with essential hypertension. When the converting enzyme inhibitor, SQ 20881, was employed as a blocking agent, however, 70 percent to 85 percent of patients with essential hypertension showed a significant response. Case et al. (1977) have performed a careful study in which the hypotensive response to the two agents was compared in a single patient population (Fig. 2.5). At the extremes of the blood pressure response spectrum, there was agreement: Those patients who showed the largest blood pressure fall following inhibition of converting enzyme also showed a substantial fall in blood pressure with saralasin. Conversely, the patients with the smallest fall in blood pressure in response to SQ 20881 showed either no response or a pressor response to saralasin, presumably reflecting its intrinsic, angiotensinlike activity. In the vast majority of patients between these two poles, however, no relationship was demonstrable. The central question is, which agent more truly defines the contribution of angiotensin?

Saralasin's well-documented partial agonist activity has been suggested to account for the difference (Case et al., 1977). As pointed out above, it is not difficult to imagine that the partial agonist activity results in an underestimate of angiotensin's role in the maintenance of essential hypertension. It is equally reasonable to ask, of course, whether SQ 20881 overestimates the importance of angiotensin as a mediator. Does the problem lie in the lack of sensitivity of saralasin or in the lack of specificity of converting enzyme inhibitors?

Significant blockade of pressor responses to exogenous angiotensin occurs with saralasin doses well below those required for intrinsic pressor activity in man (Hollenberg et al., 1976). We therefore adopted a protocol in which saralasin was infused in a gradually increased dosage, from subthreshold for intrinsic activity (30–100ng/kg/min), to the highest dose likely to be effective, 30µg/kg/min (Hollenberg et al., 1979). This approach revealed significant hypotensive responses in only 5 of 60 (8%) patients with uncomplicated essential hypertension and in only 7 of 32 (22%) patients with advanced essential hypertension likely to have been complicated by nephrosclerosis. The capacity of saralasin to identify renovascular hypertension, reviewed above, and the close correlation between the magnitude of the hypotensive response and the plasma angiotensin II concentration in responders suggested that saralasin, properly employed, does identify and provide a quantitative index of angiotensin-mediated hypertension.

Still open to debate is the specificity of the action of SQ 20881 in reducing blood pressure: The enzyme, as reviewed earlier, is also responsible in part for degradation of bradykinin (Ferreira, Bartelt, and Greene, 1970). An increase in plasma bradykinin concentration following SQ 20881 did not occur in normal subjects (Hollenberg et al., 1977), or in patients with essential hypertension who did not respond with a significant blood pressure fall (Swartz et al., 1979), but a constant increase in plasma bradykinin concentration was documented in the responders (Swartz et al., 1979; Williams and Hollenberg, 1977). Moreover, in patients with a response to SQ 20881, the control bradykinin concentration was higher.

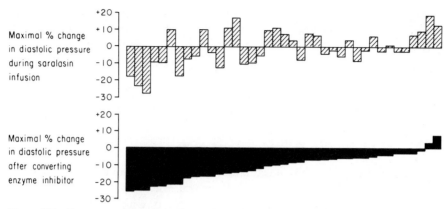

Maximal % change
in diastolic pressure
during saralasin
infusion

Maximal % change
in diastolic pressure
after converting
enzyme inhibitor

Figure 2.5   Depressor responses to the angiotensin antagonist, saralasin, and to the converting enzyme inhibitor (SQ 20881) in the same patients. Note the systematically larger and more consistent reduction in blood pressure induced by SQ 20881. If SQ 20881 operates entirely by reducing plasma angiotensin II, these data suggest that angiotensin makes an important contribution to the maintenance of the hypertension in at least 70 percent of patients with essential hypertension. Unfortunately, as discussed in the text, it is unlikely that SQ 20881 enjoys this specificity. Case et al., 1977. (Figure reproduced by permission of the authors and the publisher.)

To test the specificity of the response to SQ 20881, angiotensin II was infused intravenously in responders in a dose adjusted to return arterial blood pressure to the pre-SQ 20881 level. The working premise was that if the fall in blood pressure following SQ 20881 is entirely due to the fall in plasma angiotensin II concentration, then, when angiotensin II returns blood pressure to control the plasma angiotensin II concentration will also be restored to control levels. If, on the other hand, some additional factor is involved in the fall in blood pressure, then one may anticipate that a higher plasma angiotensin II concentration will be required to restore blood pressure. The latter was found The plasma angiotensin II concentration required to restore blood pressure is strikingly higher than it is prior to SQ 20881 administration (Swartz el al., 1979). Some response other than a fall in plasma angiotensin II concentration induced by SQ 20881 must be involved in the response. Whether the additional factor involves bradykinin, a potent vasodilator, or involves some additional action of the agent is not yet known.

In view of the nonspecificity of SQ 20881, it is quite clear that responses to the agent cannot be used as an index of angiotensin-mediated hypertension. Thus, as a diagnostic procedure, the depressor response is unlikely to be very useful. On the other hand, Re and coworkers (1978) have utilized the agent to enhance the diagnostic utility of renal vein sampling for renin activity determinations. They exploited the fact that converting enzyme inhibition elevates plasma renin activity, presumably because angiotensin II is one of the determinants of renin release. In seven patients with primarily unilateral disease, which was due to renal artery stenosis in six and hydronephrosis in one, the ratio of involved renal vein plasma renin activity increased from 2.9 to 8.4; in a control group of patients without a lateralizing lesion, the ratios were not changed systematically. Although employed in only a small series to date, this approach appears to be promising. Not only will this approach, if successful in a larger series, make it unnecessary to employ an elaborate preparation for renal vein sampling, but hypertension can be controlled during that interval without concern about introducing artifacts in the test.

The nonspecificity, while limiting the diagnostic utility of converting enzyme inhibitors, had important implications for therapy.

IMPLICATIONS FOR THERAPY

Whereas the evidence reviewed above suggests that renin-angiotensin system activity does not play a primary or central role in the pathogenesis of the elevated arterial blood pressure in most patients with essential hypertension—and is perhaps commonly the dominant factor only in patients with renal artery stenosis, advanced nephrosclerosis, and terminal chronic renal parenchymal disease—abundant evidence also suggests that this system is activated whenever therapy is instituted. Certainly, restriction of sodium intake, commonly employed as initial therapy, activates the system. As reviewed earlier, this activation results not only in an increase in plasma renin activity and circulating plasma angiotensin II concentrations, but also in an increased role in maintaining blood pressure, as indicated by an enhanced sensitivity to pharmacologic interruption of the renin-angiotensin system. Natriuretic agents are usually employed as the next step in therapy. A reactive increase in plasma renin activity is common, or perhaps universal, in response to these agents (Laragh, 1977).

To recapitulate, the reactive renin response has several implications: First, there is excellent evidence that the aldosterone response limits the natriuretic effect of the diuretic agents and is responsible, at least in part, for their tendency to produce potassium wasting and hypokalemia. Second, several groups have now shown an enhanced hypotensive response to angiotensin antagonists following institution of diuretic therapy (Gavras et al., 1976; Anderson et al., 1977); indeed, even the "low renin hypertensive" developed a significant hypotensive response when chlorthalidone was added to a sodium-restricted intake (Gavras et al., 1976).

Similarly, vasodilator agents, whatever their structure and mechanism of action, result in both renin release and in sodium retention (Laragh, 1977). It has long been recognized that the sodium retention may limit the ultimate therapeutic efficacy, especially in patients with severe hypertension (Finnerty, 1971). More recently, it has been demonstrated that the reactive renin response also participates in sustaining hypertension via the direct, vascular action of angiotensin II (Pettinger and Mitchell, 1975). Thus, whether one employs a modified diet, diuretic agent, vasodilators, or agents that influence autonomic nervous system activity, a reactive activation of the renin-angiotensin-aldosterone system participates in limiting the response to the agent. For these reasons, an agent that exerts a major action on this system at the same time it has additional actions in reducing blood pressure will have an important therapeutic advantage. Two classes of such agents have been described; the first and most widely utilized group includes the beta-adrenergic blocking agents. The second is the novel, orally effective converting enzyme inhibitor SQ 14225 (captopril), described earlier.

As pointed out previously, a striking association between the control plasma renin activity and the antihypertensive effect of propranolol suggested to Bühler and coworkers (1972) that this agent, which is unequivocally effective in controlling hypertension in some patients, acts via its well-documented capacity to lower plasma renin activity. Reasons for doubting that this is its major action—although it may represent a substantial portion of its effectiveness in individual patients—were reviewed earlier. Evidence does exist, however, that propranolol will participate in reducing the impact of a reactive renin-angiotensin system response to other therapeutic maneuvers. Thus, for example, when propranolol was removed from a propranolol-minoxodil combination, hypertension became worse, with an increase in plasma renin activity (Pettinger and Mitchell, 1975). Moreover, the hypertension became exquisitely sensitive to the angiotensin antagonist, saralasin. In this setting, the direct vascular actions of angiotensin II were likely to have been reduced by the propranolol. Similarly, propranolol will reduce aldosterone excretion in effectively treated essential hypertensives (Drayer et al., 1978). The reactive aldosterone increase in response to a restriction of sodium intake and diuretic therapy may well be blunted by beta blockers.

There has been considerably less experience reported with SQ 14225 (captopril), the orally effective angiotensin converting enzyme inhibitor in humans. Gavras et al. (1978) described effective control of blood pressure in 12 patients, for periods ranging up to 24 weeks. Despite the striking reduction in blood pressure and a diet that provided a liberal sodium intake, there was apparently no evidence of sodium retention. This may well have been due to the reduction in plasma aldosterone concentration, which they documented. Additional factors may be responsible for the striking failure of this agent to induce sodium retention, if it is viewed in the context of the influence of other effective antihypertensive regimens on sodium balance when diuretics are not employed and free access to sodium is allowed (Finnerty, 1971).

The poor correlation between the control plasma renin activity and the antihypertensive efficacy of SQ 14225 suggested that it, as was the case for SQ 20881 (Gavras et al., 1978), did not act solely via its primary action on the renin-angiotensin system. However, it seems likely that for both this agent and the beta-adrenergic blocking agents, their ability to blunt the influence of the reactive response of the renin-angiotensin system plays a role in their continued effectiveness when pressure is controlled.

IMPLICATIONS FOR THE KIDNEY

Multiple lines of evidence have suggested that angiotensin plays an important role in renal perfusion and function, as reviewed in detail elsewhere (Hollenberg, 1978). Editorial constraint prevents a detailed review of the available information concerning the impact of the relevant classes of agent on the kidney. Attention in this brief review will focus on documented human responses that are likely to have clinical implications from the information available on beta-adrenergic blocking agents. Studies in animal models have suggested that the angiotensin antagonists may well have clinical implications for kidney function, but few data are available from studies in humans. The potentially relevant information in animal models will be reviewed, therefore, in brief along with the cursory information available from studies in man.

Angiotensin antagonists

This subject has been reviewed in detail recently (Hollenberg, 1978). In animal models of states in which the renin-angiotensin system is activated and renal perfusion and glomerular filtration rate are reduced, a number of studies have documented reversal of these renal vascular responses with angiotensin antagonists.

In the simplest model, in which the renin-angiotensin system is activated and renal blood flow is reduced by restriction of sodium intake, both the angiotensin antagonists and converting enzyme inhibitors have induced an increase in renal blood flow in animals (Freeman et al., 1973; Mimran, Guiod, and Hollenberg, 1974) and in humans (Hollenberg et al., 1977). In earlier studies, an angiotensin antagonist did not increase glomerular filtration rate or sodium excretion (Freeman et al., 1973; Mimran et al., 1974), but in an elegant investigation, Kimbrough et al. (1977) documented an increase in glomerular filtration rate and sodium excretion when the agents were infused into the renal artery, thus avoiding systemic hypotension. In their study, performed in the unanesthetized dog, neither saralasin nor SQ 20881 influenced renal perfusion or function in animals on a high salt diet. In animals ingesting a diet restricted in sodium the two classes of agents induced an identical 29 percent increase in renal blood flow, with an approximately parallel increase in glomerular filtration rate (Fig. 2.6) and a brisk natriuresis. All have been confirmed (Hall et al., 1977). From these data it appears that a substantial portion of the renal response to restriction of sodium intake can be attributed to the renal response to angiotensin. Hypotension is a recurring theme in this area, because in all of the states in which the renin-angiotensin system is activated, both classes of agent induce what is often a large reduction in blood pressure (Hollenberg, 1978).

The renal vascular response in states in which more striking activation of the system occurs, including anesthesia and trauma (Burger et al., 1976), in thoracic inferior vena cava obstruction (Taub et al., 1977; Freeman et al., 1973), in experimental heart failure (Freeman et al., 1975), in hemorrhagic shock (LaChance et al., 1974), in the impaired reflow after hemorrhage hypotension (Frega et al., 1973), and in acute renal failure (Ishikawa and Hollenberg, 1976) has been reversed in part or in toto by these agents. Angiotensin, therefore, appears to contribute to sustaining both the increase in total periph-

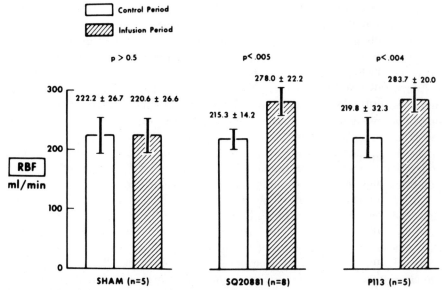

Figure 2.6A   Rise in renal blood flow (RBF) with blockade of the renin-angiotensin system with intrarenal infusion of a converting enzyme inhibitor (SQ 20881) and an angiotensin antagonist (saralasin or P113). Both agents induced a 29 percent increase in renal perfusion in dogs in balance on a sodium-restricted intake, as shown, but did not influence RBF in dogs ingesting a high salt intake. (From Kimbrough, et al., 1977; reproduced by permission of the authors and publisher.)

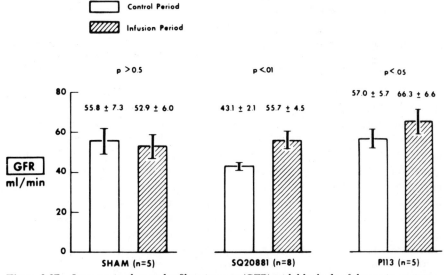

Figure 2.6B   Increase in glomerular filtration rate (GFR) with blockade of the renin-angiotensin system in the same dogs. There was also an increase in sodium excretion. These studies indicate that a substantial, if not the total, renal response to restriction of sodium intake in the healthy animal is mediated by a direct vascular action of angiotensin II.

eral resistance and the increase in renal vascular resistance in these states—which share as their common feature either a true deficit in effective plasma and extracellular fluid volume—or at least a perceived deficit owing to either relative venous dilatation during anesthesia or inadequate myocardial function in congestive heart failure, as examples.

Interpretation of the functional response of the kidney to pharmacological interruption has been complicated by several factors. A blood pressure fall during administration of these agents occurs not only in some patients with secondary hypertension but, as indicated above, also in patients with hepatic cirrhosis (Schroeder et al., 1976), Bartter's syndrome (Sasaki et al., 1976), and congestive heart failure in humans (personal observations). The resultant hypotension may well have limited the renal vascular and functional response.

Caldicott and Taub in our laboratory (unpublished observation) have shown that when an optimal renal blood flow increase is induced with saralasin, by infusing graded doses until the largest renal blood flow increase is obtained, then approximately one-third of the renal blood flow reduction induced by thoracic inferior vena caval occlusion is reversed. In parallel with the renal blood flow increase, there is a similar increase in glomerular filtration rate. Despite the increase in renal perfusion and glomerular filtration rate, a natriuresis does not occur. This result contrasts with that reported by Kimbrough et al. (1977) in which reduced sodium intake in the dog served as the stimulus; the larger stimulus induced by caval occlusion appears to recruit additional factors responsible for sodium retention.

Few data are available for humans. As in the animal models, the agents do not increase renal blood flow in normal persons when the renin-angiotensin system is suppressed by a high salt intake, but they do so when the system is activated by restriction of sodium intake (Hollenberg et al., 1977). Converting enzyme inhibition by SQ 20881 has induced a potentiated increase in renal blood flow in patients with essential hypertension (Williams and Hollenberg, 1977). We have documented (unpublished observation) a statistically and, perhaps biologically, significant increase in glomerular filtration rate in response to this agent in essential hypertension: Approximately a 25 percent increase in glomerular filtration occurred, which was largest in patients in whom glomerular filtration rate was reduced prior to study and in whom more severe hypertension was present. Natriuresis also occurred; the increase in sodium excretion did not parallel the increase in glomerular filtration rate and occurred even in patients in whom an increase in glomerular filtration rate could not be documented. More preliminary studies suggested a similar response of the kidney to SQ 14225. We have also documented an increase in glomerular filtration rate in patients with congestive heart failure who were refractory to therapy with other agents utilized for afterload reduction.

This essentially anecdotal report reflects the current state of information: Little has been published and considerable investigation remains to be done on the implication for the kidney that the angiotensin antagonists hold. If agents that block the system with a preferential action on the kidney can be developed (Taub et al., 1977), this line of investigation can be pursued safely and effectively.

Beta-adrenergic blocking agents

To the extent that these agents reduce renin release, one would anticipate that their impact on the kidney in various states would resemble the response to angiotensin antagonists. Unfortunately, as pointed out earlier, this class of agent enjoys a complicated pharmacology, and no single principle defines the actions of all of the agents.

A number of investigators have demonstrated that propranolol, the most widely studied agent, induces a reduction in renal blood flow and, where measured, in the glomerular filtration rate (Schirmeister et al., 1966; Nayler et al., 1967; Carriere, 1969; Fenyvesi and Kallay, 1970; Nies, McNeil, and Schrier 1971; Krauss et al., 1972; Ibsen and Sederberg-Olsen, 1973; Sullivan, Adams, and Hollenberg, 1976). Because a reduction in the renal blood flow and glomerular filtration rate are common with agents that reduce cardiac output (Sannerstedt and Conway 1970), as does propranolol, the renal response has been widely attributed to the systemic effects of the agent. On that basis a reduction in renal blood flow would be anticipated in response to other beta-adrenergic blocking agents, as was, indeed, demonstrated for dichloroisoproterenol, oxprenolol, and pindolol (Cooper et al., 1967; Bufano and Piacentini, 1969; Abdel-Razzak, 1977; Heierli, Thoelen, and Radielovic, 1977).

On the other hand, several investigators have presented evidence which suggests that the response to propranolol may reflect a local intrarenal rather than a systemic effect and thus be specific for the individual agents. Carriere (1969) demonstrated that the renal vasculature in the dog responds to propranolol when infused into the renal artery in doses too small to have a systemic effect, and that the local effects of propranolol are reversed with phenoxybenzamine, an observation that was quickly confirmed by Fenyvesi and Kallay (1970). Nies et al. (1971) did not report a preferential action of propranolol infused into the renal artery, and therefore concluded that the renal action must be secondary to systemic effects, in a widely cited study. Unfortunately, they employed the same dose infused into the renal artery as was shown earlier to have a systemic effect, so that an influence on the contralateral kidney during intra-arterial infusion should not have been surprising. Other investigators employed a subthreshold dose of propranolol for intra-arterial infusion and were thus able to document a preferential local action (Carriere, 1969; Fenyvesi and Kallay, 1970). Similarly, we demonstrated in humans that propranolol induces renal vasoconstriction in doses too small to reduce heart rate or measured cardiac output (Sullivan, Adams, and Hollenberg, 1976).

Propranolol not only reduces renal plasma flow; glomerular filtration rate has also been shown to be reduced in a number of reports (Schirmeister, et al., 1966, Nies et al., 1971; Ibsen and Sederberg-Olsen, 1973), presumably via mechanisms similar to those responsible for the reduction in renal blood flow. Under most circumstances, the reduction in glomerular filtration rate does not appear to have clinical significance, although it may contribute to the reduced capacity of patients receiving propranolol to handle a sodium load (Epstein and Braunwald, 1966; Krauss et al., 1972) and to the sodium retention that occurs occasionally and that may limit the antihypertensive effect (Wilkinson et al., 1974). Warren, Swainson, and Wright (1974) described three patients with moderately severe chronic renal failure in whom a rapid deterioration of renal function followed therapy with propranolol or oxprenolol. They attributed the renal response to the beta-blocking agents because of the close temporal association and the absence of any other precipitating factors for the azotemia. On the other hand, a substantial experience, including patients with moderate renal insufficiency, has failed to reveal a consistent deleterious effect of propranolol on renal function. Stephen (1966) reported a moderate increase in blood urea in only 7 of 137 patients treated with propranolol. Greenblatt and Koch-Weser (1973) noted a substantial increase in adverse reactions to propranolol in patients in whom the blood urea nitrogen exceeded 25 mg/dl, but progressive azotemia was not mentioned. Thompson and Joekes (1974) reported no systematic effect of propranolol on creatinine clearance in a study that included many patients who were already azotemic, a surprising observation in view of the already well-documented effects of propranolol on glomerular filtration rate.

Other beta-adrenergic blocking agents including pindolol (Heierli, Thoelen, and Radielovic, 1977), acebutolol and tenormine (Zech et al., 1976) also reduce glomerular filtration rate and sodium excretion. That these are not inevitable concomitants of beta-adrenergic blockade is evident from the demonstration by Gibson (1972) that practolol induces an increase in sodium excretion, urine output, and renal free water clearance. Moreover neither alprenolol (Pedersen and Mogensen, 1976) nor tolamolol (Bianchi et al., 1976), in dosages that achieve unequivocal beta-adrenergic blockade, influence either renal perfusion or filtration rates. Nadolol, in dosages that produce a substantial reduction in heart rate, induces a consistent increase in renal blood flow (Hollenberg et al., 1979). Circumstantial evidence suggests that the renal vascular response to nadolol is secondary to reduced renin release (Hollenberg et al., 1979) but definitive studies to prove this point were not performed. In all, it has not been possible to define a single theme that accounts for all of the renal responses to beta-adrenergic blocking agents.

CONCLUSION

In the decade since the first agents were observed to block the renin-angiotensin system with relative specificity and sensitivity, there has been a rapid advance in our understanding of the contribution of this system to physiology and pathophysiology. New approaches in diagnosis and therapy are on the horizon. In diagnosis, saralasin shows promise as an adjunct to our evaluation of renovascular hypertension. In therapy, the converting enzyme inhibitors show early promise not only in primary therapy but as an adjunct in blocking the multiple limbs of the renin-angiotensin system which are responsible, at least in part, for ineffectiveness of other forms of therapy. Finally, preliminary evidence suggests that our ability to block the renin-angiotensin system may well have additional implications for the kidney.

ACKNOWLEDGMENT

The original research that is reported in this essay was performed in our laboratory and supported by National Institute of Health Grants (HL 14944, GM 18674, HL 11668, 5M01 RP 31 13) and a grant from the National Aeronautics and Space Administration.

REFERENCES

Abdel-Razzak, M. (1977). Effect of some beta-adrenergic blocking drugs on renal blood flow in dogs. *Archives Internationales de Pharmacodynamie et de Therapie,* **229,** 227–234.

Anderson, G. H. Jr., Dalakos, T. G., Elias, A., Tomycz, N. & Streeten, D. H. P. (1977). Diuretic therapy and response of essential hypertension to saralasin. *Annals of Internal Medicine,* **87,** 183–187.

Anderson, G. H. Jr., Streeten, D. H. P. & Dalakos, T. G. (1977). Pressor response to 1-Sar-8-Ala angiotensin II (saralasin) in hypertensive subjects. *Circulation Research,* **40,** 243–250.

Baer, L., Parra-Carrillo, J. Z., Radichevich, I. & Williams, G. S. (1977). Detection of renovascular hypertension with angiotensin II blockade. *Annals of Internal Medicine,* **86,** 257–260.

Beckerhoff, R., Furrer, J., Vetter, W., Nussberger, J. & Siegenthaler, W. (1976). Hypotension during angiotensin blockade with saralasin. *British Medical Journal,* **2,** 849.

Beckerhoff, R., Vetter, W., Furrer, J., Zaruba, K., Vetter, H. & Siegenthaler, W. (1976). The effect of the angiotensin antagonist saralasin (1-sar-8-ala-angiotensin II) on blood pressure in secondary hypertension. *Schweizerische Medizinische Wochenschrift,* **106,** 1738–1741.

Bianchi, C., Bonadio, M., Donadio, C., Tramonti, G., Figus, S. & Papalexiou, P. (1976). Acute effects of tolamolol on renal function in hypertensive patients. *Experientia,* **32,** 1565–1566.

Brod, J., Bahlman, J., Cachovan, M., Bubrich, W. & Pretschner, P. (1978). The effect of the angiotensin antagonist saralasin on the blood pressure and haemodynamics in hypertensive non-uraemic chronic parenchymatous renal disease. *7th International Congress of Nephrology,* Montreal, p. B-11.

Brunner, H. R., Gavras, H. & Laragh, J. H. (1973). Angiotensin II blockade in man by sar¹-ala⁸-angiotensin II for understanding and treatment of high blood pressure. *Lancet,* **2,** 1045–1048.

Brunner, H. R., Kirshman, J. D., Sealey, J. E. & Laragh J. H. (1971). Hypertension of renal origin: Evidence for two different mechanisms. *Science,* **174,** 1344–1346.

Bufano, G. & Piacentini, L. (1969). Studio comparativo dell'influenza esercitata da agonisti e antagonisti beta-adrenergici sulla funzione renale del'umo normale. *Minerva Medica,* **60,** 1229–1232.

Buehler, F. R., Laragh, J. H., Baer, L., Vaughan, E. D. Jr., & Brunner, H. R.: (1972). Propranolol inhibition of renin secretion. A specific approach to diagnosis and treatment of renin-dependent hypertensive diseases. *New England Journal of Medicine,* **287,** 1209–1214.

Bühler, F. R., Burkart, F., Lutold, B. E., Bertel, O. & Pfisterer, M. (1977). Plasmakatecholamine und Hamodynamik im Verlauf der antihypertensiven Betablockade: Verschiedene muster bei Propranolol-Responders und Non-Responders. *Schweizerische Medizinische Wochenschrift,* **107,** 1589–1590.

Bumpus, F. M. (1977). In *Hypertension, Mechanisms, Diagnosis and Management,* ed. Davis, J. O., Laragh, J. H. & Selwyn, A., pp. 46–58. New York: HP Publishing Company.

Burger, B. M., Hopkins, T., Tulloch, A. & Hollenberg, N. K. (1976). The role of angiotensin in the canine renal vascular response to barbiturate anesthesia. *Circulation Research*, **38**, 196–202.

Carriere, C. (1969). Effect of norepinephrine, isoproterenol, and adrenergic blockers upon the intrarenal distribution of blood flow. *Canadian Journal of Physiology and Pharmacology*, **47**, 199–208.

Case, D. B., Wallace, J. M., Keim, H. J., Weber, M. A., Sealey, J. E. & Laragh, J. H. (1977). Possible role of renin in hypertension as suggested by renin-sodium profiling and inhibition of converting enzyme. *New England Journal of Medicine*, **296**, 641–646.

Cooper, N., Barry, W. F. Jr., Labay, P. & Boyarsky, S. (1967). Evidence of renal hemodynamic changes encountered after dichloroisoproterenol. *Investigative Urology*, **4**, 366–371.

Davis, J. O. (1977). The pathogenesis of chronic renovascular hypertension. *Circulation Research*, **40**, 439–444.

Drayer, J. I. M., Weber, M. A., Longworth, D. L. & Laragh, J. H. (1978). The possible importance of aldosterone as well as renin in the long-term antihypertensive action of propranolol. *The American Journal of Medicine*, **64**, 187–192.

Duhme, D. W., Sancho, J., Athanasoulis, C., Haber, E. & Koch-Weser, J. (1974). Hypotension during administration of angiotensin converting enzyme inhibitor SQ 20881. *Lancet*, March 9, 1974, p. 408.

Epstein, S. E. & Braunwald, E. (1966). Effect of beta-adrenergic blockade on urinary sodium excretion: Studies in normal subjects and in patients with heart disease. *Annals of Internal Medicine*, **65**, 20–27.

Erdös, E. G. (1975). Angiotensin I converting enzyme. *Circulation Research*, **36**, 247–255.

Fagard, R. (1978). In *Studies on the Renin-Angiotensin-Aldosterone System*, ed. Fagard, R., 149 pages, Leuven.

Fenyvesi, T. & Kallay, K. (1970). The presence of beta-adrenergic receptors in the renal vascular bed. *Acta Physiologica Academiae Scientiarum Hungaricae*, **38**, 159–166.

Ferreira, S. H., Bartelt, D. C. & Greene, L. J. (1970). Isolation of bradykinin potentiating peptides from *Bothrops jaracara* venom. *Biochemistry (Washington)*, **9**, 2583–2593.

Finnerty, F. A. Jr. (1971). Relationship of extracellular fluid volume to the development of drug resistance in the hypertensive patient. *American Heart Journal*, **81**, 563–565.

Freeman, R. H., Davis, J. O., Spielman, W. S. & Lohmeier, T. E. (1975). High-output heart failure in the dog: Systemic and intrarenal role of angiotensin II. *American Journal of Physiology*, **229**, 474–478,

Freeman, R. H., Davis, J. O., Vitale, S. J. & Johnson, J. A. (1973). Intrarenal role of angiotensin II. *Circulation Research*, **32**, 692–698.

Frega, N., Guerther, B., Bibona, D. & Leaf, A. (1973). The role of angiotensin II in the impaired reflow following hemorrhagic hypotension. *American Society of Nephrology*, **6**, 37.

Gavras, H. R., Brunner, H. R., Turini, G. A., Kershaw, G. R., Tifft, C. P., Cuttelod, S., Gavras, I., Vukovich, R. A. & McKinstry, D. N. (1978). Antihypertensive effect of the oral angiotensin converting enzyme inhibitor SQ 14225 in man. *New England Journal of Medicine*, **298**, 991–995.

Gavras, H. R., Brunner, H. R., Vaughan, E. D. Jr. & Laragh, J. H. (1973). Angiotensin-sodium interaction in blood pressure maintenance of renal hypertensive and normotensive rats. *Science*, **180**, 1369–1371.

Gavras, H., Ribeiro, A. R., Gavras, I. & Brunner, H. R. (1976). Reciprocal relation between renin dependency and sodium dependency in essential hypertension. *New England Journal of Medicine*, **295**, 1278–1283.

Gibson, D. G. (1972). Effects of practolol administration on cardiac and renal function in patients with chronic atrial fibrillation. *Acta Cardiologica, Suppl.*, **15**, 279–280.

Greenblatt, D. J. & Koch-Weser, J. (1973). Adverse reactions to propranolol in hospitalized medical patients: A report from the Boston Collaborative Drug Surveillance Program. *American Heart Journal*, **86**, 478–484.

Gross, F. (1977). Beta-adrenergic blockade, blood pressure, and the renin-angiotensin system. *European Journal of Clinical Investigation*, **7**, 321–322.

Haber, E. (1976). The role of renin in normal and pathological cardiovascular homeostasis. *Circulation*, **54**, 849–861.

Hall, J. E., Guyton, A. C., Trippodo, N. C., Lohmeier, T. E., McCaa, R. E. & Cowley, A. W. (1977). Intrarenal control of electrolyte excretion by angiotensin II. *American Journal of Physiology*, **232**, F538–F544.

Heierli, C., Thoelen, H. & Radielovic, P. (1977). Renal function following a single dose of pindolol in hypertensive patients with varying degrees of impairment of renal function. *International Journal of Clinical Pharmacology*, **15**, 65–71.

Holland, O. B. & Kaplan, N. M. (1976). Propranolol in the treatment of hypertension. *New England Journal of Medicine*, **294**, 930–936.

Hollenberg, N. K. (1978). Angiotensin antagonists, the renin-angiotensin system, and the kidney. *Proceedings of the 7th International Congress of Nephrology*, Montreal, 677–685.

Hollenberg, N.K. (1979). Pharmacologic interruption of the renin-angiotensin system. In *Annual Reviews of Pharmacology*, ed. George, R. & Okun, R., vol. 19. Palo Alto, Calif.: Annual Reviews.

Hollenberg, N. K., Williams, G. H., Adams, D. F., Moore, T., Brown, C., Borucki, L. J., Leung, F., Bavli, S., Solomon, H. S., Passan, D. & Dluhy, R. (1979). Response to saralasin and angiotensin's role in essential and renal hypertension. *Medicine*, **58**, 115–127

Hollenberg, N. K., Williams, G. H., Burger, B., Ishikawa, I. & Adams, D. F. (1976). Blockade and stimulation of renal, adrenal, and vascular angiotensin II receptors with 1-sar, 8-ala angiotensin II in normal man. *Journal of Clinical Investigation*, **57**, 39–46.

Hollenberg, N. K., Williams, G. H., Taub, K. J., Ishikawa, I., Brown, C. & Adams, D. F. (1977). Renal vascular response to interruption of the renin-angiotensin system in normal man. *Kidney International*, **12**, 285–293.

Ibsen, H. & Sederberg-Olsen, P. (1973). Changes in glomerular filtration rate during long-term treatment with propranolol in patients with arterial hypertension. *Clinical Science*, **44**, 129–134.

Ishikawa, I. & Hollenberg, N. K. (1976). Pharmacologic interruption of the renin-angiotensin system in myohemoglobinuric acute renal failure. *Kidney International*, **10**, S183–S190.

Khairallah, P. A., Toth, A. & Bumpus, F. M. (1970). Analogs of angiotensin II. Mechanism of receptor interaction. *Journal of Medical Chemistry*, **13**, 181.

Kimbrough, H. M. Jr., Vaughan, E. D. Jr., Carey, R. M. & Ayers, C. R. (1977). Effect of intrarenal AII blockade on renal function in conscious dogs. *Circulation Research*, **40**, 174–178.

Krauss, X. H., Schalekamp, M. A. D. H., Kolsters, G., Zaal, G. A. & Birkenhager, W. H. (1972). Effects of chronic beta-adrenergic blockade on systemic and renal hemodynamic responses to hyperosmotic saline in hypertensive patients. *Clinical Science*, **43**, 385–391.

LaChance, J. G., Arnoux, E., Brunnette, M. G. & Carriere, S. (1974). Factors responsible for the outer cortical ischemia observed during hemorrhagic hypotension in dogs. *Circulatory Shock*, **1**, 131–144.

Laragh, J. H. (1977). Vasoconstriction-volume analysis in treatment of hypertension. In, *Hypertension: Mechanisms, Diagnosis and Management*, ed. Davis, J. O., Laragh, J. H., Selwyn, A. Chap. 7. New York: H. P. Publishing Company.

Marks, L. S., Maxwell, M. H., & Kaufman, J. J. (1977). Renin, sodium, and vasodepressor response to saralasin in renovascular and essential hypertension. *Annals of Internal Medicine*, **87**, 176–182.

Marshall, G. R. (1976). Structure-activity relations of antagonists of the renin-angiotensin system. *Federation Proceedings, Federation of American Societies for Experimental Biology*, **35**, 2494–2501.

Maxwell, M. H. (1975). Cooperative study of renovascular hypertension: Current status. *Kidney International*, **8**, S153–S160.

Mimran, A., Guiod, L. & Hollenberg, N. K. (1974). Angiotensin's role in the cardiovascular and renal response to salt restriction. *Kidney International*, **5**, 248–355.

Nayler, W. G., McInnes, J., Swann, J. B., Carson, V. & Lowe, T. E. (1967). Effect of propranolol, a beta-adrenergic antagonist, on blood flow in the coronary and other vascular fields. *American Heart Journal*, **73**, 207–216.

Nies, A. S., McNeil, J. S. & Schrier, R. W. (1971). Mechanism of increased sodium reabsorption during propranolol administration. *Circulation*, **44**, 596–604.

Ogihara, T., Yamamoto, T. & Kumahara, Y. (1974). Clinical applications of synthetic angiotensin II analogue. *Japanese Circulation Journal*, **38**, 997.

Ondetti, M. A., Rubin, B. & Cushman, D. W. (1977). Design of specific inhibitors of angiotensin-converting enzyme: New class of orally active antihypertensive agents. *Science*, **196**, 441–444.

Ondetti, M. A., Williams, N. G., Sabo, E. F., Plusec, J., Weaver, E. R. & Kocy, O. (1971).

Angiotensin-converting enzyme inhibitors from the venom of *Bothrops jaracara*. Isolation, elucidation of structure, and synthesis. *Biochemistry*, **10**, 4033–4039.

Pals, D. T., Masucci, F. D., Denning, G. S. Jr., Sipos, F. & Fessler, D. C. (1971). Role of the pressor action of angiotensin II in experimental hypertension. *Circulation Research*, **29**, 673–681.

Peach, M. J. & Chiu, A. T. (1974). Stimulation and inhibition of aldosterone biosynthesis in vitro by angiotensin II and analogs. *Circulation Research (supplement)*, **34** & **35**, I7–I13.

Pedersen, E. B. & Mogensen, C. E. (1976). Effect of antihypertensive treatment on urinary albumin excretion, glomerular filtration rate, and renal plasma flow in patients with essential hypertension. *Scandinavian Journal of Clinical and Laboratory Investigation*, **36**, 231–237.

Pettinger, W. A., Keeton, T. K., Campbell, W. B. & Harper, D. C. (1976). Evidence for a renal beta-adrenergic receptor inhibiting renin release in rats. *Circulation Research*, **38**, 1–10.

Pettinger, W. A., Keeton, K., Phil, M. & Tanaka, K. (1975). Radioimmunoassay and pharmacokinetics of saralasin in the rat and hypertensive patients. *Clinical Pharmacology and Therapeutics*, **17**, 146–158.

Pettinger, W. A. & Mitchell, H. C. (1975). Renin release, saralasin and the vasodilator-beta-blocker drug interaction in man. *New England Journal of Medicine*, **292**, 1214–1217.

Re, R., Novelline, R., Escourrou, M-T., Athanasoulis, C., Burton, J. & Haber, E. (1978). Inhibition of angiotensin-converting enzyme for diagnosis of renal-artery stenosis. *New England Journal of Medicine*, **298**, 582–586.

Regoli, D., Park, W. K. & Rioux, F. (1974). Pharmacology of angiotensin. *Pharmacology Reviews*, **26**, 69–123.

Rocchini, A. P. & Barger, A. C. (1979). Renovascular hypertension in sodium-depleted dogs: Role of renin and carotid sinus reflex. *American Journal of Physiology* **236**, H101–H107.

Sannerstedt, R. & Conway, J. (1970). Hemodynamic and vascular response to antihypertensive treatment with adrenergic blocking agents: A review. *American Heart Journal*, **79**, 122–127.

Sasaki, H., Okumara, H., Ikeda, H., Kawasaki, I. & Fukiyama, K. (1976). Hypotensive response to angiotensin II analogue in Bartter's syndrome. *New England Journal of Medicine*, **294**, 611–612.

Schalekamp, M. A., Beevers, D. G., Briggs, J. D., Brown, J. J., Davies, D. L., Fraser, R., Lebel, M., Lever, A. F., Medina, A., Morton, J. J., Robertson, J. I. S. & Tree, M. (1974). Hypertension in chronic renal failure: An abnormal relation between sodium and the renin-angiotensin system. In, *Hypertension Manual*, ed. Laragh, J. H., pp. 485–508. New York: Dun-Donnelley Publishing Corporation.

Schirmeister, J., VonDecot, M., Hallauer, W. & Willman, H. (1966). Beta-receptoren und renale Hamodunamik des Menschen. *Artzneinittel Forschung*, **16**, 847–850.

Schroeder, E. T., Anderson, G. H., Goldman, S. H. & Streeten, D. H. P. (1976). Effects of angiotensin II (AII) blockade with 1-Sar-8-Ala (saralasin) in patients with cirrhosis and ascites. *Kidney International*, **9**, 511–519.

Stephen, S. A. (1966). Unwanted effects of propranolol. *American Journal of Cardiology*, **18**, 463–472.

Sullivan, J. M., Adams, D. F. & Hollenberg, N. K. (1976). Beta-adrenergic blockade in essential hypertension. *Circulation Research*, **39**, 532–536.

Swartz, S. L., Williams, G. H., Hollenberg, N. K., Moore, T. J. & Dluhy, R. G. (1979). Factors mediating the hypotensive response to converting enzyme inhibition. *Hypertension*, **1**, 106–111.

Taub, K. J., Caldicott, W. J. H. & Hollenberg, N. K. (1977). Angiotensin antagonists with increased specificity for the renal vasculature. *Journal of Clinical Investigation*, **59**, 528–535.

Thompson, F. D. & Joekes, A. M. (1974). Beta-blockade in the presence of renal disease and hypertension. *British Medical Journal*, **2**, 555–556.

Warren, D. J., Swainson, C. P. & Wright, N. (1974). Deterioration in renal function after beta-blockade in patients with chronic renal failure and hypertension. *British Medical Journal*, **2**, 193–194.

Wilkinson, R., Pickering, M., Robson, V., Elliott, R. W. & Kerr, D. N. S. (1974). The use of frusemide and propranolol in the treatment of the hypertension of chronic renal disease. *Scottish Medical Journal*, **19**, 25–30.

Williams, G. H. & Hollenberg, N. K. (1977). Accentuated vascular and endocrine response to SQ 20881 in hypertension. *New England Journal of Medicine*, **297**, 184–188.

Wilson, H. M., Wilson, J. P., Slaton, P. E., Foster, J. H., Liddle, G. W., Hollifield, J. W. (1977). Saralasin infusion in the recognition of renovascular hypertension. *Annals of Internal Medicine*, **87**, 36–42.

Zech, P., Pozet, N., Labeeuw, M., Sassard, J., Bernheim, J., Pellet, M. & Traeger, J. (1976). Acute renal effects of new beta-adrenergic receptor site blocking agents on renal function. *Proceedings of the European Dialysis Transplantation Association*, **12**, 203–209.

3

Biochemistry and pharmacology of renal prostaglandins

AUBREY R. MORRISON
PHILIP NEEDLEMAN

Biochemistry
Phospholipase A$_2$
Cyclooxygenase
Thromboxane synthetase
Renal prostacyclin synthesis
Site of PG synthesis
    Cortex
    Medulla

Metabolism
Pharmacology
Cyclooxygenase inhibition
Renal blood flow
Ureteral obstruction

Since the original reports by Kurzok and Lieb (1930), von Euler (1930), and Bergstrom and Sjovall (1960), which describe the biological effects of prostaglandins on smooth muscle, there has been a virtual explosion of information relating to the biochemistry, metabolism, and physiology of the lipids. In the last ten to fifteen years, much information on the role of prostaglandins in renal physiology has emerged. While the capacity for prostaglandin biosynthesis is ubiquitous, many organs seem to have their own characteristic end products of prostaglandin biosynthesis. In addition, certain pathological conditions can unmask pathways of endoperoxide metabolism that, while dormant under basal conditions, may be potential mediators of the pathophysiologic events. In this chapter we will concentrate on the biochemical parameters controlling prostaglandin biosynthesis and the pharmacology of these vasoactive compounds on renal vascular resistance.

BIOCHEMISTRY—SYNTHESIS

Phospholipase A$_2$

There is no evidence that prostaglandins are stored; thus, release into extracellular fluid reflects de novo biosynthesis (Piper and Vane, 1969; Piper and Vane, 1971). In addition, for endogenous prostaglandin biosynthesis to occur the free fatty acid precursor (primarily arachidonic acid) must be released by a stimulus. (Lands and Samuelsson, 1968, Isakson et al., 1977). Arachidonic acid ([all-Z]-5,8,11,14-eicosatetraenoic acid) is a polyunsaturated fatty acid and the precursor for the 2-series prostaglandins. Tissue levels of free fatty acids are very low. Most of the arachidonic acid in kidney tissue has been reported to be in the phospholipid fraction (Morgan, Tinker, and Hanahan, 1963; Crowshaw, 1973; Muller et al., 1976). This observation has been confirmed by labelling the isolated perfused rabbit kidney with [^{14}C] arachidonic acid. The [^{14}C] fatty acid was incorporated mainly into phospholipids primarily in the 2-position of phosphatidylcholine and phosphatidylethanolamine (Isakson, Raz, and Needleman, 1976; Hsueh, Isakson, and Needleman, 1977).

The release of arachidonic acid appears to involve the cleavage of phospholipids by phospholipase A_2 (Kunze and Vogt, 1971; Danon et al., 1975; Flower and Blackwell, 1976). Prostaglandin release from rabbit kidney medulla slices was inhibited in low calciuim media and increased on exposure to cobra venom phospholipase A_2 (Kalisher and Dyer, 1972). Additional experiments by Knapp et al. (1977) using the ionophore A23187 suggest that there is an obligatory requirement for Ca^{++} in the release of arachidonate metabolites from rat renal papilla minces.

Although arachidonic acid ($C_{20:4}$) is the major fatty acid in the phospholipid fractions of renal cortex and outer medulla, linoleic ($C_{18:2}$), oleic ($C_{18:1}$), and palmitic ($C_{16:0}$) acids are also present in significant quantities (Mueller et al., 1976). The substrate specificity of phospholipase was demonstrated by infusing kidneys with different [^{14}C]-labeled fatty acids (i.e., palmitate, oleate, linoleate, and arachidonate [Hseuh et al., 1977]). Each fatty acid was comparably incorporated into the phospholipid fraction of the kidney (Fig. 3.1). During the infusion of the fatty acids, only exogenous arachidonic acid produced spasmogenic compounds (Hsueh et al., 1977). Stimulation of the prelabelled tissues with the peptide hormone bradykinin released prostaglandinlike substances (PLS as measured by superfusion bioassay). However, if the perfusate collected after stimulation with bradykinin was acidified to pH 3.5 and extracted into organic solvent and subjected to thin layer chromatography only, [^{14}C] PGE_2 was present in the effluent from kidneys with [^{14}C]-labelled phospholipids. In these experiments the arachidonic, linoleic, oleic, and palmitic acids were all incorporated into the native phospholipid pools. Of these fatty acids, only arachidonate was released from the phospholipid pool in response to stimulation with bradykinin.

The apparent sequence of events occurring during hormone stimulation seems to involve activation of a specific receptor at the cell surface, which in turn activates phospholipase A_2 and then cleavage of arachidonate from the 2-position of phospholipids. The arachidonate can then be metabolized to cyclized (prostaglandins) and noncyclized products or be reacylated back into the phospholipid pool (Figure 3.2). Such a model presupposes one of two possibilities. First, either bradykinin-stimulated arachidonate release is coupled to a specific phospholipase A_2, which cleaves only arachidonate from the 2-position; or second, that the stimulus is coupled to a very discrete pool of phos-

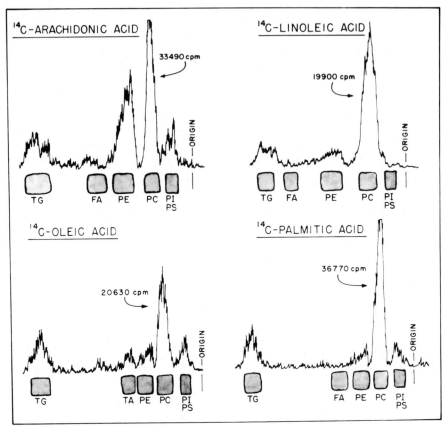

Figure 3.1   Kidneys labelled with various [^{14}C] fatty acids homogenized with lipids extracted in 20 vol chloroform:methanol (2:1). The extracted lipids are then chromatographed in chloroform:methanol:ammonia (65:35:5) for separation of phospholipids. (The following abbreviations of chromatographic standards are employed: triglycerides, TG; fatty acid, FA; phosphatidyl ethanolamine, PE; phosphatidyl choline, PC; spingomyelin, Sph; phosphatidyl inositol, PI; phosphatidyl serine, PS.) (From Hsueh et al., 1977, with permission.)

pholipids which contain only arachidonate in the 2-position such that bradykinin stimulation activates a phospholipase A$_2$, which can then only release arachidonate.

Cyclooxygenase

The biosynthesis of prostaglandin E$_2$ in renal medulla from arachidonic acid was initially investigated by Lee et al. (1967), Hamberg (1969), and Crowshaw (1971). There was very little evidence of cortical prostaglandin synthesis. However, Larsson and Anggard (1973) demonstrated that the renal cortical synthesis was about 10 percent of that in the renal medulla. Cortical prostaglandin biosynthesis has since been confirmed by several investigators (Dunn, 1976; Pong and Levine, 1976).

Intensive investigation of prostaglandin biosynthesis (Hamberg and Sa-

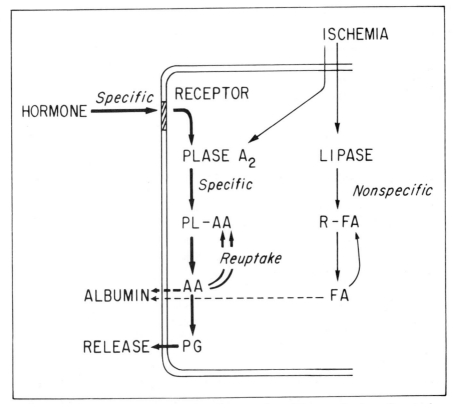

Figure 3.2 Diagrammatic representation of proposed regulatory mechanisms of prostaglandin synthesis in the cell.

muelsson, 1973; Hamberg et al., 1974; Nugteren and Hazelhof, 1973) has led to the isolation and identification of two endoperoxides (PGG_2 and PGH_2), which are unstable intermediates generated prior to the appearance of the stable prostaglandins PGE_2 and $PGF_{2\alpha}$. The group of enzymes responsible for the conversion of arachidonate to endoperoxides has been referred to as the cyclooxygenase system (endoperoxide synthetase). The steps involved in this transformation are removal of the pro-S hydrogen at C-13, isomerization of the Δ^{11} double bond into the Δ^{12} position, and insertion of oxygen at C-11 (Samuelsson, 1965; Samuelsson, 1972). This is then followed by ring closure (cyclization) and formation of a hydroperoxy group at C_{15}. This complex series of reactions leads to the unstable intermediate PGG_2 ($t_{1/2} = 5$ min in aqueous solution) which is further reduced to PGH_2 by $PGG_2 \rightarrow PGH_2$ reductase and liberation of a free radical (Egan, Paxton, and Kuehl, 1976). In the kidney the major prostaglandin end product appears to be PGE_2, which is formed by the enzyme $PGH_2 \rightarrow PGE_2$ isomerase (Miyamoto, Yamamoto, and Hayaishi, 1974; Miaymoto et al., 1976). PGD_2 is also produced by an isomerase in the kidney in vitro (Granstrom, Lands, and Samuelsson, 1968). Renal $PGF_{2\alpha}$ is believed to arise by the action of 9-ketoreductase, a cytoplasmic enzyme from PGE_2 (Lee and Levine, 1974; Lee et al., 1975; Stone and Hart, 1976). In addition, $PGF_{2\alpha}$

may also be formed by $PGH_2 \rightarrow PGF_{2\alpha}$ reductase (Hamberg and Samuelsson, 1973; Nugteren and Hazelhof, 1973). Which of the two pathways of $PGF_{2\alpha}$ biosynthesis is more important is unclear. However, the activity of 9-keto reductase in the kidney may be regulated by salt balance (Weber, Larsson and Scherer, 1977), bradykinin (Terragno and McGiff, 1975, Wong et al., 1977) and by cyclic GMP (Wong and McGiff, 1977).

Thromboxane synthetase

Recently we discovered that thromboxane A_2 is produced by hormone stimulation of the isolated perfused kidney of the rabbit with ureteral obstruction (Morrison, Nishikawa and Needleman, 1977, 1978). This arachidonate product has a biological $t_{1/2}$ of 40 secs at 37°C in aqueous media (Hamberg, Svensson, and Samuelsson, 1975) and is not found in normal rabbit kidney. Microsomes prepared from cortex and medulla of the ureter-obstructed kidney and incubated with PGH_2 produced a potent aortic constrictor (Morrison et al., 1978), the synthesis of which was blocked by imidazole a specific inhibitor of thromboxane synthetase (Needleman et al., 1977a & b; Tai and Yuan, 1978). Subsequent radiochemical experiments using [^{14}C] arachidonate as substrate indicated that the microsomes from cortex and medulla of ureter-obstructed kidney converted [^{14}C] arachidonate to PGE_2, $PGF_{2\alpha}$, PGD_2, and, in addition, a peak of radioactivity corresponding to thromboxane B_2 (stable metabolite of thromboxane A_2). The peak, which co-migrates with TxB_2 on the radiochromatogram, was completely inhibited by imidazole (Morrison et al., 1977). Similar experiments with microsomal preparations from cortex and medulla from contralateral (i.e., unobstructed) and normal rabbit kidneys have not demonstrated any evidence of thromboxane biosynthesis either in bioassay or radiochemical experiments. Thus in the rabbit kidney ureter obstruction unmasked the biosynthesis of thromboxane A_2. This potent vasoactive substance may be of critical importance in the regulation of renal vascular resistance during ureter obstruction. Recently, normal rat kidney cortical microsomes (Zenser et al., 1977) have been shown to synthesize thromboxane A_2.

Renal prostacyclin synthesis

Since the important discovery of PGI_2 (PGX, prostacyclin) synthesis in blood vessel microsomes (Moncada et al., 1976) a & b; Gryglewski et al., 1976), several investigators have demonstrated PGI_2 synthesis in almost every vascular bed studied (Bunting et al., 1976; Pace-Asciak and Rangaraj 1977; Powell and Solomon, 1977; Terragno et al. 1977). PGI_2 biosynthesis has since been demonstrated in whole kidney homogenates of rat kidney (Pace-Asciak and Rangaraj, 1977), in cortical microsomes of rat kidney using PGH_2 as substrate (Zenser et al., 1977), rabbit kidney cortex (Sun, Chapman and McGuire, 1977; Whorton et al., 1978) and in perfused rabbit kidney with exogenous arachidonate acid (Needleman et al., 1978). PGI_2 has potent antiaggregatory properties (Moncada et al., 1976b) and has been shown to stimulate renin release from renal cortical slices (Whorton et al., 1977) and intact dog kidneys (Gerber et al., 1978). In addition, PGI_2 relaxes the isolated bovine coronary artery strip (Kulkarni, Roberts, and Needleman, 1976; Raz et al., 1977; Isakson et al., 1977a), hence local production in the afferent glomerular arteriole may serve a dual function. PGI_2 may have a direct effect on modulating afferent glomerular arteriolar tone as well as on increasing renin release from the juxtaglomerular apparatus, which may then have more general effects on salt balance in the intact animal. Figure 3.3 shows the pathways of arachidonate metabolism currently believed to exist in the kidney.

Site of PG synthesis

Cortex

Early studies by Hamberg (1969) and Crowshaw (1971) indicated that the renal medulla was the major site of synthesis of prostaglandins. As previously indicated, however, several investigators have shown that the renal cortex is capable of prostaglandin biosynthesis. Studies by Whorton et al. (1978) in the rabbit suggest that the cortex is the major site of PGI_2 biosynthesis. Our studies in the ureter-obstructed rabbit kidney demonstrate that the major site of thromboxane biosynthesis is the cortex (Morrison et al., 1978). The localization of synthesis of these potent vasoactive agents (PGI_2 and thromboxane A_2) seem to be of critical importance in modulating total and regional blood flow because the resistance vessels (afferent and efferent glomerular arterioles) are cortical and 98 percent of renal blood flow passes through this area (Thurau, 1964).

We performed experiments in our laboratory using a technique of labelling the endogenous phospholipid pool with [^{14}C] arachidonic acid. Two labelling techniques were employed: (1) infusion of [^{14}C] arachidonate in a single pass through the perfused kidney in the absence of protein, or (2) recirculation of the same quantity of label in the presence of bovine serum albumin. In these experiments autoradiographic studies on the labelled kidneys showed preferential labelling of vascular structures in kidneys labelled by single pass and uniform labelling of vascular structures and renal parenchyma when labelled by recirculation with albumin (Hsueh and Needleman, 1978). Stimulation with bradykinin released comparable amounts of bioassayable (cold) prostaglandins from kidneys labelled by both methods. Bradykinin stimulation of the kidney with preferential vascular labelling (without protein carrier) produced higher absolute amounts of [^{14}C] arachidonic acid and [^{14}C] PGE_2 in the effluent than labelling by recirculation with protein. The ratio of [^{14}C] arachidonate and [^{14}C] PGE_2 in the effluent was the same in both experimental situations. Thus the specific activity of the arachidonic acid and PGE_2 were higher in the kidney labelled by infusion (preferential vascular labelling). The data suggests that the hormone-stimulated pool of phospholipid was predominantly localized to vascular structures. Thus cortical prostaglandin biosynthesis in and

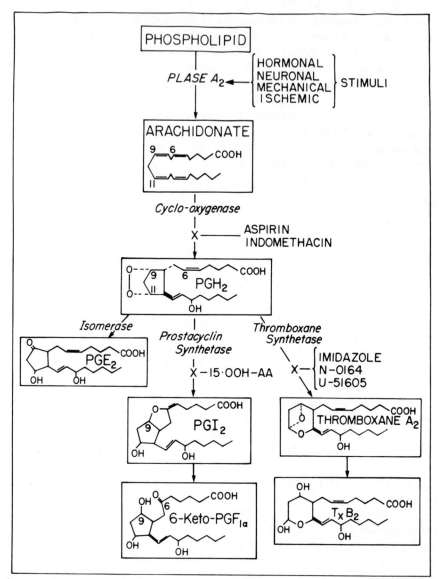

Figure 3.3 Schema of pathways of arachidonic metabolism in the kidney.

around blood vessels in response to hormonal stimulation may be modulating local vascular tone.

Medulla

Janszen and Nugteren (1971), using a histochemical method, found prostaglandins located almost exclusively in the collecting ducts. In addition, Cavallo (1976a & b) using a histochemical reaction with H_2O_2 as substrate, found a peroxidase localized in the medullary interstitial cells and in the collecting duct cells and suggested that this enzyme was related to prostaglandin synthesis. More recently Bohman (1977) has isolated medullary collecting duct cells and demonstrated that they were capable of converting arachidonate to PGE_2, $PGF_{2\alpha}$, and PGD_2. In addition, their studies indicated that one other cell type, probably the medullary interstitial cell, contributed significantly to prostaglandin biosynthesis. In earlier studies, Muirhead et al. (1972; 1973) grew monolayers of renomedullary interstitial cells in tissue culture derived from isogeneic grafts of transplanted renal medulla. These cultured renomedullary cells synthesized both prostaglandins and a nonprostanoic moiety termed antihypertensive neutral renal lipid. More recently, using the same culture techniques, Zusman and Kaiser (1977a & b) have demonstrated the capacity of the renal interstitial cells to synthesize prostaglandins in response to arginine vasopressin, angiotensin II, and bradykinin.

Thus, there appears to be at least three different regions capable of PG biosynthesis in the kidney: (1) the glomerulus and afferent arteriole (i.e., vascular synthesis); (2) the medullary collecting duct; and (3) the medullary interstitial cell.

METABOLISM

The initial biological inactivation of prostaglandin is catalyzed by a 15-hydroxy prostaglandin dehydrogenase (Anggard and Samuelsson, 1964, 1966; Hamberg and Samuelsson, 1971). Lee et al. (1975) have shown that two classes of the enzyme exist in swine kidney cortex and medulla. The $NADP^+$-dependent (type II) activity is slightly higher in medulla than cortex. The cortex, however, has a tenfold higher activity of the NAD^+-dependent (type I) dehydrogenase than the medulla (Larsson and Anggard, 1973; Lee et al. 1975). The PGDH type II seems to have a much lower affinity for PGE_2 than does PGDH type I (Hansen, 1976). The activity of the type I enzyme in rat kidney has been shown to be dependent on de novo protein synthesis and that enzyme activity declines with a $t_{1/2}$ of 45 to 75 minutes, after a single dose of cycloheximide (Blackwell, Flower, and Vane, 1975). The 15-keto compound formed is rapidly converted to a 13, 14-dihydro-15-keto compound by a Δ^{13} reductase. Further metabolism proceeds via beta oxidation to give the dinor and tetranor compounds and by ω oxidation to afford $\omega 1$ and $\omega 2$ hydroxy compounds. Thus the main metabolites of PGE_2 and $PGF_{2\alpha}$ are 7α-hydroxy-5, 11-α-diketotetranorprostane-1, 16 dioic acid, and 5α, 7α-dihydroxy-11-ketotetranorprostane 1, 16 dioic acid, respectively.

Metabolism of thromboxane A_2 in kidney involves the spontaneous reduction of the oxatane bridge resulting in the formation of thromboxane B_2. Thromboxane B_2 has been shown to be further metabolized in primate kidney with the appearance in the urine of several metabolites of thromboxane B_2 (Roberts et al., 1977a & b) as determined by gas chromatography mass spectroscopy. PGI_2 spontaneously degrades to 6-keto-$PGF_{1\alpha}$ (Johnson et al., 1976).

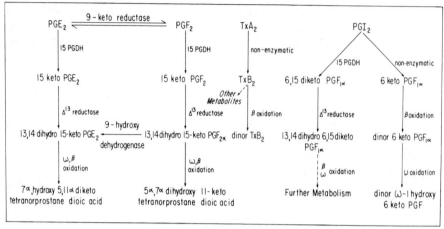

Figure 3.4 Schema of metabolic pathways of the biologically active renal prostaglandins.

This compound has been shown to be further metabolized to dinor 6 keto-$PGF_{1\alpha}$ and dinor ω-1-hydroxy-6-keto-$PGF_{1\alpha}$ (Pace-Asciak, Domazet & Carrara, 1977) by rat kidney and these compounds were excreted as the major metabolites of 6-keto-$PGF_{1\alpha}$. However, recent evidence that PGI_2 is a good substrate for the 15-hydroxy prostaglandin dehydrogenase with about the same K_m and V_{max} as PGE_2 would suggest that this may be an important pathway of PGI_2 metabolism (Wong et al., 1978). In addition, Needleman et al. (1978) have shown that PGI_2 is rapidly metabolized to an inactive metabolite in a single pass through the kidney, suggesting enzymatic degradation. Figure 3.4 shows the metabolism of the biologically active prostaglandin in the kidney. Many drugs including aspirin, indomethacin, furosemide, ethacrynic acid, and probenecid inhibit 15-hydroxydehydrogenase (Hansen, 1976) but at high doses which could also inhibit cyclooxygenase.

PHARMACOLOGY

Renal vascular tone is determined by the interrelationships among the exogenous (i.e., circulating or administered) vasoactive substances, the autonomic neuronal traffic to the resistance vessels, and the biosynthesis and release of endogenous vasoactive materials. While it is conceivable that exogenous prostaglandins may mimic the systemic effects of endogenous prostaglandins, great caution must be exercised in interpreting data obtained from infusion of exogenous prostaglandins. First, exogenous prostaglandins may not achieve the same concentration at the specific locus of activity as would be possible if they were released directly at their sites of synthesis. Second, administration of a prostaglandin exogenously presupposes that the infused PG is the active species responsible for the physiological changes observed from endogenous release. Several examples of the inadequacy of relying on exogenous PG as mirror images of endogenous release exist. For example, infusion of exogenous

PGE_2 into the vascular bed of the kidney does not parallel the effects on renal resistance and blood flow distribution when compared with the effects observed with infusions of the precursor fatty acid (Arendshort et al., 1974b; Weber et al., 1976b). Similarly, while infusion of arachidonic acid into the kidney is a potent stimulus to renin release, PGE_2 does not directly release renin (Weber et al., 1976a & b). These observations would then suggest that modulating endogenous synthesis by providing the precursor fatty acid or by inhibition of total synthesis or selective modification of pathways of endoperoxide metabolism, would provide more meaningful data and would more closely approximate the in vivo situation.

Cyclooxygenase inhibition

Acetylsalicylic acid (ASA) and other nonsteroidal anti-inflammatory drugs exert their anti-inflammatory action by inhibition of prostaglandin synthesis (Vane, 1971). These drugs have been shown to exert their effects on prostaglandin biosynthesis at the level of cyclooxygenase. The IC_{50} for aspirin and indomethacin on rabbit kidney microsomal synthetase is 2,800 and 3.7 μM, respectively (Flower and Vane, 1974). The use of these inhibitors of prostaglandin biosynthesis has resulted in significant information about the role of endogenous prostaglandin biosynthesis in renal physiology. Several stimuli are known to release endogenous prostaglandins from the kidney: Angiotensin II (McGiff et al., 1970b), norepinephrine (Needleman et al., 1974; McGiff et al., 1972b), bradykinin (McGiff et al., 1972b), nerve stimulation (Dunham and Zimmerman, 1970), and ischemia (McGiff et al., 1970b). The change in renal resistance to these stimuli, all of which (with the exception of bradykinin) reduce renal blood flow, is augmented when the kidney is pretreated with indomethacin suggesting that the major prostaglandin released in response to these stimuli is a vasodilator prostaglandin.

Renal blood flow

Several investigators have studied the effect of endogenous prostaglandin biosynthesis on the total and regional blood flow in intact animals. These experiments suggest that in awake trained animals inhibition of prostaglandin biosynthesis with indomethacin had no effect on resting renal blood flow (Swain et al., 1975; Zins, 1975). When animals were studied under anesthesia and acute surgical trauma, conditions that would be expected to activate the renin-angiotensin and adrenergic nervous systems, then indomethacin did reduce total renal blood flow in the dog (Feigen et al., 1976; Herbaczynska-Cedro and Vane, 1973; Lonigro et al., 1973; Venuto et al., 1975) and caused a redistribution of blood flow toward outer cortical areas (Kirschenbaum, 1974; Larsson and Anggard, 1974; Chang et al., 1975). These experiments suggest that under resting conditions the basal synthesis of prostaglandins is low and does not contribute significantly to renal vascular resistance. When the system is perturbed or stressed, however, prostaglandin biosynthesis may be critical to the modulation of renal vascular resistance. In contrast to cyclooxygenase inhibition, infusions of arachidonic acid ($C_{20:4}$) into the renal artery of dogs causes an increase in renal blood flow with redistribution towards the inner cortical and juxtamedullary areas (Anggard and Larsson, 1974, Chang et al., 1975). This effect was blocked by ETYA (5,8,11,14 eicosateraynoic acid), an inhibitor of both cyclooxygenase and lipoxygenase pathways (Tannenbaum et al., 1975).

Ureteral obstruction

Experiments by Schramm and Carlson (1975) using a model of acute ureteral obstruction in the cat suggested that endogenous prostaglandin biosynthesis is stimulated by tying off the ureter and acutely blunted by the vasoconstrictor effect of nerve stimulation and exogenous norepinephrine. These modulating effects of acute ureteral obstruction are abolished in part by pretreatment of the kidney with indomethacin, suggesting that a vasodepressor prostaglandin is released in response to the obstruction that blunted the effects of exogenous norepinephrine and renal nerve stimulation. Similar experiments in the dog with unilateral ureteral obstruction showed that ligation of the ureter initiates a transient rise in renal blood flow (fall in resistance),

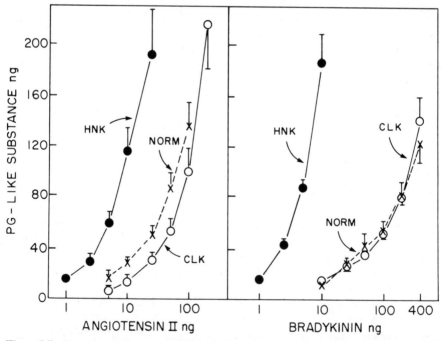

Figure 3.5   Dose response curves (DRC) for hydronephrotic (HNK) normal and contralateral (CLK) kidneys perfused ex vivo to agonists angiotensin II (A_{II}) and bradykinin (BK). PG-like activity (PLS) was calculated from a standard curve of the rat fundal stomach strip standardized to exogenous PGE_2. (From Nishikawa et al., 1977, with permission.)

which lasts for about 4 to 5 hours (Vaughn, Shenasky, and Gillenwater, 1971) and is followed by persistent renal vasoconstriction. Pretreatment of the animal with indomethacin and subsequent ligation of the ureter is associated with a fall in total renal blood flow and the characteristic ipsilateral renal vasodilation does not occur (Allen, Vaughn, and Gillenwater, 1978). Furthermore, the ureteral pressure remains significantly lower than that in nonindomethacin-treated animals, suggesting that intact prostaglandin biosynthesis is necessary for the renal vasodilation to occur in response to ureteral occlusion.

In the rabbit, unilateral ureteral occlusion for three days causes an enhanced basal and hormone (angiotensin II, bradykinin, and norepinephrine)-stimulated prostaglandin biosynthesis (Nishikawa, Morrison, and Needleman, 1977), as evidenced by a shift to the left of dose response curves in the perfused, ureter-obstructed kidney as compared with the contralateral normal kidney (Fig. 3.5). The renal venous effluent obtained after agonist stimulation from a perfused rabbit kidney prelabelled with [^{14}C] arachidonate, was extracted and chromatographed and found to contain primarily ^{14}C-PGE$_2$. Similar enhanced hormone-stimulated PGE$_2$ release is obtained in a strain of rats that develop congenital hydronephrosis (Nishikawa et al., 1977). It could be shown that the basal resistance in the surgical model of unilateral ureteral ligation in the rabbit is dependent in part on endogenous vasodepressor prostaglandin biosynthesis since indomethacin treatment increases basal perfusion pressure significantly (Table 3.1). Furthermore, whereas indomethacin does not significantly alter the angiotensin II-induced changes in renal resistance in the contralateral (unobstructed) kidney, it markedly enhances and prolongs the change in resistance to angiotensin II in the ureter-obstructed kidney. Because

Table 3.1   Effect of Indomethacin on renal perfusion pressure[a]

	HNK		CLK	
	Indo		Indo	
Treatment	−	+	−	+
	Basal perfusion Pressure mm Hg			
Control	47 ± 1	62 ± 5	45 ± 3	48 ± 3
	Δ PPmmHg			
AIIng				
10	23 ± 10	39 ± 6	27 ± 7	21 ± 3
100	30 ± 8	78 ± 6	56 ± 3	48 ± 13
400	70 ± 9	91 ± 9	75 ± 3	76 ± 7
		n = 4		n = 4

[a] Ipsilateral isolated rabbit kidney perfused ex vivo at constant flow of 15 ml/min in Krebs Hensleit buffer at 37° C (95% O_2–5% CO_2). Changes in perfusion pressure are a measure of alterations in renal resistance. Experiments are carried out in hydronephrotic (HNK) and contralateral (CLK) kidneys before and after 15 min. pretreatment with indomethacin (INDO) infused through the kidney at a rate of 10μg/min. Basal perfusion pressure (PP) is recorded in the mm Hg and increment of pressure (ΔPP) measured in response to angiotensin II (AII) injected through the kidney (Nishikawa et al., 1977).

the major determinants of renal resistance reside in the cortical afferent and efferent glomerular arterioles, prostaglandinlike material released in response to the agonist angiotensin II must then be modulating cortical vascular tone.

Comparisons of in vitro cortical biosynthesis in hydronephrotic and in normal kidneys were carried out by incubating microsomal preparations with [14C] arachidonate. There was a significant difference in cortical conversion of [14C] arachidonate into [14C] PGE$_2$ between hydronephrotic and normal kidneys, presumably reflecting enhanced cyclooxygenase activity (Table 3.2). Local PG synthesis in and around cortical blood vessels may be enough to mediate the alterations in renal resistance observed in animal models of hydronephrosis.

While the production of vasodepressor prostaglandins may explain the fall in resistance seen in the initial phases of ureteral obstruction in the cat (Schramm and Carlson, 1975) and dog (Vaughn et al., 1971), it does not explain the progressive fall in the renal blood flow and GFR observed in the dog by eighteen hours of ureteral obstruction (Moody et al., 1975). It has been suggested that in the rat (Arendshorst, Finn, and Gottschalk, 1974a) the major cause for reduction in renal blood flow and GFR is preglomerular vasoconstriction. This implies that if an endogenous mediator of the preglomerular vasocontriction exists, its biological effects must override the vasodepressor prostaglandins produced under basal conditions and presupposes that it is vasoconstrictor prostaglandin. We obtained evidence for such an endogenous vasoconstrictor when we observed that variable alterations in the renal perfusion pressure with bradykinin stimulation depends on the duration of the perfusion experiment. For example, with low doses of hormone, the perfusion pressure falls, but with higher doses, especially late in the perfusion experiment, there occurs a biphasic response: an initial fall in resistance followed by a rise (Fig. 3.6). This observation led us to include a rabbit aorta as part of our bioassay system in the superfusion cascade in search of a vasoconstrictor substance. Bradykinin (100 ng) administered to the hydronephrotic kidney causes the release into the venous effluent of a substance that contracts the rabbit aorta. This contractile activity is abolished by indomethacin pretreatment of the kidney. Even high doses of bradykinin (2μg) through the contralateral (un-

Table 3.2 Percentage of [14C] AA converted to [14C] PGE$_2$ per mg microsomal protein[a]

Time mins.	Normal cortex (4)	HNK cortex (10)
5′	0.45 ± .18	1.3 ± .22
10′	1.5 ± .21	3.25 ± .51
15	2.7 ± .65	5.3 ± .88

[a] Cortical microsomes (1 mg protein) from hydronephrotic and normal kidneys incubated in phosphate buffer ph 7.9 with [14C] arachidonic acid, 300,000 cpm (1μg) in the presence of L-epinephrine 1.2 mM as cofactor. Reaction was carried out for 5, 10, and 15 mins. At end of incubation the reaction mixture was acidified to pH 3.0, extracted with ethyl actetate, and subjected to thin layer chromatography. The results were expressed as percentage of total [14C] AA converted to [14C] PGE$_2$ and represent the mean ± S.E.

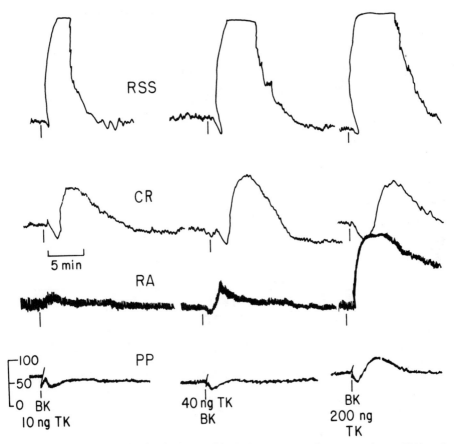

Figure 3.6 Dose dependency of release of PGE_2 (contraction of rat stomach strip RSS and chick rectum CR) and thromboxane A_2 (contraction of rabbit aorta RA). At low doses 10 ng BK, perfusion pressure (therefore resistance) falls and no contraction of aorta is noted. At higher doses 200 ng BK, there is a biphasic response in perfusion pressure with an initial fall followed by an increase. This is associated with release of thromboxane A_2 as indicated by contraction of aorta.

obstructed) kidney does not release a rabbit aorta contractile substance (RCS) into the renal venous effluent. The rate of disappearance ($t_{1/2}$ 30 sec. at 37°) of contractile activity released from the ureter-obstructed kidney by bradykinin is identical to the rate of disappearance of authentic TXA_2 and not PGH_2 (Figure 3.7). These experiments suggest that the hydronephrotic kidney releases thromboxane A_2 with peptide hormone stimulation. Similarly, we could demonstrate that angiotensin II, bradykinin, arachidonate, and ATP all release thromboxane from the hydronephrotic kidney in a dose-dependent manner (Morrison et al., 1978).

The major vascular determinants of renal resistance are the afferent and efferent glomerular arterioles, which are cortical in distribution (Thurau, 1964). With complete occlusion of the ureter during rabbit kidney perfusion experi-

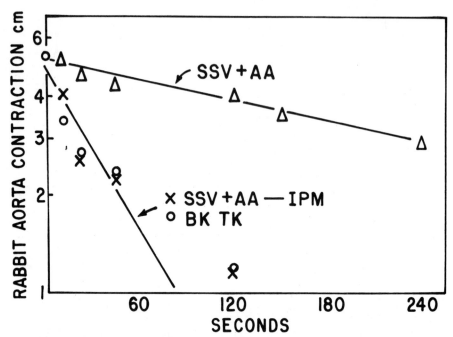

Figure 3.7 Disappearance curves of released rabbit aorta-contracting substance from the hydronephrotic kidney stimulated with bradykinin BK. Biological activity is monitored by contraction of rabbit aorta. △———△ shows disappearance curve for endoperoxide generated by incubating sheep seminal vesicles (SSV) with arachidonic acid (AA). X———X shows disappearance curve for thromboxane A_2 generated by incubating SSV and AA (source of endoperoxide) with indomethacin-treated platelet microsomes (IPM)—source of thromboxane synthetase. o———o shows disappearance curve for RCS released into venous effluent of the HNK.

ments, bulk flow of fluid along the tubules is negligible. Ligation of the ureter during perfusion does not alter the enhanced sensitivity, nor the alterations in renal resistance produced by exogenous AII (Nishikawa et al., 1977) during perfusion, which suggests that PG synthesized in the medulla is not transported to the cortex via the tubules. It has also been suggested that the vasa recta may be the transport channels whereby PG synthesized in the medulla may reach the cortex (Frolich et al., 1972). The vasa recta are mainly associated with juxtamedullary nephrons, which constitute about 20 percent of the nephron population (Schmidt-Nielson and O'Dell, 1961). To affect cortical resistance, PG transported from the medulla by the vasa recta would have to reach the corticomedullary area and then diffuse into the cortex, an area that is rich in 15-prostaglandin dehydrogenase activity (Larsson and Anggard, 1973). Thus it appears unlikely that the vasa recta are a major route of transport of PG from medulla to cortex.

The observation of significant cortical biosynthesis in this model of hydronephrosis suggests that PG are being synthesized locally and acting as modulators of local vascular tone. The temporal changes in PG biosynthesis in ureteral obstruction with the unmasking of cortical synthesis of thromboxane

A_2 suggest that release of this potent vasoconstrictor may be involved in the circulatory adjustments occurring in chronic ureteral obstruction. Indeed, this constriction may mediate the preglomerular vasoconstriction, which has been recognized as the hallmark of chronic ureteral obstruction. The enhanced cortical synthesis of PGE_2, and the unmasking of thromboxane A_2 biosynthesis in the ureter-obstructed kidney taken in concert with the autoradiographic data, certainly suggest that biosynthesis of hormone-stimulated PGE_2 and thromboxane A_2 is localized to the glomerular and afferent arterioles and their biosynthesis may be modulating their intrinsic tone.

Yarger and Harris (1978) have recently demonstrated that imidazole, an inhibitor of thromboxane synthetase, significantly increases renal blood flow and GFR in the ureter-obstructed kidney of the rat, which suggests that inhibition of thromboxane A_2 biosynthesis is the cause of the increase in renal blood flow and GFR.

Although firm statements concerning the role of endogenous PG biosynthesis—statements based on isolated, perfused organs or on in vitro enzyme assays in modulating renal vascular resistance in pathologic states—may be premature, sufficient evidence does exist to suggest that resting and hormone-stimulated endogenous prostaglandin biosynthesis may be critical to the final expression of renal vascular resistance in ureteral obstruction. Furthermore, these alterations lend themselves to pharmacological manipulation. With the development of more selective potent inhibitors of various pathways of endoperoxide metabolism, the contribution of endogenous PG biosynthesis to renal vascular resistance can be more thoroughly evaluated.

ACKNOWLEDGMENT

This work was supported by NIH grants HE 14397, HL 20787, and postdoctoral fellowship AM 05480-01.

REFERENCES

Allen, J. T., Vaughan, E. D., Jr. & Gillenwater, J. Y. (1978). The effect of indomethacin on renal blood flow and ureteral pressure in unilateral ureteral obstruction in awake dogs. *Investigative Urology*, **15**, 324–327.

Anggard, E. & Samuelsson, B. (1964). Prostaglandin and related factors 28. Metabolism of prostaglandin E_1 in guinea-pig lung: The structures of two metabolites. *Journal of Biological chemistry*, **239**, 4097–4102.

Anggard & Samuelsson, B. (1966). Purification and properties of a 15-hydroxy prostaglandin dehydrogenase from swine lung. *Archiv. Kemi*, **25**, 293–300.

Anggard, E. & Larson, C. (1974). Stimulation and inhibition of prostaglandin biosynthesis: Opposite effects on blood pressure and intra renal blood flow distribution. In *Prostaglandin Synthetase Inhibitors*, ed. Robinson, H. J. & Vane, J. R., 311–315.

Arendshorst, W. J., Finn, W. R. & Gottschalk, C. W. (1974a). Nephron stop flow pressure response to obstruction for 24 hrs. in the rat kidney. *Journal of Clinical Investigation*, **53**, 1497–1500.

Arendshorst, W. J., Johnston, P. A. & Selkurt, E. E. (1974b). Effect of prostaglandin E_1 on renal hemodynamics non-diuretic and volume-expanded dogs. *American Journal of Physiology*, **226**, 218–225.

Bergstrom, S. & Sjovall (1960). The isolation of prostaglandin F from sheep prostatic glands. *Acta Chemica Scandinavia*, **14**, 1693–1900.

Blackwell, G. J., Flower, R. H. & Vane, J. R. (1975). Rapid reduction of prostaglandin 15-hydroxydehydrogenase activity in rat tissues after treatment with protein synthesis inhibitors. *British Journal of Pharmacology*, **55**, 233–238.

Bohman, S. O. (1977). Demonstration of prostaglandin synthesis in collecting duct cells and other cell types of the rabbit renal medulla. *Prostaglandins*, **14**, 729–744.

Bunting, S., Gryglewski, R., Moncada, S. & Vane, J. R. (1976). Arterial walls generate from prostaglandin endoperoxides a substance (Prostaglandin X) which relaxes strips of mesenteric and coeliac arteries and inhibits platelet aggregation. *Prostaglandins*, **12**, 897–913.

Cavallo, T. (1976a). Fine structural localization of endogenous peroxidase activity in ureter medullary interstitial cells of rat kidney. *Laboratory Investigation*, **34**, 223–228.

Cavallo, T. (1976b). Cytochemical localization of endogenous peroxidase activity in renal medullary collecting tubules and papillary mucosa of the rat. *Laboratory Investigation*, **34**, 223–228.

Chang, L. C. T., Splawinski, J. A., Oates, J. A. & Nies, A. S. (1975). Enhanced renal prostaglandin production in the dog II. Effects of intrarenal hemodynamics. *Circulation research*, **36**, 204–207.

Crowshaw, K. (1971). Prostaglandin biosynthesis from endogenous precursors in rabbit kidney. *Nature New Biology*, **231**, 240–242.

Crowshaw, K. (1973). The incorporation of [1-^{14}C] arachidonic acid into the lipids of rabbit renal slices and conversion to prostaglandins E_2 and F_{2a}. *Prostaglandins*, **3**, 607–620.

Danon, A., Chang, L. C. T., Sweetman, B. J., Nies, A. S. & Oates, J. A. (1975). Synthesis of prostaglandins by the rat renal papilla *in vitro*. Mechanism of stimulation by angiotensin II. *Biochemica et Biophysica Acta*, **388**, 71–83.

Dunham, E. W. & Zimmerman, B. G. (1970). Release of prostaglandin like material from dog kidney during nerve stimulation. *American Journal of Physiology*, **219**, 1279–1285.

Dunn, M. J. (1976). Renal prostaglandin synthesis in the spontaneously hypertensive rat. *Journal of Clinical Investigation*, **58**, 862–870.

Egan, R. W., Paxton, J. & Kuehl, F. A., Jr. (1976). Mechanism for irreversible self-deactivation of prostaglandin synthetase. *Journal of Biological Chemistry*, **251**, 7329–7335.

Feigen, L. P., Lainer, E., Chapnick, B. M. & Kadowitz, P. J. (1976). The effect of indomethacin on renal function in pentobarbital anesthetized dogs. *Journal of Pharmacology and Experimental Therapeutics*, **198**, 457–463.

Flower, R. J. & Vane, J. R. (1974). Some pharmacologic and biochemical aspects of prostaglandin biosynthesis and its inhibition. Prostaglandin Synthetase Inhibitors, ed. Robinson, H. J. & Vane, J. R. pp. 9–18. New York: Raven Press.

Flower, R. J. & Blackwell, G. J. (1976). The importance of phosphilipase A_2 in prostaglandin biosynthesis. *Biochemical Pharmacology*, **25**, 285–291.

Frolich, J. C., Sweetman, B. J., Carr, K., Splawinski, J., Watson, J. T., Anggard, E. & Oates, J. A. (1972). Occurrence of prostaglandins in human urine. In *International Conference of Prostaglandins Advances in the Biosciences* Vol. 9. pp. 321–330. Vieweg: Pergamon Press.

Gerber, J. G., Branch, R. A., Nies, A. S., Gerkens, J. F., Shand, D. G., Hollifield, J. & Oates, J. A. (1978). Prostaglandin and renin release II Assessment of renin secretion following infusion of PGE_2, E_2 and D_2 into the renal artery of anaesthetized dogs. *Prostaglandins*, **15**, 81–88.

Granstrom, E., Lands, W. F. M. & Samuelsson (1968). Biosynthesis of 9α, 15-dihydroxy-11-ketoprost-13-lenoic acid. *Journal of Biological Chemistry*, **243**, 4104–4108.

Gryglewski, R. J., Bunting, S., Moncada, S., Flower, R. J. & Vane, J. R. (1976). Arterial walls are protected against deposition of platelet thrombi by a substance (Prostaglandin X) which they make from prostaglandin endoperoxides. *Prostaglandins*, **12**, 685–713.

Hamberg, M. (1969). Biosynthesis of prostaglandins in the renal medulla of rabbit. *FEBS Letters*, **5**, 127–130.

Hamberg, M. & Samuelsson, B. (1971). Metabolism of prostaglandin E_2 in guinea-pig liver II. Pathways in the formation of the major metabolites. *Journal of Biological Chemistry*, **246**, 1073–1077.

Hamberg, M., Svensson, J., Wakabayashi, T. & Samuelsson, B. (1974). Isolation and structure of two prostaglandin endoperoxides that cause platelet aggregation. *Proceedings of the National Academy of Sciences U.S.A.*, **71**, 345–349.

Hamberg, M. & Samuelsson, B. (1973). Detection and isolation of an endoperoxide intermediate in prostaglandin biosynthesis. *Proceedings of the National Academy of Sciences U.S.A.*, **70**, 899–903.

Hamberg, M., Svensson, J. & Samuelsson, B. (1975). Thromboxanes: A new group of biologically active compounds derived from prostaglandin endoperoxides. *Proceedings of the National Academy of Sciences U.S.A.*, **72**, 2994–2998.

Hansen, H. S. (1976). 15-hydroxy prostaglandin dehydrogenase. A review. *Prostaglandins*, **12**, 647–679.

Herbaczynska-Cedro, K. & Vane, J. R. (1973). Prostaglandins as mediators of reactive hyperemia in kidney. *Nature*, **247**, 492.

Hsueh, W., Isakson, P. C. & Needleman, P. (1977). Hormone selective lipase activation. *Prostaglandins*, **13**, 1073–1091.

Hsueh, W. & Needleman, P. (1978). Presented at Federation of American Societies of Experimental Biology.

Isakson, P. C., Raz, A., & Needleman, P. (1976). Selective incorporation of [^{14}C] arachidonic acid into the phospholipids of intact tissues and subsequent metabolism to [^{14}C]-prostaglandins. *Prostaglandins*, **12**, 739–748.

Isakson, P. C., Raz, A., Denny, S. E., Wyche, A. & Needleman, P. (1977a). Hormonal stimulation of arachidonate release from isolated perfused organs: Relationship to prostaglandin biosynthesis. *Prostaglandins*, **14**, 853–871.

Isakson, P. C., Raz, A., Denny, S. E., Pure, E. & Needleman, P. (1977b). A novel prostaglandin is the major product of arachidonic acid metabolism in rabbit heart. *Proceedings of the National Academy of Sciences*, **74**, 101–105.

Itskovitz, H. D., Terragno, N. A. & McGiff, J. C. (1974). Effect of a renal prostaglandin on distribution of blood flow in the isolated canine kidney. *Circulation Research*, **34**, 770–776.

Janszen, F. H. A. & Nugteren, D. H. (1971). Histochemical localization of prostaglandin synthetase. *Histochemie*, **27**, 159–164.

Johnson, R. A., Morton, D. R., Kinner, J. H., Gorman, R. R., McGuire, J.R., Sun, F. F., Whittaker, N., Bunting, S., Salmon, J. A., Moncada, S. & Vane, J. R. (1976). The chemical characterization of prostaglandin X (prostacyclin). *Prostaglandins*, **12**, 915–928.

Kalisker, A. & Dyer, D. C. (1972). *In vitro* release of prostaglandins from the renal medulla. *European Journal of Pharmacology*, **19**, 305–309.

Kirschenbaum, M. A., White, N., Stein, J. H. & Ferris, T. (1974). Redistribution of renal cortical blood flow during inhibition of prostaglandin synthesis. *American Journal of Physiology*, **227**, 801–805.

Knapp, H. R., Olez, O., Roberts, L. J., Sweetman, B. J., Oates, J. A. & Reed, P. (1977). Ionophores stimulate prostaglandin and thromboxane biosynthesis. *Proceedings of the National Academy of Sciences U.S.A.*, **74**, 4251–4255.

Kulkarni, P. S., Roberts, R. & Needleman, P. (1976). Paradoxical endogenous synthesis of a coronary dilating substance from arachidonate. *Prostaglandins*, **12**, 337–353.

Kunze, H. & Vogty, W. (1971). Significance of phospholipase A for prostaglandin formation. *Annals of the New York Academy of Sciences*, **180**, 123–125.

Kurzok, R. & Lieb, C. (1930). Biochemical studies of human semen II. The action of semen on the human uterus. *Proceedings of the Society of Experimental Biology and Medicine*, **28**, 268–272.

Lands, W. E. M. & Samuelsson, B. (1968). Phospholipid precursors of prostaglandins. *Biochimica et Biophysica Acta*, **164**, 426–429.

Larsson, C. & Anggard, E. (1973). Regional differences in the formation and metabolism of prostaglandins in the rabbit kidney. *European Journal of Pharmacology*, **21**, 30–36.

Lee, J. B., Crowshaw, K., Takman, B. H., Ahrep, K. & Gougontas, J. Z. (1967). The identification of prostaglandins E_2, $F_{2\alpha}$ and A_2 from rabbit kidney medulla. *Biochemical Journal*, **105**, 1251–1260.

Lee, S. C. & Levine, L. (1974). Prostaglandin metabolism I. Cytoplasmic reduced nicotinamide adenine dinucleotide phosphate dependent and microsomal reduced nicotinamide adenine dinucleotide tissues. *Journal of Biological Chemistry*, **249**, 1369–1375.

Lee, S. C., Pong, S. S. Katzen, D., Wu, K-Y & Levine, L. (1975). Distribution of prostaglandin E-9-ketoreductase and types I and II 15-hydroxy prostaglandin dehydrogenase in swine kidney medulla and cortex. *Biochemistry*, **14**, 142–145.

Lonigro, A. J., Itskovitz, H. D., Crowshaw, K. & McGiff, J. C. (1973). Dependency of renal blood flow on prostaglandin synthesis in the dog. *Circulation research*, **32**, 712–717.

McGiff, J. C., Crowshaw, K., Terragro, N. A. & Lonigro, A. J. (1970a). Release of a prostaglandin like substance into renal venous blood in response to angiotensin II. *Circulation Research*, **27–28**, I-121–130. Supplement 1.

McGiff, J. C., Crowshaw, K., Terragno, N. A., Lonigro, A. J., Shand, J. C., Williamson, M. A., Lee, J. B. & Ng, K. K. F. (1970b). Prostaglandin-like substances appearing in the canine renal venous blood during renal ischemia. Their partial characterization by pharmacologic and chromatographic procedures. *Circulation Research*, **27**, 765–782.

McGiff, J. C., Crowshaw, K., Terragno, N. A., Malik, K. U. & Lonigro, A. J. (1972a). Differential effect of noradrenaline and renal nerve stimulation on vascular resistance in the dog kidney and release of prostaglandin E-like substance. *Clinical Science*, **42**, 223–233.

McGiff, J. C., Terragno, N. A., Malik, K. U. & Lonigro, A. J. (1972b). Release of prostaglandin E-like substance from canine kidney by bradykinin. *Circulation Research*, **31**, 36–43.

Miller, M. M., Kaiser, E., Bauer, P., Scheiber, V. & Hohenegger, M. (1976). Lipid composition of the rat kidney. *Nephron*, **17**, 41–50.

Miyamoto, T., Yamamoto, S. & Hayaishi, O. (1974). Prostaglandin synthetase system—Resolution into oxygenase and isomerase components. *Proceedings of the National Academy of Science*, U.S.A., **71**, 3645–3648.

Miyamoto, F., Ogino, N., Yamamoto, S. & Hayaishi, O. (1976). Purification of prostaglandin endoperoxide synthetase from bovine vesicular gland microsomes. *Journal of Biological Chemistry*, **251**, 2629–2636.

Moncada, S., Gryglewski, R. J., Bunting, S. & Vane, J. R. (1976a). An enzyme isolated from arteries transforms prostaglandin endoperoxides to an unstable substance that inhibits platelet aggregation. *Nature (London)*, **263**, 663–665.

Moncada, S., Gryglewski, R. J., Bunting, S. & Vane, J. R. (1976b). A lipid peroxide inhibits the enzyme in blood vessel microsomes that generate from prostaglandin endoperoxides the substance (prostaglandin X) which prevents platelet aggregation. *Prostaglandins*, **12**, 715–737.

Moody, T. E., Vaughn, E. D., Jr. & Gillenwater, J. Y. (1975). Relationship between renal blood flow and ureteral pressure during eighteen hours of total unilateral occlusion. Implication for changing sites of renal resistance. *Investigative Urology*, **13**, 246–251.

Morgan, T. E., Tinker, D. O. & Hanahan, D. J. (1963). Phospholipid metabolism in kidney I. Isolation and identification of lipids of rabbit kidney. *Archives of Biochemistry and Biophysis*, **103**, 54–64.

Morrison, A. R., Nishikawa, K. & Needleman, P. (1977). Unmasking of thromboxane A_2 synthesis by ureter obstruction in the rabbit kidney. *Nature (London)*, **267**, 259–260.

Morrison, A. R., Nishikawa, K. & Needleman, P. (1978). Thromboxane A_2 biosynthesis in the ureter obstructed isolated perfused kidney of the rabbit. *Journal of Pharmacology and Experimental Therapeutics*, **205**, 1–8.

Muirhead, E. E., Brooks, B., Pitcock, J. A. & Stephenson, P. (1972). The renomedullary antihypertensive function in accelerated (malignant) hypertension: With observations on the renomedullary interstitial cells. *Journal of Clinical Investigation*, **51**, 181–190.

Muirhead, E. E., Germain, G. S., Leach, B. E., Brooks, B. & Stephenson, P. (1973). Renomedullary interstitial cells (RIC). Prostaglandins (PG) and the antihypertensive function of the kidney. *Prostaglandins*, **3**, 581–594.

Needleman, P., Douglas, J. R., Jakschik, B., Stoelklein, P. B. & Johnson, E. M., Jr. (1974). Release of renal prostaglandin by catecholamines. Relationship to renal endocrine function. *Journal of Pharmacology and Experimental Therapeutics*, **188**, 453–460.

Needleman, P., Bryan, B., Wyche, A., Bronson, S. D., Eakins, K., Ferrendelli, J. A., & Minkes, M. (1977a). Thromboxane synthetase inhibitors as pharmacological tools: Differential biochemical and biological effects on platelet suspension. *Prostaglandins*, **14**, 897–907.

Needleman, P., Raz, A., Ferrendelli, J. A. & Minkes, M. (1977b). Application of imidazole as a selective inhibitor of thromboxane synthesis in human platelets. *Proceedings of the National Academy of Science U.S.A.*, **74**, 1716–1720.

Needleman, P., Bronson, S. D., Wyche, A., Sivakoff, M. & Nicolaou, K. C. (1978). Cardiac and renal prostaglandin I_2 biosynthesis and biological effects in isolated perfused rabbit tissues. *Journal of Clinical Investigation*, **61**, 839–849.

Nishikawa, K., Morrison, A. & Needleman, P. (1977). Exaggerated prostaglandin biosynthesis and its influence on renal resistance in the isolated hydronephrotic rabbit kidney. *Journal of Clinical Investigation*, **59**, 1143–1150.

Nugteren, D. H. & Hazelhof, E. (1973). Isolation and properties of intermediates in prosta-glandin biosynthesis. *Biochimica et Biophysica Acta,* **326,** 448–461.

Pace-Asciak, C. R. & Rangaraj, G. (1976). The 6-keto prostaglandin $F_{1\alpha}$ pathway in the lamb ductus arteriosus. *Biochimica et Biophysica Acta,* **486,** 583–585.

Pace-Asciak, C. R. & Rangaraj, G. (1977). Distribution of prostaglandin biosynthetic path-ways in several rat tissues. Formation of 6-keto prostaglandin $F_{1\alpha}$. *Biochimica et Biophy-sica Acta,* **486,** 579–582.

Pace-Asciak, C. S., Domazet, Z. & Carrara, M. (1977). Catabolism of 6-keto prostaglandin $F_{1\alpha}$ by the rat kidney cortex. *Biochimica et Biophysica Acta,* **487,** 400–404.

Piper, P. J. & Vane, J. R. (1969). Release of additional factor in anaphylaxis and its antago-nism by antiinflammatory drugs. *Nature (London),* **223,** 29–35.

Piper, P. H. & Vane, J. R. (1971). The release of prostaglandins from lung and other tissues. *Annals of the New York Academy of Sciences,* **180,** 363–385.

Pong, S. S. & Levine, L. (1976). Biosynthesis of prostaglandins in rabbit renal cortex. *Re-search Communications of Chemical Pathology and Pharmacology,* **13,** 115–123.

Powell, W. S. & Solomon, S. (1977). Formation of 6-oxo prostaglandin $F_{1\alpha}$ by arteries of the fetal calf. *Biochemical and Biophysical Research Communications,* **75,** 815–822.

Raz, A., Isakson, P. C., Minkes, M. S. & Needleman, P. (1977). Characterization of a novel metabolic pathway of arachidonate in coronary arteries which generates a potent endo-genous vasodilator. *Journal of Biological Chemistry,* **252,** 1123–1126.

Roberts, L. J., II, Sweetman, B. J., Morgan, J. L., Payne, N. A. & Oates, J. A. (1977a). Identi-fication of the major urinary metabolite of thromboxane B_2 in the monkey. *Prostaglandins,* **13,** 631–645.

Roberts, L. J., II, Sweetman, B. J., Payne, A. & Oates, J. A. (1977b). Metabolism of throm-boxane B_2 in man. Identification of the major urinary metabolite. *Journal of Biological Chemistry,* **252,** 7415–7417.

Samuelsson, B. (1972). Biosynthesis of prostaglandins. *Federation Proceedings, Federation of American Societies for Experimental Biology,* **31,** 1442–1450.

Samuelsson, B. (1965). On the incorporation of oxygen in the conversion of 8,11,14 eicosa-trienoic acid to prostaglandin E_1. *Journal of the American Chemical Society,* **87,** 3011–3013.

Schmidt-Nielsen, B. & O'Dell, R. (1961). Structure and concentrating mechanism in the mammalian kidney. *American Journal of Physiology,* **200,** 1119–1124.

Schramm, L. P. & Carlson, D. E. (1975). Inhibition of renal vasoconstriction by elevated ureteral pressure. *American Journal of Physiology,* **228,** 1126–1133.

Stone, K. J. & Hart, M. (1976). Inhibition of renal PGE_2 9-keto reductase in rabbit kidney. *Prostaglandins,* **12,** 197–207.

Sun, F. F., Chapman, J. P. & McGuire, J. C. (1977). Metabolism of prostaglandin endoperox-ide in animal tissues. *Prostaglandins,* **14,** 1055–1074.

Swain, J. A., Heyndrickx, G. D., Boettcher, D. H. & Vatner, S. F. (1975). Prostaglandin con-trol of renal circulation in the unanesthetized dog and baboon. *American Journal of Phys-iology,* **229,** 826–830.

Tai, H. H. & Yuan, B. (1978). On the inhibitory potency of imidazole and its derivatives on thromboxane synthetase. *Biochemical and Biophysical Research Communications,* **80,** 236–242.

Tannenbaum, J., Splawinski, J. A., Oates, J. A. & Nies, A. S. (1975). Enhanced renal prosta-glandin production in the dog I. Effects on renal function. *Circulation Research,* **36,** 197–203.

Terragno, N. A., Terragno, D. A. & McGiff, J. C. (1975). Prostaglandins synthesis by bovine mesenteric arteries and veins. *Circulation Research,* **36–37,** Supplement I, I-76–80.

Terragno, N. A., Terragno, A., McGiff, J. C. & Rodriquez, D. J. (1977). Synthesis of Prosta-glandins by the ductus arteriosus of the bovine fetus. *Prostaglandins,* **14,** 721–727.

Thurau, K. (1964). Renal hemodynamics. *American Journal of Medicine,* **36,** 698–719.

Vane, J. R. (1971). Inhibition of prostaglandin synthesis as a mechanism of action for aspirin-like drugs. *Nature New Biology,* **231,** 232–235.

Vaughn, E. D., Shenashy, J. H., II, & Gillenwater, J. Y. (1971). Mechanism of acute hemo-dynamic response to ureteral occlusion. *Investigative Urology,* **9,** 109–118.

Venuto, R. C., O'Dorisio, T., Ferris, T. G. & Stein, J. H. (1975). Prostaglandins and renal function II. The effect of prostaglandin inhibition on autoregulation of blood flow in the intact kidney of the dog. *Prostaglandins,* **9,** 817–828.

Von Euler, U. S. (1935). A depressor substance in the vesicular gland. *Journal of Physiology (London)*, **84**, 219.

Weber, P. C., Larsson, C. & Scherer, B. (1977). Prostaglandin E_2 9-keto reductase as a mediator of salt intake-related prostaglandin-renin interaction. Nature (London), **266**, 65–66.

Weber, P. C., Larsson, C., Anggard, E., Hamberg, M., Covey, E. J., Nicolaou, K. C., & Samuelsson, B. (1976a). Stimulation of renin release from rabbit renal cortex by arachidonic acid and prostaglandin endoperoxides. *Circulation Research*, **39**, 868–874.

Weber, P. C., Larsson, C., Hamberg, M., Anggard, E., Covey, E. J. & Samuelsson, B. (1976b). Effects of stimulation and inhibition of the renal prostaglandin synthetase system on renin release *in vivo* and *in vitro*. *Clinical Science and Molecular Medicine*, **51**, 271s–274s.

Whorton, A. R., Misono, K., Hollifield, J., Frolich, J. C., Inagami, T., & Oates, J. A. (1977). Prostaglandins and renin release: I stimulation of renin release from rabbit renal cortical slices. *Prostaglandins*, **14**, 1095–1104.

Whorton, A. R. Smigel, M., Oates, J. A. & Frolich, J. C. (1978). Regional differences in prostacyclin formation by the kidney: Prostacyclin is a major prostaglandin of renal cortex. *Biochemica et Biophysica Acta*, **529**, 176–180.

Wong, P. & McGiff, J. C. (1977). Enzymic regulation of prostaglandin levels in blood vessels: Relationship to cyclic GMP. *Federation Proceedings, Federation of American Societies for Experimental Biology*, **36**, 673.

Wong, P. Y. K., Terragno, D. A., Terragno, N. A. & McGiff, J. C. (1977). Dual effects of bradykinin on prostaglandin metabolism: Relationship to the dissimilar vascular actions of kinins. *Prostaglandins*, **13**, 1113–1125.

Wong, P. & Sun, F. (1978). Presented at Winter Prostaglandin Conference Sarasota, Fla.

Yarger, W. E. & Harris, R. H. (1978). Thromboxane A_2 (TxA_2) and prostaglandin E_2 (PGE_2): Vasoactive agents in hydronephrotic kidneys (HK) *in vivo*. *Clinical Research*, **26**, 546A.

Zenser, T. V., Herman, C. A., Gorman, R. R. & Davis, B. B. (1977). Metabolism and action of the prostaglandin endoperoxide PGH_2 in rat kidney. *Biochemical and Biophysical Research Communications*, **79**, 357–363.

Zusman, R. M. & Kaiser, H. R. (1977a). Prostaglandin biosynthesis by rabbit renomedullary interstitial cells in tissue culture stimulation by angiotensin II, bradykinin and arginine vasopressin. *Journal of Clinical Investigation*, **60**, 215–223.

Zusman, R. M. & Kaiser, H. R. (1977b). Prostaglandin E_2 biosynthesis by rabbit renomedullary interstitial cells in tissue culture. Mechanism of stimulation by vasoactive peptides. *Journal of Biological Chemistry*, **252**, 2069–2071.

4

Renal prostaglandins: Influences on excretion of sodium and water, the renin-angiotensin system, renal blood flow, and hypertension

MICHAEL J. DUNN

INTRODUCTION

Renal prostaglandins have been studied under most conceivable circumstances and have been ascribed potential roles in many renal processes. With some exceptions, investigations of the importance of renal prostaglandins began less than one decade ago. Proper biochemical techniques including mass spectroscopy, radioimmunoassay, and various forms of chromatography have recently been added to bioassay methodology in prostaglandin research. Some of the prostaglandins (prostacyclin or prostaglandin I_2 [PGI_2]) and the thromboxanes were described and characterized within the last five years. The field is thus unsettled, lacking unanimity, and full of excitement.

In this chapter we will consider the possible physiologic roles of renal prostaglandins in the control of salt and water excretion, and we will review the interactions of prostaglandins, renin, angiotension II, and kinins. Finally, we shall confront the confusing literature about prostaglandins and regulation of blood pressure. When possible, clinical applications will be discussed; however, the focus of most investigations has been to understand the normal physiology, biochemistry, and pharmacology of the renal prostaglandins.

PROSTAGLANDINS AND RENAL EXCRETION OF SODIUM

The role of renal prostaglandins as regulators of renal excretion of sodium is uncertain. Despite extensive investigation, it remains difficult to assign any substantial influence of the prostaglandins on renal sodium homeostasis (Dunn and Hood, 1977). This is unexpected since most prostaglandins are potent natriuretic compounds and hence have often been assigned a physiologic function as regulators of renal tubule sodium reabsorption.

Tubular sodium transport

Most prostaglandins synthesized in the kidney are natriuretic, both in humans and in animals. The most potent natriuretic prostaglandins are PGE_2 (prostaglandin E_2) and PGI_2 (Bolger 1978; Fulgraff and Brandenbusch, 1974: Fulgraff, Bradenbusch, and Heintze, 1974; Lee et al., 1971) whereas $PGF_{2\alpha}$ (prostaglandin $F_{2\alpha}$) is natriuretic only at dosages threefold to fivefold higher (Fulgraff and Brandenbusch, 1974). Stimulation of renal synthesis of prostaglandins by infusion of arachidonic acid promptly induced a natriuresis in dogs (Chang et al., 1975) and in rats (Weber et al., 1975). The natriuretic actions of prostaglandins result from their vasodilatory properties and also from a possible direct effect on membrane sodium transport. In general, the extent and the duration of natriuresis correlate with the renal vasodilatation (Carriere, Fribourg, and Guay, 1971; Martinez-Maldonado et al., 1972). However, simultaneous infusion of acetylcholine and PGE_2 increased sodium excretion without increasing RBF above that with infusion of acetylcholine alone (Shea, Eisner, and Slotkoff, 1978). These results suggest a direct inhibitory influence of PGE_2 upon tubular reabsorption of sodium. Direct assessment of this question using the isolated and perfused rabbit nephron has yielded conflicting results. If rabbits were pretreated with desoxycorticosterone acetate, 5 mg/day from 4 to 11 days, PGE_2 inhibited net sodium transport and transepithelial potential in cortical and outer medullary collecting tubules (Stokes and Kokko, 1977). Other workers using rabbit-collecting tubules from animals not pretreated with desoxycorticosterone acetate reported no inhibitory actions of PGE_2 on sodium reabsorption (Fine and Trizna, 1977). Direct exposure of renal slices and suspensions of rabbit cortical or medullary tubules to various prostaglandins including PGE_2 demonstrated no changes of sodium or water transport between the cells and the medium (Dunn and Howe, 1977).

Three experimental approaches have been used to assess the importance of the renal prostaglandins in the control of sodium excretion: (1) measurement of prostaglandins in urine, renal venous blood, or renal tissue after manipulation of sodium intake; (2) evaluation of the effects of inhibitors of fatty acid cyclooxygenase on renal sodium excretion; (3) assessment of the inhibition of diuretic-induced natriuresis by inhibitors of fatty acid cyclooxygenase.

Alterations of sodium balance

The first approach based on the measurement of prostaglandins has not yielded consistent data, possibly because of significant limitations of the prostaglandin assays as well as the extreme variability of experimental conditions (species studied, acute or chronic experiments, level of sodium and potassium intake, anesthesia, etc.). PGE_2, $PGF_{2\alpha}$, or PGA_2 were measured in renal venous blood (Papanicolaou et al., 1975; Shimizu, Yamamoto, and Yoshitoshi, 1973; Terashima, Anderson and Jubiz, 1976), renal tissue (Attallah and Lee, 1973; Tobian and O'Donnell, 1976), peripheral plasma (Zusman et al., 1973), and urine (Kaye et al., 1978; Lifschitz et al., 1978; Scherer, Siess, and Weber, 1977; Weber, Larsson, and Scherer, 1977a) in humans (Kaye et al., 1978; Papanicolaou et al., 1975; Zusman et al., 1973), rabbits (Attallah and Lee, 1973; Lifschitz et al., 1978; Scherer et al., 1977; Weber et al., 1977a), dogs (Shea et al., 1978; Terashima et al., 1976), and rats (Tobian and O'Donnell, 1976). These various authors have reported that volume expansion with saline or increased oral intake of sodium increased renal venous PGE_2 (Papanicolaou et al., 1975; Shimizu et al., 1973; Terashima et al., 1976), reduced renal tissue (Tobian and O'Donnell, 1976) and urine PGE_2 (Weber et al., 1977a; Scherer et al., 1977), increased urine PGE_2 (Kaye et al., 1978), did not alter urine $PGF_{2\alpha}$ (Lifschitz et al., 1978), decreased PGA_2 in peripheral plasma (Zusman et al., 1973) and in renal papilla (Attallah and Lee, 1973), and did not change urine $PGF_{2\alpha}$ (Scherer et al., 1977; Weber et al., 1977a). At present it is impossible to reconcile these results into a coherent hypothesis. A systematic approach will be required, preferably using normal volunteers, to evaluate acute and chronic effects of parenteral and oral sodium loads with constant intake of potassium upon urinary excretion of PGE_2 and $PGF_{2\alpha}$. Since urinary excretion of prostaglandins reflects renal synthesis (Dunn, Laird, and Dray, 1978; Frohlich et al., 1975), this approach is preferable and avoids the problems of renal venous collections at a single point in time as well as the confounding influences of platelet release of prostaglandins when blood is collected (Dunn and Hood, 1977).

Inhibition of prostaglandin synthesis

The second approach, namely, administration of inhibitors of prostaglandin cyclooxygenase and measurement of renal sodium excretion, has yielded only somewhat greater unanimity. Acute administration of aspirin (Susic and Sparks, 1975) or indomethacin (Dusing, Melder, and Kramer, 1976, 1977; Leyssac et al., 1975) to anesthetized or conscious rats and anesthetized or conscious dogs (Altsheler et al., 1977) reduced urine volume and sodium excretion especially after sodium loading. In other experiments with trained conscious dogs, meclofenamate increased (Kirschenbaum and Stein, 1976) or had no effect (Gagnon and Felipe, 1977) on sodium excretion. Zambraski & Dunn (1979) found no change of sodium excretion when conscious dogs were given indomethacin or meclofenamate. In acutely prepared, anesthetized dogs, aspirin (Berg and Bergan, 1976; Ramsay and Elliot, 1967) and indomethacin (Kövér and Tost, 1977) reduced urine sodium and volume. Chronic treatment of rabbits with indomethacin did not alter the renal response to three different sodium intakes (Lifschitz et al., 1978). Acute parenteral administration of indomethacin increased papillary (interstitial) concentration of sodium in rats, which suggests a natriuretic role for renal prostaglandins (Ganguli et al., 1977). Normal and hypertensive subjects did not retain sodium during 4 days of indomethacin treatment (200 mg per day) (Patak et al., 1975). However, other workers have reported that indomethacin, 150 mg per day for 3 days reduced renal sodium excretion on normal or low sodium intake in normal men or in patients with renal disease (Arisz et al., 1976; Donker et al., 1976). Furthermore, acute intravenous administration of acetylsalicylic acid, 750 mg, to patients with chronic renal failure reduced sodium excretion by 80 percent (Berg, 1977). All experiments with inhibitors of cyclooxygenase have the theoretical disadvantage that the observed results may be secondary to actions of the drugs apart from reduction of prostaglandin synthesis (Dunn and Hood, 1977).

Diuretics, sodium excretion, and prostaglandins

A third approach to the question of the relationship of renal prostaglandins to sodium excretion has produced the most consistent results. Although some investigators have failed to demonstrate a negative or inhibitory interaction between inhibitors of prostaglandin cyclooxygenase and diuretic-induced natriuresis (Bailie, Crosslan, and Hook 1976; Berg, 1977; Weber et al., 1977b; Williamson, Bourland, and Marchand, 1974, 1975a), most workers have found that "loop diuretics" (ethacrynic acid, furosemide, bumetanide) have reduced natriuretic potency after inhibition of prostaglandin synthesis. These diuretics increase renal blood flow after acute administration (Olsen, 1977; Williamson et al., 1974, 1975a). This increment of renal blood flow is accompanied by increased prostaglandin synthesis (Scherer et al., 1978; Williamson et al., 1975b) and is reduced or inhibited by indomethacin (Olsen, 1977; Williamson et al., 1974, 1975a). Although acute intravenous administration of furosemide increased urinary excretion of PGE in both normotensive (Scherer et al., 1978) and hypertensive subjects (Abe et al., 1977), the increment of urine PGE was twofold greater in the normotensive controls (Abe et al., 1977). In conscious rabbits indomethacin blunted the acute natriuresis of furosemide (Oliw et al., 1976). Anesthetized (Berg and Bergan, 1976; Kövér and Tost, 1977) and conscious dogs (Berg and Loew, 1977; Olsen, 1975) showed a diminished natriuresis after furosemide or bumetanide if pretreated with acetylsalicylic acid or indomethacin. Indomethacin reduces natriuresis after furosemide in normal and hypertensive subjects (Patak et al., 1975). Although aspirin reduced urine sodium in healthy subjects, it did not affect the natriuresis after furosemide (Berg, 1977). It is impossible to separate the effects of these inhibitors on renal blood flow from any possible action on tubular prostaglandin production and natriuresis. It is possible that much of the antinatriuretic action is secondary to decreasing renal blood flow.

Several reports have called attention to the important inhibitory interactions of fatty acid cyclooxygenase inhibitors and furosemide in patients with renal disease. In four patients with the nephrotic syndrome, indomethacin 150 mg daily blunted the natriuresis of large doses of furosemide (500–2000 mg per day) (Tiggeler, Koene, and Wijdeveld, 1977). Glomerular filtration rate also decreased by 20 to 40 percent in two series of patients with nephrotic syndrome treated with indomethacin to reduce proteinuria (Arisz et al., 1976; Tiggeler et al., 1977) and by 15 percent in patients with chronic renal failure (Donker et al., 1976). Aspirin has a similar inhibitory action on the natriuretic efficacy of furosemide in patients with chronic renal failure (Berg, 1977).

In conclusion, one can state that despite the potent natriuretic properties of PGE_2 and PGI_2, it remains unproved that increased renal production of prostaglandins, in vivo, mediates the physiological response to sodium loading. In fact, some workers have reported decreased renal excretion of PGE_2 as urine sodium increases. Inhibition of fatty acid cyclooxygenase with aspirin, indomethacin, or meclofenamate has variable effects upon sodium excretion and the response to saline loading. However, these drugs exert a rather consistent antagonistic action on diuretic-induced natriuresis. This antagonism of furosemide, ethacrynic acid, and bumetanide seems to be exaggerated in patients with renal disease, especially the nephrotic syndrome. This may partially depend upon the extent of the secondary elevation of renin and angiotensin II and hence upon the severity of the decrease in effective circulating volume.

PROSTAGLANDINS, ADH, AND WATER EXCRETION

Evidence is progressively accumulating which supports an important interaction between renal prostaglandin synthesis and the action of ADH (antidiuretic hormone [vasopressin]) upon the collecting tubule. Because PGE_2 and $PGF_{2\alpha}$ are synthesized in renal medullary interstitial cells and collecting tubule cells (Bohman, 1977; Janszen and Nugteren, 1971; Smith and Wilkin, 1977), many workers have sought a role for these prostaglandins in physiologic processes of the renal medulla, especially water reabsorption under the control of ADH.

Prostaglandins and cyclic AMP

Infusion of PGE into one renal artery of dogs under hydropenic and under nonhydropenic conditions produces an increment in free water excretion (Martinez-Maldonado et al., 1972). Although intra-arterial infusion of PGE_1 exerted both proximal and distal effects, these authors concluded that PGE_1 depressed the permeability of the collecting tubule to water in vivo (Martinez-Maldonado et al., 1972). Orloff, Handler, and Bergstrom (1965) had previously shown that PGE_1 inhibited the ADH-stimulated increment of water flux in the toad bladder. Since the toad bladder behaves in many ways similar to the mammalian collecting tubule, these results accurately presaged future developments in this area. PGE antagonized the ADH-stimulation of water reabsorption in the isolated, perfused rabbit collecting tubule (Grantham and Orloff, 1968). This antagonism appears to occur at the adenylate cyclase since PGE does not alter the permeability responses to cyclic AMP (cyclic adenosine 3'5' monophosphate) or theophylline in the toad bladder (Olsen, 1977) or collecting tubule (Grantham and Orloff, 1968). PGE_1 did inhibit the vasopressin-mediated increments of cyclic AMP in toad bladder (Lipson and Sharp, 1971), rabbit collecting tubule (Grantham and Orloff, 1968), hamster medulla and papilla (Maruma and Edelman 1971), and rat inner medullary slices (Beck et al., 1971).

Inhibitors of prostaglandin synthesis and urine concentration

If prostaglandins reduce vasopressin-stimulated water transport, then inhibition of prostaglandin production should potentiate water reabsorption after vasopressin administration. The prostaglandin cyclooxygenase inhibitors, indomethacin, meclofenamate, and aspirin enhance ADH stimulation of water reabsorption in vivo in rats (Berl et al., 1977; Leyssac et al., 1975; Lum et al., 1977), dogs (Anderson et al., 1975; Fejes-Töth, Maggar, and Walter, 1977), and humans (Berl et al., 1977). Indomethacin also potentiates the in vitro response (water flux) of the toad bladder to vasopressin (Albert and Handler, 1974; Flores and Sharp, 1972; Zusman, Keiser, and Handler, 1977). Figure 4.1 taken from Anderson et al. (1975) illustrates the potentiation by meclofenamate of low doses of vasopressin upon the renal concentrating mechanism. Additionally, since indomethacin increases papillary osmolality, the osmotic driving forces for water reabsorption are also increased (Gerkins et al., 1978; Higashihara and Kokko, 1978; Stoff et al., 1978).

Interactions of prostaglandins and vasopressin

These data, in the aggregate, suggest that renal prostaglandins (especially PGE_2) operate as an inhibitory or negative feedback pathway to modulate the action of vasopressin on the collecting tubule. If this is the case, then vasopressin should stimulate renal prostaglandin synthesis. Using renal medullary in-

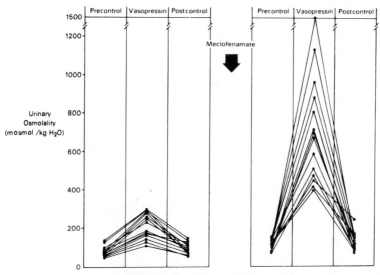

Figure 4.1 Inhibition of prostaglandin synthesis in which meclofenamate potentiates the water reabsorption after low dose vasopressin in the dog. Indomethacin produces similar effects. (From Anderson et al., 1975)

terstitial cells in culture, Zusman et al. (1977) have demonstrated that prostaglandin synthesis (only PGE_2 was measured) was enhanced by vasopressin. In vitro, vasopressin also increased production of PGE by rabbit renal medullary slices (Kalisker and Dyer, 1972). In vivo, vasopressin enhances renal production of PGE_2 (Dunn et al., 1978; Walker et al., 1978) and PGF_a (Dunn et al., 1978) in normal and homozygous diabetes insipidus rats. Furthermore, the untreated diabetes insipidus animals excrete 80 percent less PGE_2 and PGF_2 than the control animals. Figure 4.2 depicts these results. The data confirm that vasopressin, endogenously produced or exogenously administered, stimulates renal synthesis of prostaglandins in vivo. Recent work using toad bladder (Zusman et al., 1977) and renal cells in culture (Zusman and Keiser, 1977) demonstrated that vasopressin activates phospholipase (acylhydrolase), thereby deacylating membrane phospholipids. The increased availability of arachidonic acid, the substrate for the fatty acid cyclooxygenase, increased the synthesis of PGE_2. It may be important to note that vasopressin enhances prostaglandin synthesis at much lower concentrations than is necessary for maximal stimulation of water flux (Zusman et al., 1977). Figure 4.3 summarizes our current understanding of the interrelationships between vasopressin, PGE_2, and water permeability of the mammalian collecting tubule. Activation of phospholipase by vasopressin releases arachidonic acid, which yields more PGE_2. PGE_2 acts as an inhibitory modulator of vasopressin at or near the adenylate cyclase receptor. Blockade of PGE_2 biosynthesis enhances the action of vasopressin to produce cyclic AMP and hence increases water reabsorption. The effects of PGE_2 are most important with low concentrations

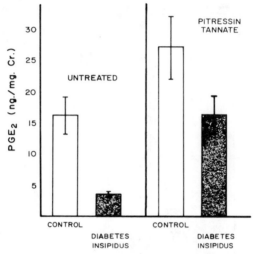

Figure 4.2 Control rats excreted substantially more PGE_2 than the Brattleboro homozygous diabetes insipidus rats. Pitressin tannate in oil, 200 milliunits per rat, increased urinary excretion of PGE_2 in both groups and the treated diabetes insipidus animals excreted as much PGE_2 as the untreated controls. (From Dunn et al., 1978)

of vasopressin; maximum concentrations of vasopressin are largely unaffected by the prostaglandin feedback loop.

RENIN AND ANGIOTENSIN

Prostaglandins as modulators of renal vasoconstriction

The interactions between the renin-angiotensin system and renal prostaglandin synthesis are complex and bidirectional. Nonetheless the evidence is persuasive that these biochemical systems are interrelated physiologically in both health and disease.

McGiff and his coworkers (1970) showed that infusions of angiotensin II in the dog increased renal venous concentrations of PGE-like material. Subsequent work has confirmed these findings and also demonstrated that $PGF_{2\alpha}$ as well as PGE_2 increases in renal venous blood and in urine of dog (Dunn et al., 1978) and humans (Frohlich et al., 1975) after infusions of angiotensin II. The extent of the renal vasoconstriction following infusions of angiotensin II is modulated by the synthesis and release of PGE_2 and perhaps PGI_2 from vascular and renal tissue. The synthesis of these vasodilatory prostaglandins reduces the constrictor and ischemic actions of angiotensin II (Aiken and Vane, 1973; Satoh and Zimmerman, 1975; Terragno, Terragno, and McGiff, 1977). Norepinephrine has similar actions (Needleman et al., 1974). It is also well established that blockade of prostaglandin synthesis enhances the extent and the duration of vasoconstriction after infusion of angiotensin II (Aiken and Vane, 1973; Finn

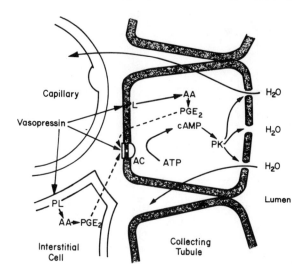

Figure 4.3 This schema summarizes the interactions of vasopressin, PGE_2, and the collecting tubule. (phospholipids, PL; arachidonic acid, AA; adenylate cyclase, AC; adenosine triphosphate, ATP; adenosine triphosphate, ATP; cyclic AMP, cAMP; protein kinase, PK; stimulate, →; inhibit, ---→.) It is conjectural that vasopressin occupies different receptors on the tubular cell membrane in order to activate adenylate cyclase and phospholipase. (Redrawn from Dunn and Hood et al., 1977)

and Arendshorst, 1976; Satoh and Zimmerman, 1975, Swain et al., 1975). Figure 4.4 depicts data from the work of Dunn, Liard, and Dray (1978), who evaluated the importance of renal PGE_2 synthesis for the maintenance of renal blood flow during ischemia. In the dog the compensatory return of renal blood flow towards control levels, after the onset of renal arterial constriction or renal arterial infusion of angiotensin II, was a function of the increment of renal synthesis of PGE_2 (Dunn et al., 1978). However the stimulation of prostaglandin synthesis by angiotensin II is not solely the result of vasoconstriction and ischemia. Studies using renal slices of rat papilla (Danon et al., 1975), rabbit renal medullary interstitial cells in culture (Zusman and Keiser, 1977), and human vascular endothelial and smooth muscle cells in culture (Alexander and Gimbrone, 1976; Gimbrone and Alexander, 1975) have demonstrated a direct stimulatory action of angiotensin II on prostaglandin production. Furthermore, this effect in vitro is secondary to increased deacylation of phospholipids providing greater amounts of substrate, arachidonic acid, to the prostaglandin cyclooxygenase (Zusman and Keiser, 1977).

Kallikrein, kinins, and prostaglandins

Besides vasoconstriction and a direct effect on membrane phospholipase, angiotensin II induces chronic changes of the kallikrein-kinin system, which may chronically increase renal prostaglandin synthesis (Nasjletti and Colina-Chourio, 1976). Aldosterone and other mineralocorticoids stimulate kallikrein excretion (Margolius et al., 1974) and spironolactone, an aldosterone antago-

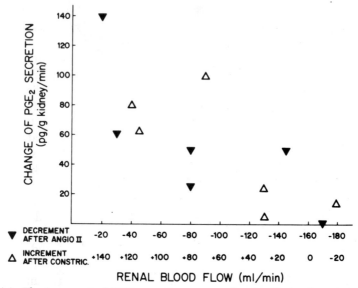

Figure 4.4 The increment of PGE₂ secretion was correlated with the decrement of renal blood flow after angiotensin II infusion and the extent of recovery of renal blood flow after partial renal arterial constriction. Angiotensin II 50 ng/min into the canine renal artery, minimally reduced blood flow when PGE₂ secretion (renal venous PGE₂) was greatest. The compensatory recovery of blood flow after renal arterial constriction was greatest when PGE₂ secretion was increased. (From Dunn et al., 1978)

nist, reduces kallikrein excretion (Seino et al., 1977). The kallikrein-kinin system stimulates renal prostaglandin production (Dunn et al., 1978; McGiff et al., 1972; Nasjletti and Colina-Chourio, 1976) probably by activating membrane phospholipase and deacylating phospholipid to arachidonic acid (Zusman and Keiser, 1977). Figure 4.5 summarizes these interrelations of renin, angiotensin, aldosterone, kallikrein, and renal synthesis of various prostaglandins. The physiological importance of these pathways is unknown. Modulation of angiotensin-induced vasoconstriction is the best documented action of renal PGE₂; however, it appears that PGE₂ and PGF₂ₐ may mediate some of bradykinin's actions (McGiff et al., 1976; Nasjletti and Colina-Chourio, 1976) on the kidney, especially the natriuresis; the renal vasodilatation and water diuresis are largely independent of PGE₂ production (Blasingham and Nasjletti, 1977).

Control of renin release

Prostaglandins and prostaglandin precursors are potent stimuli of renin release. Arachidonic acid, infused into the renal artery of rats (Weber et al., 1975), rabbits (Larsson, Weber, and Anggard, 1974), and dogs (Bolger et al., 1976), increases renal venous renin activity. This is not a direct effect of arachidonic acid because agents that antagonize prostaglandin cyclooxygenase and thereby block conversion to endoperoxides and prostaglandins will nullify the renin stimulation (Bolger et al., 1976; Larsson et al., 1974). In experiments with rabbit renal cortical slices in vitro, Weber et al. (1976) reported enhancement of renin synthesis by arachidonic acid and the endoperoxides, but not by PGE_2. Furthermore, these workers observed inhibition of renin release by $PGE_{2\alpha}$. Contrary results have been reported with stimulation of renin synthesis by both PGE_2 and $PGF_{2\alpha}$ superfused over rat renal cortical slices (Franco, Tan, and Mulrow, 1977). PGI_2 (prostacyclin) added to renal cortical slices (Franco et al., 1977; Whorton et al., 1977) or infused into the renal artery (Bolger et al., 1978) is a potent stimulus of renin secretion. Most (but not all) studies using intrarenal infusions of PGE (E_1 and E_2) have confirmed in vivo that renin synthesis is stimulated (Werning et al., 1971; Yun et al., 1977). This is probably a direct action on the juxtaglomerular cells since the nonfiltering kidney, with no distal delivery of filtrate to the macula densa, responds to PGE_2 (Yun et al., 1977) and PGI_2 (Bolger et al., 1978) with enhancement of renin release. Studies of the effects of indomethacin and other inhibitors of prostaglandin cyclooxygenase reinforce these interpretations of the role of prostaglandins in control of renin synthesis and release. These inhibitors reduce basal and stimulated plasma renin activity in humans (Donker et al., 1976; Patak et al., 1975; Rumpf et al., 1975; Speckart et al., 1977; Tan and Mulrow, 1977) and in animals (Bailie et al., 1976; Larsson et al., 1974; Leyssac et al., 1975; Yun et al., 1977). The decrement of plasma renin activity is greatest when indomethacin is administered after activation of renin synthesis. This has been dramatically shown in patients with Bartter's syndrome. Figure 4.5 presents these data in summary fashion. It remains a puzzle that most renal prostaglandins exert a positive rather than a negative feedback influence on renal renin synthesis. Since these systems cannot be continually self-reinforcing some important regulatory step or steps must be operative to interrupt the cycle.

Bartter's syndrome

Clinical research on the pathophysiology of Bartter's syndrome has enhanced our understanding of the interrelations of renin-angiotensin, aldosterone, kallikrein-kinin, and prostaglandins. Bartter's syndrome is a rare and often familial disorder characterized by renal losses of sodium and potassium, severe hypokalemia and metabolic alkalosis, elevated plasma renin activity with juxtaglomerular cellular hyperplasia, increased aldosterone secretion and excretion, and resistance to the pressor action of angiotensin II despite normotension. Renal production of PGE is increased when measured as enhanced urinary excretion of PGE_2 (Bowden et al., 1978; Gill et al., 1976; Halushka et al., 1977). Many reports have documented the benefits of therapy with inhibitors of prostaglandin synthesis (indomethacin, ibuprofen, aspirin) (Bowden et al., 1978; Donker et al., 1977; Fichman et al., 1976; Gill et al., 1976; Halushka et al., 1977; Norby et al., 1976; Verberckmoes et al., 1976). Inhibition of prostaglandin synthesis induces a positive balance of sodium and potassium, increases serum potassium, reduces plasma renin activity, and enhances the pressor responsiveness to angiotensin II. Indomethacin appears to be more ef-

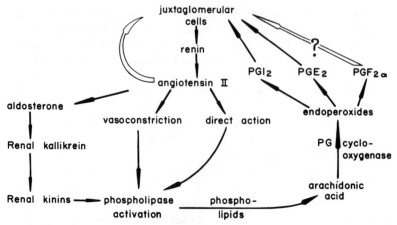

Figure 4.5 This schematic summary attempts to interrelate the renin-angiotensin and kinin systems with phospholipid deacylation, prostaglandin synthesis, and subsequent actions of prostaglandins on the juxtaglomerular cells. Stimulation, (→); inhibition, (→); conflicting studies, (?).

ficacious than ibuprofen or aspirin, perhaps because of more complete inhibition of PGE_2 synthesis (Bowden et al., 1978). Urinary kallikrein excretion (Halushka et al., 1977; Lechi et al., 1976; Vinci et al., 1976) and plasma bradykinin (Vinci et al., 1976) were increased in untreated patients and therapy with indomethacin significantly reduced both urinary PGE_2 and kallikrein (Halushka et al., 1977; Vinci et al., 1976). The levels of urine kallikrein and PGE_2 were highly correlated (Halushka et al., 1977). Figure 4.6 taken from Bowden et al. (1978) depicts the effects of indomethacin therapy in a patient with Bartter's syndrome.

It is unknown whether the overproduction of prostaglandins is a primary or secondary abnormality in Bartter's syndrome. Although decrements of extracellular potassium increased PGE_2 production by renal medullary interstitial cells in culture, studies in vivo have been unable to demonstrate any increase of urinary PGE_2 or $PGF_{2\alpha}$ in potassium-depleted rats (Hood and Dunn, 1978). Contrariwise, potassium depletion in dogs may exert stimulatory effects on renal PGE_2 synthesis (Galvez et al., 1977).

Patients who have severe secondary hyperreninemia and hyperaldosteronism owing to hepatic failure and to ascites appear to have elevated plasma and urine concentrations of PGE_2 (Zipser et al., 1977). It is likely that PGE_2 serves an important modulating function to minimize the renal hemodynamic effects of angiotensin II since inhibition of prostaglandin synthesis is followed by substantial reductions of glomerular filtration rate, renal plasma flow, and urine volume (Zipser et al., 1977). Similar but less dramatic results have been reported in patients with the nephrotic syndrome who receive indomethacin (Arisz et al., 1976).

In summary, it seems fair to conclude that the renin-angiotensin system, the kallikrein-kinin system, and renal prostaglandin synthesis are interconnected

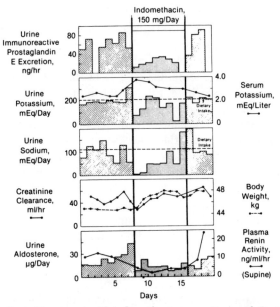

Figure 4.6 The effect of treatment with indomethacin in a patient with Bartter's syndrome is shown. The basal urine PGE is elevated. Seven patients showed similar short-term responses to inhibitors of prostaglandin cyclooxygenase. (From Bowden et al., 1978)

in important ways. Vasodilatory prostaglandins reduce the constrictor actions of angiotensin II. Bradykinin mediates some of its actions via stimulation of prostaglandin synthesis. Kallikrein and urinary PGE_2 are both elevated in Bartter's syndrome. PGI_2 and PGE_2 stimulate renal renin production, and hyperreninemic conditions in humans may often elicit increases of renal PGE_2 synthesis. Indomethacin and related compounds significantly reduce renal renin release and plasma renin activity.

HYPERTENSION

There has been extensive and continuing interest in a possible role of renal prostaglandins as a cause of, or as a compensatory response to, hypertension. Diverse hypertensive models have been used, including essential hypertension in humans and rats, one and two kidney renal arterial constriction models in rats and rabbits, and high salt-intake models (with or without mineralocorticoid or angiotensin II). The continuing interest can be ascribed to the multiple actions of the prostaglandins and thromboxanes, which can alter blood pressure. These actions include vasodilatation (PGE_2, PGD_2, PGI_2), vasoconstriction ($PGF_{2\alpha}$, TXA_2 [thromboxane A_2]), natriuresis (PGE_2, PGI_2), renin stimulation (PGE_2, PGI_2, endoperoxides) and inhibition of adrenergic transmission (PGE_2). Consideration of antihypertensive (or prohypertensive) effects of the renal prostaglandins should include recognition that it is unlikely that these effects would be exerted at extrarenal sites. Since the lungs efficiently degrade PGE_2 and $PGF_{2\alpha}$, renal venous prostaglandins rarely reach the arterial circulation. PGI_2 is an exception since pulmonary degradation is minimal after a single pulmonary passage (Gerkins et al., 1978; Spannhake et al., 1978). Hence PGI_2 given intravenously is tenfold more potent than PGE_2 as a vasodepressor substance (Armstrong et al., 1978; Fitzpatrick et al., 1978). It seems more logical to search for local, intrarenal actions and effects that would modulate blood pressure (McGiff and Vane, 1975). If one accepts the hypotheses of Guyton and coworkers (1972), then the kidney has a certain primacy in the control of blood pressure. Failure to excrete salt normally and thereby to maintain a normal pressure–natriuresis curve will cause hypertension. Renal arteriolar vasoconstriction may play an important role in the genesis of "essential" hypertension, especially if tubular reabsorption of sodium, chloride, and water are enhanced. Table 4.1 summarizes most of the published studies on hypertension and renal prostaglandin production.

Decreased renal synthesis of PGE in hypertension

Since most prostaglandins are vasodepressor, some of the earliest hypotheses suggested a renal deficiency of prostaglandins as a cause of hypertension (Lee et al., 1971). Some evidence exists in support of this theory. Renal medulla and papilla removed from renovascular and spontaneously hypertensive rats released less PGE than control slices (Pugsley, Beilin, and Peto, 1975; Sirois and Gagnon, 1974). Perfused kidneys from renovascular hypertensive rats released less PGE into the perfusate (Leary, Ledingham, and Vane, 1974). Studies of urinary excretion of PGE in patients with essential hypertension have also yielded some uniformity of results. Using a bioassay, Papanicolaou et al. (1975) found decreased concentrations of PGE in the urine. Using radioimmunoassay of PGE, Abe et al. (1977) found hypertensive patients to have only 50 percent as much urinary PGE as 19 normotensive controls. Furthermore, furosemide stimulated renal excretion of PGE in the controls whereas the hypertensives had smaller increments of urine PGE, and these increments were restricted to males. Figure 4.7 summarizes these findings (Abe et al., 1977). Tan and Mulrow (1978), also using a radioimmunoassay for PGE, documented lower urinary values in hypertensive patients, especially those with low renin hypertension.

Prostaglandins in Kyoto hypertensive rats

The Japanese Wistar Kyoto rat (SHR, a spontaneously hypertensive rat), inbred successively by Okamoto and coworkers, provides a valuable model of essential hypertension independent of salt intake or renal manipulations. We have studied these rats and have measured renal medullary microsomal concentration of prostaglandin (fatty acid) cyclooxygenase (Dunn, 1976), renal venous and urinary concentration of PGE_2 and $PGF_{2\alpha}$, and zonal distribution of

Table 4.1 Summary of prostaglandins in human and experimental hypertension (modified Dunn and Hood et al., 1977)

Author	Hypertensive Model	Sample	Assay	Prostaglandin
Tobian and Azar (1971)	high Na Diet (rat)	renal papilla	bioassay[a]	↑ PGE release
Sirois and Gagnon (1974)	renovascular and SHR	renal papilla	bioassay	↑ PGE release
Pugsley et al. (1975)	renovascular (rat)	renal medulla	GC-electron capture	↑↓ PGE release
Leary et al. (1974)	renovascular (rat)	perfused kidney	RIA	↓ PGE release
Nekrasova and Lantsberg (1969)	renovascular (rabbit)	renal medulla	vasodepressor[b]	↓ PG content
Nekrasova et al. (1970)	renovascular (man)	renal medulla	vasodepressor	↓ PG content
Zusman et al. (1973)	SHR	plasma and kidney	RIA	↑ PGA content
Tobian and O'Donnell (1976)	SHR	whole kidney	bioassay	↑ PGF$_{2\alpha}$
Dunn (1976)	SHR	renal medulla	RIA	PGF$_{2\alpha}$ unchanged
Ahnfelt-Ronne (1977)	SHR	urine	RIA	↑ PGF$_{2\alpha}$ excretion
Juncos and Strong (1973)	renovascular (man)	renal venous	RIA[c]	↓ PG concn
Edwards et al. (1969)	renovascular (man)	renal venous	vasodepressor	↑ PG concn
Hornych et al. (1976)	essential and renovascular (man)	peripheral plasma	RIA	↑ PGA concn
Hornych et al. (1975)	renal parenchymal disease (man)	peripheral plasma	RIA	↑ PGA concn
Papanicolaou et al. (1975)	essential (man)	urine	bioassay	↓ PGE concn
Tan et al. (1978)	essential (man)	urine	RIA	↓ PGE$_2$ excretion
Abe et al. (1977)	essential (man)	urine	RIA	↓ PGE excretion

[a] Bioassay includes all in vitro muscle strip assays.

[b] Rat vasodepressor assay in vivo; results are expressed as total prostaglandin (PG).

[c] RIA for PGA and PGE converted to PGB. ↑, increase; ↓, decrease.

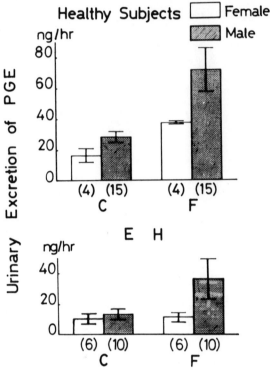

Figure 4.7   The renal excretion of PGE in healthy subjects and essential hypertensives (EH) is shown during control (C) and furosemide (F) periods. Females consistently excreted less PGE than males and hypertensives less than normotensive controls. Number of measurements, ( ) (From Abe et al., 1977)

renal blood flow measured by microsphere technique (Wait and Dunn, 1979). Figure 4.8 shows a comparison of the activity or concentration of prostaglandin cyclooxygenase in microsomes obtained from normotensive and hypertensive rat renal medullae. The renal medullae from hypertensive rats consistently synthesized more PGE_2 and $PGF_{2\alpha}$ (not shown) than normotensive Wistar Kyoto controls. These differences were more marked after the third month of age. Pace-Asciak (1976) has reported that Japanese SHR have decreased levels of prostaglandin 15-hydroxydehydrogenase in their kidneys. Armstrong et al. (1976) reported similar findings in New Zealand hypertensive rats. If renal synthesis of PGE_2 was increased and degradation was diminished, we theorized that renal venous and urinary levels of PGE_2 should be increased in vivo. We have measured renal venous concentrations of PGE_2 and $PGF_{2\alpha}$ as well as 24-hour urinary excretion of PGE_2 and $PGF_{2\alpha}$ in Japanese SHR. There were no differences in 24-hour urinary excretion of PGE_2 and $PGF_{2\alpha}$ between Wistar Kyoto controls and SHR. Renal venous concentrations of PGE_2 and $PGF_{2\alpha}$ collected immediately after the 24-hour urine sampling revealed no differences between hypertensive and normotensive rats. These results are puzzling because of the aforementioned work showing increased synthetic and decreased degradative enzymes.

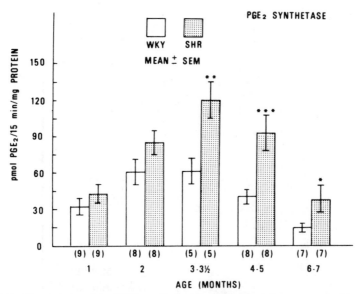

Figure 4.8 The activity of the PGE$_2$ synthetase (cyclooxygenase) was measured in rat renal medullary microsomes using ^{14}C-arachidonic acid and thin layer chromatographic separation of end products. Wistar Kyoto (WKy) normotensive rats were compared to spontaneously hypertensive rats (SHR). The number of rats is given beneath each column. The values are expressed as picomoles of PGE$_2$ produced per mg of microsomal protein per 15 min. incubation. *p<0.05; **p<0.02; ***p<0.01. (From Dunn, 1976)

If intrarenal concentrations of prostaglandins were increased, especially in the medulla in the hypertensive kidney, one would expect alterations of renal blood flow with enhanced flow to deeper portions of the cortex, especially to juxtamedullary nephrons. Using microsphere injections, Wait and Dunn (1979) measured inner and outer cortical distribution of renal blood flow. Figure 4.9 shows the results. Zonal distribution of renal blood flow between outer (zones 1 and 2) and inner (zones 3 and 4) cortex was unaltered although the SHR had greater fractional flow to the outermost cortical areas (zone 1) with proportionally less flow to zone 2. These studies, therefore, do not suggest increased in vivo production of PGE$_2$ in the kidney of SHR.

Renal medullary interstitial cells

Muirhead and his coworkers (1972a & b, 1973, 1975) have pioneered an alternative approach towards understanding the importance of renal vasodepressor factors and hypertension. They have demonstrated that transplantation or implantation of renal medullary tissue (Muirhead et al., 1972a & b, 1975) or renal medullary interstitial cells propagated in culture (Muirhead et al., 1975) reduce the blood pressure towards or to normal in rats, rabbits, and dogs with renoprival, renovascular, and angiotensin-salt hypertensions (Muirhead et al., 1972a & b, 1973, 1975). Muirhead et al. do not believe that renomedullary prostaglandins mediate this vasodepressor response since indomethacin does not reduce the beneficial effects of the implanted tis-

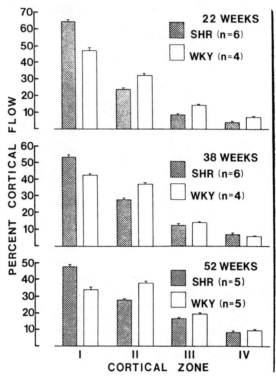

Figure 4.9   The fractional distribution of cortical renal blood flow was determined with radio-labelled microspheres. Zones I & II are outer cortical and zones III & IV are inner cortical and juxtamedullary. Normotensive (WKy) and hypertensive (SHR) differed only in zones I & II with SHR consistently showing greater superficial cortical flow. (From Wait and Dunn, 1979)

sue or cells. The putative vasodepressor substance has been called antihypertensive, neutral, renomedullary lipid.

Effects of indomethacin on blood pressure

If renal prostaglandins participate primarily or secondarily in various types of hypertension, then inhibitors of prostaglandin synthesis may aggravate or ameliorate the increased pressure. Most studies have shown a mild pressor action of indomethacin and no reports document a vasodepressor effect of cyclooxygenase blockade. Indomethacin, and related inhibitors given acutely and intravenously raise the blood pressure of normotensive (Davis and Horton, 1972; Larsson and Anggard, 1973) and hypertensive rabbits (Romero and Strong, 1977) renovascular hypertensive rats (Pugsley et al., 1975; Scholkens and Steinbach, 1975) and SHR (Levy, 1977), anesthetized normotensive dogs (Feigen *et al.*, 1976; Herbaczynska-Cedro and Vane, 1973) but not conscious unanesthetized dogs (Fejes-Tóth et al., 1977; Kirschenbaum and Stein, 1976, Zambraski & Dunn, 1979). In humans, indomethacin raised mean blood

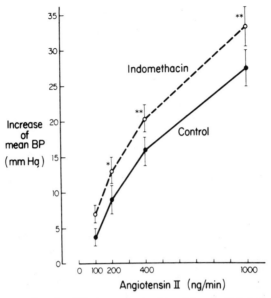

Figure 4.10   Ten normal male volunteers received angiotensin II infusions, intravenously, before and after indomethacin 150 mg in 3 doses over 16 hrs. °p<0.025, °°p<0.01. There was no weight gain owing to indomethacin. Indomethacin potentiated the angiotensin II pressor response curve. (From Negus et al., 1976)

pressure 5 mmHg after 3 days of treatment with 150 mg per day in normal and hypertensive subjects (Patak et al., 1975). Indomethacin, 25 mg given intravenously to 12 healthy volunteers, increased mean arterial blood pressure 10 mmHg within 10 minutes (Wennmalm, 1978). The extent of the pressor response after indomethacin should depend upon the extent of prior vasoconstriction mediated either by angiotensin II or by the alpha-adrenergic nervous system. Inhibition of vascular and renal synthesis of prostaglandins, in the presence of a compensatory increase of these prostaglandins to offset vasoconstriction, should enhance blood pressure. This hypothesis is supported by the demonstration that indomethacin potentiates the angiotensin pressor response curve in normal subjects (Negus, Tannen, and Dunn, 1976) (Figure 4.10). This is not surprising since angiotensin II stimulates vascular (Gimborne and Alexander, 1975) and renal (Dunn et al., 1978; McGiff et al., 1970) production of prostaglandins, which in turn act as a negative feedback pathway to modulate the vasoconstriction (Dunn et al., 1978; McGiff et al., 1970).

It is impossible to offer any unifying hypothesis about renal prostaglandins and experimental or clinical hypertension. Different species and different models undoubtedly elicit different prostaglandin responses. Some experimental models apparently increase renal synthesis and decrease degradation of vasodilatory prostaglandins in response to the elevated blood pressure. Other experimental models show opposite changes. Clinical studies of essential hypertension in humans have reported decreased urine concentrations of PGE. The importance of this observation is unknown.

ACKNOWLEDGMENT

This work was supported by the NIH (HL 22563), and an American Heart Association Grant In Aid.

REFERENCES

Abe, K., Yasujima, M., Chiba, S., Irokawa, N., Ito, T. & Yoshinaga, K. (1977). Effect of furosemide on urinary excretion of prostaglandin E in normal volunteers and patients with essential hypertension. *Prostaglandins*, **14**, 513–521.

Ahnfelt-Ronne, I. & Arrigoni-Martelli, E. (1977). Renal prostaglandin metabolism in spontaneously hypertensive rats. *Biochemical Pharmacology*, **26**, 485–488.

Aiken, J. W. & Vane, J. R. (1973). Intrarenal prostaglandin release attenuates the renal vasoconstrictor activity of angiotensin. *Journal of Pharmacology and Experimental Therapeutics*, **184**, 678–687.

Albert, W. C. & Handler, J. S. (1974). Effect of PGE, indomethacin and polyphloretin phosphate on toad bladder response to antidiuretic hormone. *American Journal of Physiology*, **226**, 1382–1386.

Alexander, R. W. & Gimbrone, M. A. (1976). Stimulation of prostaglandin E synthesis in cultured human umbilical vein smooth muscle cells. *Proceedings of the National Academy of Sciences (U.S.A.)* **73**, 1617–1620.

Altsheler, P., Rosenbaum, R., Klahr, S. & Slatopolsky, E. (1977). Effects of prostaglandin synthetase inhibitors (PSI) on the renal excretion of sodium in normal and uremic dogs. *Clinical Research*, **25**, 424A.

Anderson, R. J., Berl, T., McDonald, K. M. & Schrier, R. W. (1975). Evidence for an *in vivo* antagonism between vasopressin and prostaglandin in the mammalian kidney. *Journal of Clinical Investigation*, **56**, 420–426.

Arisz, L., Donker, A. J., Brentjens, J. R. & Van DerHem, G. K. (1976). The effect of indomethacin on proteinuria and kidney function in the nephrotic syndrome. *Acta Medica Scandinavica*, **199**, 121–125.

Armstrong, J. M., Blackwell, G. J., Flower, R. J., McGiff, J. C., Mullane, K. M. & Vane, J. R. (1976). Genetic hypertension in rats is accompanied by a defect in renal prostaglandin catabolism. *Nature* (London), **260**, 582–586.

Armstrong, J. M., Lattimer, N., Moncada, S. & Vane, J. R. (1978). Comparison of the vasodepressor effects of prostacyclin and 6-oxo-prostaglandin F_{1a} with those of prostaglandin E_2 in rats and rabbits. *British Journal of Pharmacology*, **62**, 125–130.

Attallah, A. & Lee, J. B. (1973). Radioimmunoassay of prostaglandin A. Intrarenal PGA_2 as a factor mediating saline-induced natriuresis. *Circulation Research*, **33**, 696–703.

Bailie, M. D., Crosslan, K. & Hook, J. B. (1976). Natriuretic effect of furosemide after inhibition of prostaglandin synthesis. *Journal of Pharmacology and Experimental Therapeutics*, **199**, 469–476.

Beck, N. P., Kaneko, T., Zor, U., Field, J. B. & Davis, B. B. (1971). Effects of vasopressin and prostaglandin E_1 on the adenyl cyclase-cyclic $3',5'$-adenosine monophosphate system of the renal medulla of the rat. *Journal of Clinical Investigation*, **50**, 2461–2465.

Berg, K. J. (1977). Acute effects of acetylsalicylic acid in patients with chronic renal insufficiency. *European Journal of Clinical Pharmacology*, **11**, 111–116.

Berg, K. J. & Bergan, A. (1976). Effects of different doses of acetylsalicylic acid on renal function in the dog. *Scandinavian Journal of Clinical and Laboratory Investigation*, **36**, 779–786.

Berg, K. J. & Loew, D. (1977). Inhibition of furosemide-induced natriuresis by acetylsalicylic acid in dogs. *Scandinavian Journal of Clinical and Laboratory Investigation*, **37**, 125–131.

Berg, K. J. (1977). Acute effects of acetylsalicylic acid on renal function in normal man. *European Journal of Clinical Pharmacology*, **11**, 117–123.

Berl, T., Raz, A., Wald, H., Horowitz, J. & Czaczkes, W. (1977). Prostaglandin synthesis inhibition and the action of vasopressin: Studies in man and rat. *American Journal of Physiology*, **232**, F529–F537.

Blasingham, C. & Nasjletti, A. (1977). Effects of prostaglandin synthesis inhibition on the renal actions of bradykinin in the dog. *Physiologist*, **20**, 10.

Bohman, S. O. (1977). Demonstration of prostaglandin synthesis in collecting duct cells and other cell types of the rabbit renal medulla. *Prostaglandins*, **14**, 729–744.

Bolger, P. M., Eisner, G. M., Ramwell, P. W. & Slotkoff, L. M. (1976). Effect of prostaglandin synthesis on renal function and renin in the dog. *Nature* (London), **259**, 244–245.

Bolger, P. M., Eisner, G. M., Ramwell, P. W., Slotkoff, L. M. & Corey, E. J. (1978). Renal actions of prostacyclin. *Nature* (London), **271**, 467–469.

Bowden, R. E., Gill, J. R., Radfan, N., Taylor, A. A. & Keiser, H. R. (1978). Prostaglandin synthetase inhibitors in Bartter's syndrome. Effect on immunoreactive prostaglandin E excretion. *Journal of the American Medical Association*, **239**, 117–121.

Carriere, S., Friborg, J. & Guay, J. P. (1971). Vasodilators, intrarenal blood flow, and natriuresis in the dog. *American Journal of Physiology*, **221**, 92–98.

Chang, L. C., Splawinski, J. A., Oates, J. A. & Nies, A. S. (1975). Enhanced renal prostaglandin production in the dog. II. Effects on intrarenal hemodynamics. *Circulation Research*, **36**, 204–207.

Danon, A., Chang, L. C., Sweetman, S. J., Nies, A. S. & Oates, J. A. (1975). Synthesis of prostaglandins by the rat renal papilla *in vitro;* mechanism of stimulation by angiotensin II. *Biochimica et Biophysica Acta*, **388**, 71–83.

Davis, H. A. & Horton, E. W. (1972). Output of prostaglandins from the rabbit kidney, its increase on renal nerve stimulation and its inhibition by indomethacin. *British Journal of Pharmacology*, **46**, 658–675.

Donker, A. J., Arisz, L., Brentjens, J. R., Van DerHem, G. K. & Hollemans, H. J. (1976). The effect of indomethacin on kidney function and plasma renin activity in man. *Nephron*, **17**, 288–296.

Donker, A. J., deJong, P. E., Statius van Eps, L. W., Brentjens, J. R., Bakker, K. & Doorenbos, H. (1977). Indomethacin in Bartter's syndrome. *Nephron*, **19**, 200–213.

Dunn, M. J. (1976). Renal prostaglandin synthesis in the spontaneously hypertensive rat. *Journal of Clinical Investigation*, **58**, 862–870.

Dunn, M. J., Greeley, H. P., Horner, J. & Valtin, H. (1978). Renal excretion of prostaglandin E_2 (PGE$_2$) and F_{2a} (PGF$_{2a}$) in Brattleboro homozygous diabetes insipidus (DI) rats. *American Journal of Physiology*, **235**: E624–E627.

Dunn, M. J. & Hood, V. L. (1977). Prostaglandins and the kidney. *American Journal of Physiology*, **233** (3), F169–F184.

Dunn, M. J. & Howe, D. (1977). Prostaglandins lack a direct inhibitory action on electrolyte and water transport in the kidney and erythrocyte. *Prostaglandins*, **13**, 417–429.

Dunn, M. J., Liard, J. F. & Dray, F. (1978). Basal and stimulated rates of renal secretion and excretion of prostaglandins E_2, F_a, and 13, 14-dihydro-15-keto F_a in the dog. *Kidney International*, **13**, 136–143.

Dusing, R., Melder, B. & Kramer, H. J. (1976). Prostaglandins and renal function in acute extracellular volume expansion. *Prostaglandins*, **12**, 3–10.

Dusing, R., Opitz, W. D. & Kramer, H. J. (1977). The role of prostaglandins in the natriuresis of acutely salt-loaded rats. *Nephron*, **18**, 212–219.

Edwards, W. G., Strong, C. G. & Hunt, J. C. (1969). A vasodepressor lipid resembling prostaglandin E_2 (PGE$_2$) in the renal venous blood of hypertensive patients. *Journal of Laboratory and Clinical Medicine*, **74**, 389–399.

Feigen, L. P., Klainer, E., Chapnick, B. M. & Kadowitz, P. J. (1976). The effect of indomethacin on renal function in pentobarbital-anesthetized dogs. *Journal of Pharmacology and Experimental Therapeutics*, **198**, 457–463.

Fejes-Tóth, G., Magyar, A. & Walter, J. (1977). Renal response to vasopressin after inhibition of prostaglandin synthesis. *American Journal of Physiology*, **232**, F416–F423.

Fichman, M. P., Telfer, N., Zia, P., Speckart, P., Golub, M. & Rude, R. (1976). Role of prostaglandins in the pathogenesis of Bartter's syndrome. *American Journal of Medicine*, **60**, 785–797.

Fine, L. G. & Trizna, W. (1977). Influence of prostaglandins on sodium transport of isolated medullary nephron segments. *American Journal of Physiology*, **232**, F383–F390.

Finn, W. F. & Arendshorst, W. J. (1976). Effect of prostaglandin synthetase inhibitors on renal blood flow in the rat. *American Journal of Physiology*, **231**, 1541–1545.

Fitzpatrick, T. M., Alter, I., Corey, E. J., Ramwell, P. W., Rose, J. C. & Kot, P. A. (1978). Cardiovascular responses to PGI$_2$ (prostacyclin) in the dog. *Circulation Research*, **42**, 192–194.

Flores, A. G. & Sharp, G. W. (1972). Endogenous prostaglandins and osmotic water flow in the toad bladder. *American Journal of Physiology*, **223**, 1392–1397.

Franco, R., Tan, S. Y. & Mulrow, P. (1977). Renin release in an *in vitro* superfusion system of rat kidney slices: effect of prostaglandins. *Clinical Research*, **25**, 594A.

Frolich, J. C., Wilson, T. W., Sweetman, B. J., Smigel, M., Nies, A. S., Carr, K., Watson, J. T. & Oates, J. A. (1975). Urinary prostaglandins: Identification and origin. *Journal of Clinical Investigation*, **55**, 763–770.

Fulgraff, G. & Brandenbusch, G. (1974). Comparison of the effects of the prostaglandins A_1, E_2, and F_{2a} on kidney function in dogs. *Pflügers Archiv*, **349**, 9–17.

Fulgraff, G., Brandenbusch, G. & Heintze, K. (1974). Dose-response relation of the renal effects of PGA_1, PGE_2 and PGF_{2a}. *Prostaglandins*, **8**, 21–30.

Gagnon, J. & Felipe, I. (1977). Effects of prostaglandin synthetase inhibition on Na excretion in the conscious, volume expanded dog. *Physiologist*, **20**, 31.

Galvez, O. G., Bay, W. H., Roberts, B. W. & Ferris, T. F. (1977). The hemodynamic effects of potassium deficiency in the dog. *Circulation Research Supplement I*, **40**, 11–16.

Ganguli, M., Tobian, L., Azar, S. & O'Donnell, M. (1977). Evidence that prostaglandin synthesis inhibitors increase the concentration of sodium and chloride in rat renal medulla. *Circulation Research, Supplement I*, **40**, 135–139.

Gerkins, J. F., Freisinger, G. C., Branch, R. A., Shand, P. G., Gerber, J. G. & Oates, J. A. (1978). Pulmonary, renal, and hepatic extraction of PGI_2—a potential circulating hormone. *Clinical Research*, **26**, 13A.

Gill, J. R., Frolich, J. C., Bowden, R. E., Taylor, A. A., Keiser, H. R., Hannsjorg, W. S., Oates, J. A. & Bartter, F. C. (1976). Bartter's syndrome: A disorder characterized by high urinary prostaglandins and a dependence of hyperreninemia on prostaglandin synthesis. *American Journal of Medicine*, **61**, 43–51.

Gimbrone, M. A. & Alexander, R. W. (1975). Angiotensin II stimulation of prostaglandin production in cultured human vascular endothelium. *Science*, **189**, 219–220.

Grantham, J. J. & Orloff, J. (1968). Effect of prostaglandin E_1 on the permeability response of the isolated collecting tubule to vasopressin, adenosine 3′,5′-monophosphate and theophylline. *Journal of Clinical Investigation*, **47**, 1154–1161.

Guyton, A. C., Coleman, T. G., Cowley, A. W., Scheel, K. W., Manning, R. D. & Norman, R. A. (1972). Arterial pressure regulation. Overriding dominance of the kidneys in long-term regulation and in hypertension. *American Journal of Medicine*, **52**, 584–594.

Halushka, P. V., Wohltmann, H., Privitera, P. J., Hurwitz, G., & Margolius, H. S. (1977). Bartter's syndrome: Urinary prostaglandin E-like material and kallikrein; indomethacin effects. *Annals of Internal Medicine*, **87**, 281–286.

Herbaczynska-Cedro, K. & Vane, J. R. (1973). Contribution of intrarenal generation of prostaglandin to autoregulation of renal blood flow in the dog. *Circulation Research*, **33**, 428–436.

Higashihara, E. & Kokko, J. (1978). The effect of prostaglandin (PG) inhibition on transport of water across various nephron segments of Munich-Wistar rats. *Clinical Research*, **26**, 465A.

Hood, V. L. & Dunn, M. J. (1978). Urinary excretion of prostaglandin E_2 and prostaglandin F_{2a} in potassium deficient rats. *Prostaglandins*, **15**, 273–280.

Hornych, A., Bedrossian, J., Bariety, J., Menard, J., Corvol, P., Safar, M., Fontaliran, F. & Milliez, P. (1975). Prostaglandins and hypertension in chronic renal disease. *Clinical Nephrology*, **4**, 144–150.

Hornych, M., Weiss, Y., Safar, M., Menard, J., Corvol, P., Fontaliran, F., Bariety, J. & Milliez, P. (1976). Prostaglandins A and B in the peripheral blood of hypertensive patients. *European Journal of Clinical Investigation*, **6**, 314.

Janszen, F. H. & Nugteren, D. H. (1971). Histochemical localization of prostaglandin synthetase. *Histochemistry*, **27**, 159–164.

Juncos, L. I. & Strong, C. G. (1973). Radioimmunoassay of renal venous prostaglandins in renal hypertension. In *Mechanisms of Hypertension*, ed. Sambhi, M. P. Pp. 278–287. New York: American Elsevier.

Kalisker, A. & Dyer, D. C. (1972). *In vitro* release of prostaglandins from the renal medulla. *European Journal of Pharmacology*, **19**, 305–309.

Kaye, Z., Mayeda, S., Zipser, R., Zia, P. & Horton, R. (1978). The effects of sodium on renal prostaglandins in normal man. *Clinical Research*, **26**, 140A.

Kirschenbaum, M. A. & Stein, J. H. (1976). The effect of inhibition of prostaglandin synthesis on urinary sodium excretion in the conscious dog. *Journal of Clinical Investigation*, **57**, 517–521.

Köver, G. & Tost, H. (1977). The effect of indomethacin on kidney function: Indomethacin and furosemide antagonism. *Pflügers Archiv*, **372**, 215–220.

Larsson, C. & Anggard, E. (1973). Arachidonic acid lowers and indomethacin increases the blood pressure of the rabbit. *Journal of Pharmacy and Pharmacology*, **25**, 653–655.

Larsson, C., Weber, P. & Anggard, E. (1974). Arachidonic acid increases and indomethacin decreases plasma renin activity in the rabbit. *European Journal of Pharmacology*, **28**, 391–394.

Leary, W. P., Ledingham, J. G. & Vane, J. R. (1974). Impaired prostaglandin release from the kidneys of salt-loaded and hypertensive rats. *Prostaglandins*, **7**, 425–432.

Lechi, A., Cori, G., Lechi, C., Mantero, F. & Scuro, A. (1976). Urinary kallikrein excretion in Bartter's syndrome. *Journal of Clinical Endocrinology and Metabolism*, **43**, 1175–1178.

Lee, J. B., Kannegeisser, H., O'Toole, J. & Westura, E. (1971). Hypertension and the reno-medullary prostaglandins: A human study of the hypotensive effects of PGE_1. *Annals of the New York Academy of Sciences*, **180**, 218–240.

Levy, J. V. (1977). Changes in systolic arterial blood pressure in normal and spontaneously hypertensive rats produced by acute administration of inhibitors of prostaglandin biosynthesis. *Prostaglandins*, **13**, 153–160.

Leyssac, P. P., Christensen, P., Hill, R. & Skinner, S. L. (1975). Indomethacin blockade of renal PGE-synthesis: Effect on total renal and tubular function and plasma renin concentration in hydropenic rats and on their response to isotonic saline. *Acta Physiologica Scandinavica*, **94**, 484–496.

Lifschitz, M. D., Patak, R. V., Fadem, S. Z. & Stein, J. H. (1978). Chronic changes in renal sodium excretion and renal prostaglandin E production in the rabbit. *Clinical Research*, **26**, 64A.

Lipson, L. C. & Sharp, G. W. (1971). Effect of prostaglandin E_1 on sodium transport and osmotic water flow in toad bladder. *American Journal of Physiology*, **220**, 1046–1052.

Lum, G. M., Aisenbrey, G. A., Dunn, M. J., Berl, T., Schrier, R. W. & McDonald, K. M. (1977). *In vivo* effect of indomethacin to potentiate the renal medullary cyclic AMP response to vasopresssin. *Journal of Clinical Investigation*, **59**, 8–13.

Margolius, H., Horowitz, D., Pisano, J. & Keiser, H. (1974). Urinary kallikrein in hypertension: Relationship to sodium intake and sodium-retaining steroid. *Circulation Research*, **35**, 820–825.

Martinez-Maldonado, M., Tsaparas, M. N., Eknoyan, G. & Suki, W. N. (1972). Renal actions of prostaglandins: Comparison with acetylcholine and volume expansion. *American Journal of Physiology*, **222**, 1147–1152.

Marumo, F. & Edelman, I. S. (1971). Effects of Ca^{++} and prostaglandin E_1 on vasopressin activation of renal adenyl cyclase. *Journal of Clinical Investigation*, **50**, 1613–1620.

McGiff, J. C., Crowshaw, K., Terragno, N. A. & Lonigro, A. J. (1970). Release of a prostaglandin-like substance into renal venous blood in response to angiotensin II. *Circulation Research*, **26–27**, Supplement, I, 121–130.

McGiff, J. C., Itskovitz, H. D., Terragno, A. & Wong, P. Y.-K. (1976). Modulation and mediation of the action of the renal kallikrein-kinin system by prostaglandins. *Federation Proceedings, Federation of American Societies for Experimental Biology*, **35**, 175–180.

McGiff, J. C., Terragno, N. A., Malik, K. U. & Lonigro, A. J. (1972). Release of a prostaglandin E-like substance from canine kidney by bradykinin. *Circulation Research*, **31**, 36–43.

McGiff, J. C. & Vane, J. R. (1975). Prostaglandins and the regulation of blood pressure. *Kidney International*, **8**, S262–S270.

Muirhead, E. E. (1973). Vasoactive and antihypertensive effects of prostaglandins and other renomedullary lipids. In *The Prostaglandins: Pharmacological and Therapeutic Advances*, ed. Cuthbert, M. F. Pp. 201–251. Philadelphia: Lippincott.

Muirhead, E. E., Brooks, B., Pitcock, J. A. & Stephenson, P. (1972a). Renomendullary antihypertensive function in accelerated (malignant) hypertension. Observations on renomedullary interstitial cells. *Journal of Clinical Investigation*, **51**, 181–190.

Muirhead, E. E., Germain, G., Leach, B. E., Pitcock, J. A., Stephenson, P., Brooks, B., Brosius, W. L., Daniels, E. G. & Kinman, J. W. (1972b). Production of renomedullary prostaglandins by renomedullary interstitial cells grown in tissue culture. *Circulation Research*, **30–31**, Supplement, II: 161–171.

Muirhead, E. E., Germain, G. S., Armstrong, F. B., Brooks, B., Leach, B. E., Byers, L. W., Pitcock, J. A. & Brown, P. (1975). Endocrine-type antihypertensive function of renomedullary interstitial cells. *Kidney International*, **8**, S271–S282.

Nasjletti, A. & Colina-Chourio, J. (1976). Interaction of mineralocorticoids, renal prostaglandins and the renal kallikrein-kinin system. *Federation Proceedings, Federation of American Societies for Experimental Biology,* **35,** 189–193.

Needleman, P., Douglas, J. R., Jakschik, B., Stoechlein, P. B. & Johnson, E. M. (1974). Release of renal prostaglandins by catecholamines: Relationship to renal endocrine function. *Journal of Pharmacology and Experimental Therapeutics,* **188,** 453–460.

Needleman, P., Kauffman, A. H., Douglas, J. R., Jr., Johnson, E. M., Jr. & Marshall, G. R. (1973). Specific stimulation and inhibition of renal prostaglandin release by angiotensin analogs. *American Journal of Physiology,* **224,** 1415–1419.

Negus, P., Tannen, R. L. & Dunn, M. J. (1976). Indomethacin protentiates the vasoconstrictor actions of angiotensin II. *Prostaglandins,* **12,** 175–180.

Nekrasova, A. A. & Lantsberg, L. A. (1969). Role of renal prostaglandins in the pathogenesis of hypertension. *Kardiologiya,* **9,** 86–93.

Nekrasova, A. A., Paleseva, F. M. & Khundadze, S. S. (1970). Content of depressor prostaglandin-like substances and renin activity in the kidneys of patients with renovascular hypertension. *Kardiologiya,* **10,** 88–92.

Norby, L., Lentz, R., Flamenbaum, W. & Ramwell, P. (1976). Prostaglandins and aspirin therapy in Bartter's syndrome. *Lancet II,* 604–606.

Oliw, E., Kövér, G., Larsson, C., and Ånggard, E. (1976). Reduction by indomethacin of furosemide effects in the rabbit. *European Journal of Pharmacology,* **38,** 95–100.

Olsen, U. B. (1975). Indomethacin inhibition of bumetanide diuresis in dogs. *Acta Pharmacologica et Toxicologica,* **37,** 65–78.

Olsen, U. B. (1977). The pharmacology of bumetanide: A Review. *Acta Pharmacologica et Toxicologica,* **41, Supplement III,** 1–29.

Orloff, J., Handler, J. S. & Bergstrom, S. (1965). Effect of prostaglandin (PGE₁) on the permeability response of toad bladder to vasopressin, theophylline and adenosine 3′,5′-monophosphate. *Nature* (London) **205,** 397–398.

Pace-Asciak, C. R. (1976). Decreased renal prostaglandin catabolism precedes onset of hypertension in the developing spontaneously hypertensive rat. *Nature* (London) **263,** 510–512.

Papanicolaou, N., Safar, M., Hornych, A., Fontaliran, F., Weiss, Y., Bariety, J. & Milliez, P. (1975). The release of renal prostaglandins during saline infusion in normal and hypertensive subjects. *Clinical Science and Molecular Medicine,* **49,** 459–463.

Papanicolaou, N., Mountakalakis, T., Safar, M., Bariety, J. & Milliez, P. (1976). Deficiency of renomedullary prostaglandin synthesis related to the evolution of essential hypertension. *Experientia,* **32,** 1015–1017.

Patak, R. V., Mookerjee, B. K., Bentzel, C. J., Hysert, P. E., Babeu, M. & Lee, J. B. (1975). Antagonism of the effects of furosemide by indomethacin in normal and hypertensive man. *Prostaglandins,* **10,** 649–659.

Pugsley, D. J., Beilin, L. J. & Peto, R. (1975). Renal prostaglandin synthesis in the Goldblatt hypertensive rat. *Circulation Research,* **36–37, Supplement I,** 81–88.

Ramsay, A. G. & Elliot, H. C. (1967). Effect of acetylsalicylic acid on ionic reabsorption in the renal tubule. *American Journal of Physiology,* **213,** 323–327.

Romero, J. C. & Strong, C. G. (1977). The effect of indomethacin blockade of prostaglandin synthesis on blood pressure of normal rabbits and rabbits with renovascular hypertension. *Circulation Research,* **40,** 35–41.

Rumpf, K. W., Frenzel, S., Lowetz, H. D. & Scheler, F. (1975). The effect of indomethacin on plasma renin activity in man under normal conditions and after stimulation of the renin-angiotensin system. *Prostaglandins,* **10,** 641–648.

Satoh, S. & Zimmerman, B. G. (1975). Influence of the renin-angiotensin system on the effect of prostaglandin synthesis inhibitors in the renal vasculature. *Circulation Research,* **36, Supplement I,** 89–96.

Scherer, B., Siess, W. & Weber, P. C. (1977). Radioimmunological and biological measurement of prostaglandins in rabbit urine: Decrease of PGE₂ excretion at high NaCl intake. *Prostaglandins,* **13,** 1127–1139.

Scherer, B., Schnermann, J., Sofroniev, M. & Weber, P. (1978). Prostaglandin analysis in urine of humans and rats by different radioimmunoassays: Effect on PG excretion by PG-synthetase inhibitors, laparotomy and furosemide. *Prostaglandins,* **15,** 255–266.

Scholkens, B. A. & Steinbach, R. (1975). Increase of experimental hypertension following inhibition of prostaglandin biosynthesis. *Archives Internationales de Pharmacodynamie, et de Therapie,* **214,** 328–334.

Seino, M., Abe, K., Sakurai, Y., Irokawa, N., Yasujima, M., Chiba, S., Otsuka, Y. & Yoshinaga, K. (1977). Effect of spironolactone on urinary kallikrein excretion in patients with essential hypertension and in primary aldosteronism. *Tohoku Journal of Experimental Medicine*, **121**, 111–119.

Shea, P. T., Eisner, G. M. & Slotkoff, M. (1978). Evidence for a direct tubular effect of prostaglandin E_2 induced natriuresis. *Clinical Research*, **26**, 43A.

Shimizu, K., Yamamoto, M. & Yoshitoshi, Y. (1973). Effects of saline infusion on prostaglandin-like materials in renal venous blood and medulla of canine kidney. *Japanese Heart Journal*, **14**, 140–145.

Sirois, P. & Gagnon, D. J. (1974). Release of renomedullary prostaglandins in normal and hypertensive rats. *Experientia*, **30**, 1418–1419.

Smith, W. L. & Wilkin, G. P. (1977). Distribution of prostaglandin-forming cyclo-oxygenases in rat, rabbit, and guinea pig kidney as determined by immunofluorescence. *Federation Proceedings, Federation of American Societies for Experimental Biology*, **36**, 309.

Spannhake, E. W., Chapnick, B. M., Feigen, L. P., Nelson, P. K., Hyman, A. L., Carter, M. K. & Kadowitz, P. J. (1978). Pulmonary and systemic vasodilator effects of prostacyclin. *Federation Proceedings, Federation of American Societies for Experimental Biology*, **37**, 731.

Speckart, P., Zia, P., Zipser, R. & Horton, R. (1977). The effect of sodium restriction and prostaglandin inhibition on the renin-angiotensin system in man. *Journal of Clinical Endocrinology and Metabolism*, **44**, 832–837.

Stoff, J., Silva, P., Rosa, R. & Epstein, F. (1978). Effect of indomethacin on water excretion in diabetes insipidus: Possible action of prostaglandins independent of antidiuretic hormone. *Clinical Research*, **26**, 477A.

Stokes, J. B. & Kokko, J. P. (1977). Inhibition of sodium transport by prostaglandin E_2 across the isolated, perfused rabbit collecting tubule. *Journal of Clinical Investigation*, **59**, 1099–1104.

Susic, D. & Sparks, J. C. (1975). Effects of aspirin on renal sodium excretion, blood pressure and plasma and extracellular fluid volume in salt-loaded rats. *Prostaglandins*, **10**, 825–831.

Swain, J. A., Heyndricks, G. R., Boettcher, D. H. & Vatner, S. F. (1975). Prostaglandin control of renal circulation in the unanesthetized dog and baboon. *American Journal of Physiology*, **229**, 826–830.

Tan, S. Y. & Mulrow, P. J. (1977). Inhibition of the renin aldosterone response to furosemide by indomethacin. *Journal of Clinical Endocrinology and Metabolism*, **45**, 174–176.

Tan, S. Y., Sweet, P. & Mulrow, P. (1978). Impaired renal production of prostaglandin E_2: A newly identified lesion in human essential hypertension. *Prostaglandins*, **15**, 139–150.

Terashima, R., Anderson, F. L. & Jubiz, W. (1976). Prostaglandin E release in the dog: Effect of sodium. *American Journal of Physiology*, **231**, 1429–1432.

Terragno, N. A., Terragno, D. A. & McGiff, J. C. (1977). Contribution of prostaglandins to the renal circulation in the conscious, anesthetized and laparotomized dogs. *Circulation Research*, **40**, 590–595.

Tiggeler, R. G., Koene, R. A. & Wijdeveld, P. G. (1977). Inhibition of furosemide-induced natriuresis by indomethacin in patients with the nephrotic syndrome. *Clinical Science and Molecular Medicine*, **52**, 149–151.

Tobian, L. & Azar, S. (1971). Antihypertensive and other functions of the renal papilla. *Transactions of the Association of American Physicians*, **84**, 281–288.

Tobian, L. & O'Donnell, M. (1976). Renal prostaglandins in relation to sodium regulation and hypertension. *Federation Proceedings, Federation of American Societies for Experimental Biology*, **35**, 2388–2392.

Verberckmoes, R., Van Damme, B., Clement, J., Amery, A. & Michielsen, P. (1976). Bartter's syndrome with hyperplasia of renomedullary cells: Successful treatment with indomethacin. *Kidney International*, **9**, 302–307.

Vinci, J. M., Telles, D. A., Bowden, R. E., Izzo, J. L., Keiser, H. R., Radfar, N., Taylor, A. A., Gill, J. R. & Bartter, F. C. (1976). The kallikrein-kinin system in Bartter's syndrome and its response to prostaglandin synthetase inhibition. *Clinical Research*, **24**, 414A.

Wait, R. B. & Dunn, M. J. (1979). Age-related changes in renal and intrarenal blood flow in the spontaneously hypertensive rat. Submitted for publication.

Walker, L., Whorton, R., Smigel, M., France, R. & Frolich, J. C. (1978). Antidiuretic hormone increases renal prostaglandin synthesis in vivo. *American Journal of Physiology*, **235**: F180–185.

Weber, P., Holzgreve, H., Stephan, R. & Herbst, R. (1975). Plasma renin activity and renal sodium and water excretion following infusion of arachidonic acid in rats. *European Journal of Pharmacology*, **34**, 299–304.

Weber, P. C., Larsson, C., Anggard, E., Hamberg, M., Corey, E. J., Nicolaou, K. C. & Samuelsson, B. (1976). Stimulation of renin release from rabbit renal cortex by arachidonic acid and prostaglandin endoperoxides. *Circulation Research*, **39**, 868–874.

Weber, P. C., Larsson, C. & Scherer, B. (1977a). Prostaglandin E_2-9-ketoreductase as a mediator of salt intake-related prostaglandin-renin interaction. *Nature* (London) **266**, 65–66.

Weber, P. C., Scherer, B. & Larsson, C. (1977b). Increase of free arachidonic acid by furosemide in man as the cause of prostaglandin and renin release. *European Journal of Pharmacology*, **41**, 329–332.

Wennmalm, A. (1978). Influence of indomethacin on the systemic and pulmonary vascular resistance in man. *Clinical Science and Molecular Medicine*, **54**, 141–145.

Werning, C., Vetter, W., Weichmann, P., Schweikert, H. U., Steil, D. & Siegenthaler, W. (1971). Effect of prostaglandin E_1 on renin in the dog. *American Journal of Physiology*, **220**, 852–856.

Whorton, A. R., Misono, K., Hollifield, J., Frolich, J. C., Inagami, T. & Oates, J. A. (1977). Prostaglandins and renin release: I. Stimulation of renin release from rabbit renal cortical slices by PGI_2. *Prostaglandins*, **14**, 1095–1104.

Williamson, H. E., Bourland, W. A. & Marchand, G. R. (1974). Inhibition of ethacrynic acid-induced increase in renal blood flow by indomethacin. *Prostaglandins*, **8**, 297–301.

Williamson, H. E., Bourland, W. A. & Marchand, G. R. (1975a). Inhibition of furosemide-induced increase in renal blood flow by indomethacin. *Proceedings of the Society for Experimental Biology and Medicine*, **148**, 164–165.

Williamson, H. E., Bourland, W. A., Marchand, G. R., Farley, D. B. & van Orden, D. E. (1975b). Furosemide-induced release of prostaglandin E to increase renal blood flow. *Proceedings of the Society for Experimental Biology and Medicine*, **150**, 104–106.

Yun, J., Kelly, G., Bartter, F. & Smith, H. (1977). Role of prostaglandins in the control of renin secretion in the dog. *Circulation Research*, **40**, 459–464.

Zambraski, E. J. & Dunn, M. J. (1979). Renal prostaglandin E_2 secretion and excretion in conscious dogs. *American Journal of Physiology*, in press.

Zipser, R., Hoefs, J., Speckart, P., Zia, P. & Horton, R. (1977). Evidence for a critical role of prostaglandins in renin release, vascular reactivity and renal function in liver disease. *Clinical Research*, **25**, 305A.

Zusman, R. M., Forman, B. H., Schneider, G., Caldwell, B. V., Speroff, L. & Mulrow, P. J. (1973). The effect of chronic sodium loading and sodium restriction on plasma and renal concentrations of prostaglandin A in normal Wistar and spontaneously hypertensive Aoki rats. *Clinical Science and Molecular Medicine*, **45**, 325s–329s.

Zusman, R. M. & Keiser, H. R. (1977). Prostaglandin biosynthesis by rabbit renomedullary interstitial cells in tissue culture: Stimulation by vasoactive peptides. *Journal of Clinical Investigation*, **60**, 215–223.

Zusman, R. M. & Keiser, H. R. (1977). Prostaglandin E_2 biosynthesis by rabbit renomedullary interstitial cells in tissue culture. *Journal of Biological Chemistry*, **252**, 2069–2071.

Zusman, R. M., Keiser, H. R. & Handler, J. S. (1977). Vasopressin-stimulated prostaglandin E biosynthesis in the toad urinary bladder. Effect on water flow. *Journal of Clinical Investigation*, **60**, 1339–1347.

Zusman, R. M., Spector, D., Caldwell, B. V., Speroff, L., Schneider, G. & Mulrow, P. J. (1973). The effect of chronic sodium loading and sodium restriction on plasma prostaglandin A, E, and F concentrations in normal humans. *Journal of Clinical Investigation*, **52**, 1093–1098.

5

The renal kallikrein-kinin system

HARRY S. MARGOLIUS
JOHN B. BUSE

INTRODUCTION

The enzyme kallikrein was discovered in mammalian urine over 70 years ago. Although the urinary enzyme was initially thought to originate in the pancreas (the word kallikrein is formed from the Greek term for that organ), it is now generally considered to be identical to kallikrein synthesized in the kidney. Over the last decade, interest in renal kallikrein and the kinin formed from its action has increased markedly. This is the result of work that has purified and characterized components of the kallikrein-kinin system; localized some of them within the kidney; and implicated kallikrein and kinins in various renal functions, in hypertensive and other diseases of renal origin, and even in the mechanism of action of some drugs.

This review will describe some of the findings that are making exploration of the renal kallikrein-kinin system relevant to contemporary trends in nephrology, and perhaps more importantly, some of the questions that need to be answered about the system and its function in health and disease. For more definitive treatments of specific aspects of this subject, the reader can turn to selected key articles, some recent reviews and symposia (McGiff et al., 1976; Nustad et al., 1978; Pisano, 1975; Obika, 1978), and the recently published compendium edited by Erdös (1979).

BIOCHEMISTRY OF THE SYSTEM

Kallikreins are serine-containing proteinases that liberate kinin peptides from kininogen substrates by limited proteolysis (Fig. 5.1). They have been considered to have negligible proteolytic activity upon other proteins. All mammals thus far studied have two types of kallikrein: plasma and glandular. The latter, to which this description will be limited, is found in exocrine glands and in the kidney. The glandular kallikreins differ from the plasma enzyme in molecular weight and other physicochemical characteristics, immunologically, enzymatically, and as affected by various inhibitors.

Glandular kallikreins have been highly purified from such organs and secretions as the porcine pancreas (Fiedler, 1976); the guinea pig coagulating gland (Moriwaki et al., 1974a); the rat salivary glands (Brandtzaeg et al., 1976) and kidney (Nustad, Vaaje and Pierce, 1975); the dog kidney (Moriwaki et al., 1976); and the urine of horse (Prado, Prado and Brandi, 1962), rabbit (Porcelli et al., 1974), rat (Nustad and Pierce, 1974; Oza et al., 1976), pig (Tschesche et al., 1976), and humans (Hial, Diniz and Mares-Guia, 1974; Matsuda et al., 1976). Human sweat (Fränki, Jansén, and Hopsu-Havu, 1970) and salivary (Fujimoto, Moriya, and Moriwaki, 1973) kallikreins have also been purified. In general, the glandular kallikreins are acidic glycoproteins with isoelectric points near 4.0 and molecular weights from 24,000 to 43,600 daltons. The pancreas (Fiedler, 1976), intestine (Frey et al., 1968) and urine (Corthorn et al., 1977) contain a proenzyme, called pre- or prokallikrein, which can be activated by tryptic hydrolysis.

Multiple forms of kallikrein have been identified in such sites as hog pancreas (Fiedler, 1976) and rat urine (Nustad and Pierce, 1974; Chao and Mar-

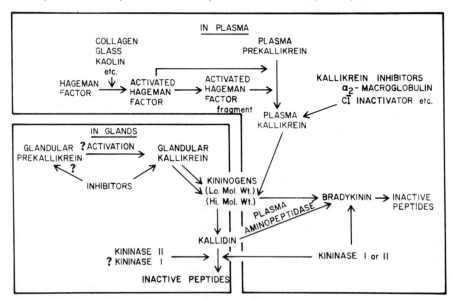

Figure 5.1 The kallikrein-kinin systems.

golius, 1979) using various column chromatographic techniques, polyacrylamide gel electrophoresis, and isoelectric focusing. The amino acid compositions of several purified glandular kallikreins are known, and the amino acid sequence of a highly purified porcine pancreatic kallikrein is known almost completely (Fiedler, 1976). It is possible that differences between isozymic forms reside in the content of charged carbohydrate moieties rather than in the amino acid composition of the molecules. Antibodies have been raised against several purified glandular kallikreins (Oza et al., 1976; Ole-Moi Yoi, Austen, and Spragg, 1977; Chao and Margolius, 1979; Nustad and Pierce, 1974) and in general, cross react well with kallikrein within other glands of the same species (Pisano, 1975; Brandtzaeg et al., 1976). However, no immunological cross-reactivity is apparent between plasma and glandular kallikreins within the same species (Nustad, Gautvik and Pierce, 1976; Ole-Moi Yoi et al., 1977).

Glandular kallikreins release the decapeptide lysylbradykinin (kallidin) from kininogens, in contrast to plasma kallikrein, which forms bradykinin (Pierce and Webster, 1961) (Fig. 5.2). The glandular enzyme cleaves two dissimilar peptide bonds, a methionyl-lysine bond and an arginyl-serine bond within kininogens (Pierce, 1968), suggesting that the enzyme may have two different active sites (Webster, Mares-Guia, and Diniz, 1970).

Like trypsin, kallikreins can hydrolyze N-α-substituted esters of arginine or lysine with a pH optimum of 8.5–9.0 (Webster and Pierce, 1961). Most of the esterolytic assays for glandular kallikreins use synthetic substrates such as N-α-tosyl-L-arginine methyl ester (Tos-Arg-OMe) or N-α-benzoyl-L-arginine ethyl ester (Bz-Arg-OEt). Although several of these esterolytic assays, especially those using radio-labelled substrates, are quite sensitive (Beaven, Pierce, and Pisano, 1970), they have limited specificity as other proteases such as trypsin or plasmin can cleave the ester. However, because of their simplicity, they can be used to assay large numbers of samples for kallikrein activity if other proteases are not present in sufficient quantity to cleave the protected arginine ester at an alkaline pH. In human urine, approximately 95 percent of the alkaline Tos-Arg-OMe esterase activity is due to urinary kallikrein (Vinci et al., 1978) but only about 50 percent of the esterase activity in raw urine is due to rat urinary kallikrein (Nustad and Pierce, 1974), necessitating pretreatment steps before assay (Beaven et al., 1970). Total Tos-Arg-OMe esterase activity in rat renal homogenates is probably also not entirely due to kallikrein, but one recent study showed that Tos-Arg-OMe esterase and kallikrein biological activity paralleled one another as renal plasma membranes were purified (Ward et al., 1975). A new chromogenic amide substrate (benzoyl-val-leu-arg-nitroanilid, Kabi, Sweden) may be a sensitive and more specific substrate for glandular kallikreins than those widely used at present.

Renal and urinary kallikrein levels can also be assayed by their ability to release a kinin from a plasma kininogen substrate. Although these various bioassays of generated kinin remain the benchmarks for the presence of kallikrein activity, most are too time consuming and tedious for repetitive or routine

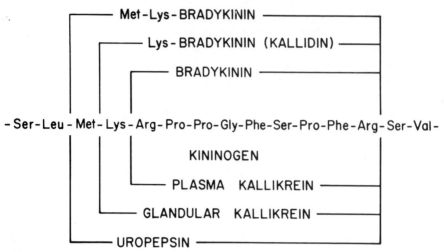

Figure 5.2 The sites of action of kinin-forming enzymes and the amino acid sequences of three mammalian kinins.

measurements. However, some newer and more convenient bioassay techniques have been developed and are surveyed in a recent review (Ward and Margolius, 1979).

Of greater interest is the newly developed radioimmunoassay technology that either replaces kallikrein measurement by bioassay or measures immunoreactive kallikrein directly. The former assays (Carretero et al., 1976) use antibodies generated against bradykinin or kallidin which cross-react well with these kinins or the undecapeptide methionyllysylbradykinin. The amount of kallikrein present in a sample is expressed in terms of the amount of kinin generated in the presence of an excess of kininogen. Usually there is also significant cross-reactivity between the antibody and kininogen and steps must be taken to remove it prior to assay. However, a recently developed kinin radioimmunoassay for kallikrein activity in urine or tissue (Shimamoto et al., 1979a) shows no kininogen-antibody cross-reactivity and may be a significant technical improvement. Direct radioimmunoassays for human and rat urinary kallikrein (Oza, 1977; Carretero et al., 1978; Shimamoto et al., 1979b) have also been reported. These assays eliminate the need to purify and use kininogen substrates or inactivate the kinin-destroying kininases. They may also be more specific than radioimmunoassays measuring kinin generation, since it has been shown that other proteolytic enzymes (urokinase, trypsin) can attack kininogens (Hial, Keiser, and Pisano, 1976). This point can only be established, however, by comparing the cross-reactivity of a particular kallikrein antibody with enzymes such as plasmin, thrombin, and trypsin. The sensitivity of these assays is now at the subnanogram level (Carretero et al., 1978; Shimamoto et al., 1979b). Despite some actual or potential problems with specificity, the reader should carry away the notion that a broad range of techniques is now available to measure kallikrein with acceptable specificity and high sensitivity.

These methodologic advances have been responsible for much of the growing interest in the role of glandular kallikrein.

There are at least four different plasma protein inhibitors of plasma kallikrein, including α_2-macroglobulin, C1 inactivator, α_1-antitrypsin, and antithrombin III. It is of considerable theoretical interest (and perhaps physiological importance) that α_2-macroglobulin, which is believed to regulate kinin release by plasma kallikrein, does not bind to the glandular enzyme (Vahatera and Hamburg, 1976) or even prevent kinin formation in circumstances where the action of plasma kallikrein is inhibited. Only one endogenous renal kallikrein inhibitor has been described thus far (Geiger and Mann, 1976). However, several natural or synthetic kallikrein inhibitors are just beginning to be used to assess the role of kallikrein in renal function. These include aprotinin, diisopropylflurophosphate analogues, and several aromatic trisamidines.

The kininogen substrates for kallikreins are acidic glycoproteins that are present in—and have been purified from—human, bovine, and porcine plasma (Pierce and Guimarães, 1976). Methods for kininogen measurement have generally been indirect, utilizing tryptic hydrolysis to maximally generate kinin, which is then bioassayed in an isolated tissue or vascular bed—or more recently with kinin radioimmunoassays. At least two functionally different kininogens exist (Pisano, 1975). The high molecular weight form (80,000–200,000 daltons) is a good substrate for both plasma and glandular kallikreins, whereas the low molecular weight form (50,000–80,000 daltons) seems to be a preferred substrate for glandular kallikrein (Pierce and Guimarães, 1976). Kallikreins have been considered generally to have negligible proteolytic activity on other serine proteinase substrates (e.g., casein), but revision of this concept may be necessary as kallikrein may prove to be capable of converting prorenin to renin (Sealey et al., 1978).

The composition of the three kinins present in urine is shown in Figure 5.2. They possess widespread pharmacologic activity and cause vasodilation, increased capillary permeability, edema, intense local pain, and contraction or relaxation of a variety of extravascular smooth muscles in microgram or smaller amounts. Many other pharmacologic properties have been described, and those with potential relevance to renal function will be mentioned below. In any event, the varied physiologic and biochemical effects that result from activation of the kallikrein-kinin system are almost universally considered to be the result of the formation of bradykinin or lysylbradykinin. This may or may not be true, and the issue probably will be unsettled until the development of specific kinin-receptor blockers, the lack of which has been a great liability to progress in defining various roles for kallikrein and kinins.

Although glandular kallikrein can attack kininogen to release lysylbradykinin, the processes and factors that regulate the formation and release of kinins by glandular kallikrein are essentially undescribed. Such is not the case with respect to the formation and generation of plasma kinin. The sequence of events resulting in plasma kinin formation, which begins with Hageman factor activation and is followed by subsequent plasma prekallikrein activation by a

Hageman factor fragment, kinin cleavage from a plasma kininogen, and subsequent inhibition of both formed kallikreins and kinin by kallikrein inhibitors and kininases, respectively, is widely known and has been described in recent reviews (Pisano, 1975; Coleman, 1974). It is uncertain if this sequence of events bears any relation to the normal maintenance of blood flow through any organ, to pathologic alterations in systemic vascular resistance, or to any variable of measured renal function. The methods used for kinin measurement have been previously mentioned.

Characterization of kinin-binding sites began by using homogenized smooth muscle from pregnant bovine uterus (Odya and Goodfriend, 1977). The binding sites were differentiated from nonspecific binding by comparing their interaction with a potent labelled agonist (^{125}I-tyr^1-lysylbradykinin) to their interaction with a labelled analogue of low biological activity (^{125}I-tyr^5-bradykinin). Sites in the bovine uterus homogenates had an apparent affinity for bradykinin that matched the contractile responsiveness of strips cut from the intact organ. The apparent k_D and the ED_{50} were both between $2-5 \times 10^{-9}$M. The relative affinities of these sites for different analogues of bradykinin generally matched the relative potencies of the analogues in bioassays. Binding sites with some characteristics of receptors have also been found in bovine lung and the medulla or porcine kidneys. It is not known if a biological or biochemical response is coupled to the binding phenomenon in these tissues.

Kallidin can be rapidly converted to bradykinin in plasma by cleavage of its N-terminal lysine through the action of an aminopeptidase. This enzyme has been purified from plasma and liver, but the significance of its action is still unclear. It has been stated that probably only a fraction of liberated kallidin is converted to bradykinin at the N-terminal end before it is inactivated at the C-terminal end (Erdös, 1976). Hydrolysis of any one of the remaining peptide bonds in kinins rapidly inactivates these substances. The enzymes that have this hydrolytic capability are known as kininase I and II (Erdös, 1976). Kininase I is a carboxypeptidase (also called carboxypeptidase N or arginine carboxypeptidase) with an estimated molecular weight of 280,000 and subunits of 90,000 and 45,000 daltons. These subunits seem to retain enzymic activity but are less stable than the native enzyme. Whether kininase I has a role in limiting the action of a glandular or renal kallikrein (and the kinin it produces) is unknown.

Much of the interest in kininase II is due to the facts that it also converts angiotensin I to angiotensin II and specific inhibitors are available to explore its functions in vitro and in vivo (Erdös, 1976; Ondetti, Rubin, and Cushman, 1977). The enzyme is a peptidyl dipeptide hydrolase with estimated molecular weights ranging from 140,000 to 480,000 daltons which cleaves phe^8-arg^9 from bradykinin and his^9-leu^{10} from angiotensin I. These actions result in destruction of biologically active kinin and formation of angiotensin II. Bradykinin, however, seems to be the preferred substrate with a lower K_m than angiotensin I (Erdös, 1976). The enzyme requires a divalent cation cofactor for activity, is activated by chloride ion, and is a glycoprotein (Erdös, 1975). Kininase II also cleaves a variety of synthetic peptide substrates, allowing investigators to quantitate its activity with chemical methods (Erdös, 1975).

Among the earliest inhibitors of kininase II were EDTA, O-phenanthroline and 8-hydroxyquinoline, which bind the metal cofactor. During an investigation of the actions of some of these agents, Ferreira (1965) discovered that the venom of the crotalid snake, *Bothrops jararaca*, contained a factor or factors that potentiated some of the pharmacologic actions of bradykinin, including the hypotensive response. The first characterized was a pentapeptide, bradykinin-potentiating factor, BPF_{5A}, and subsequently the synthesis of the nonapeptide (Cheung and Cushman, 1973), BPF_{9a} or SQ20881 was achieved. This more potent substance inhibits hydrolysis of bradykinin and angiotensin I without being a substrate for kininase II, itself. This parenterally active inhibitor has been widely used in in vitro studies of kininase II–angiotensin I converting enzyme, and in vivo to examine the role of angiotensins in the maintenance of elevated systemic vascular resistance in hypertensive states in animals or humans (Miller et al., 1972; Collier, Robinson, and Vane, 1973). Interest in this agent has now been superseded by SQ14225 (captopril), a mercaptopropanolyl derivative of proline that is not only more potent than SQ20881 as an enzyme inhibitor, but is also active orally (Ondetti, Rubin, and Cushman, 1977; Gavras et al., 1978). That these compounds will be responsible for the generation of new insights into the activity of the kallikrein-kinin as well as the renin-angiotensin system is already a certainty.

LOCALIZATION OF SYSTEM COMPONENTS

Several investigators have looked for glandular kallikrein in plasma and its activity has been detected in venous perfusates of cat salivary glands or the isolated rat kidney (Hilton, 1970; Roblero et al., 1976). However, definitive evidence for the presence of glandular kallikrein in plasma of normal subjects or animals is lacking.

On the other hand, the presence of glandular kallikrein in urine, sweat, saliva, and gastrointestinal contents has led to several recent efforts to determine the origin of the enzymes present in these fluids. Rat kidney slices can synthesize kallikreins which are biochemically and immunologically indistinguishable from those that appear in rat urine (Nustad et al., 1975). As noted by Nustad et al. (1978), it is now generally accepted that the glandular kallikreins present in secretions of exocrine glands and kidney are products of the organs themselves. Over the past few years, definitive evidence has been gathered with several techniques localizing kallikrein within the kidney. Earlier indirect efforts based upon kallikrein excretion rates in mercuric chloride-treated dogs suggested a proximal tubular localization for kallikrein (Frey et al., 1968) but Ward et al. (1975) found no kallikrein activity in the brush-border plasma membranes isolated from rat kidney proximal tubules or in tumors derived from the pars recta of rat proximal tubules (Ward et al., 1976). On the

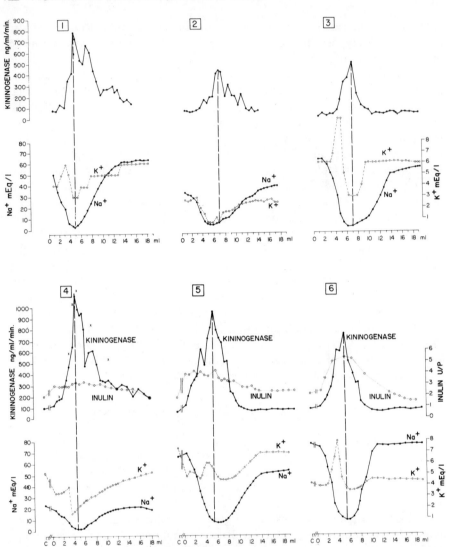

Figure 5.3 Six stop-flow patterns for kallikrein, inulin, sodium, and potassium. One and two were done in the same dog. The vertical broken line was used to relate the maximum kallikrein with sodium and potassium patterns. Kallikrein indicated by "X" in stop-flow 4 was measured by radioimmunoassay. (From Scicli et al., 1976, with permission of the publisher and author)

other hand, Scicli et al. (1976) using the "stop-flow" technique, found the highest concentrations of dog urinary kallikrein in urine fractions with lowest sodium. They concluded that the enzyme is secreted into the urine at the level of the distal nephron (Fig. 5.3) by either the tubule itself or by some structure located at this part of the nephron, such as the macula densa. More direct evidence has been obtained by Ørstavik et al. (1976) using a fluorescent antibody against purified rat urinary kallikrein, and Simson et al. (1979) using an im-

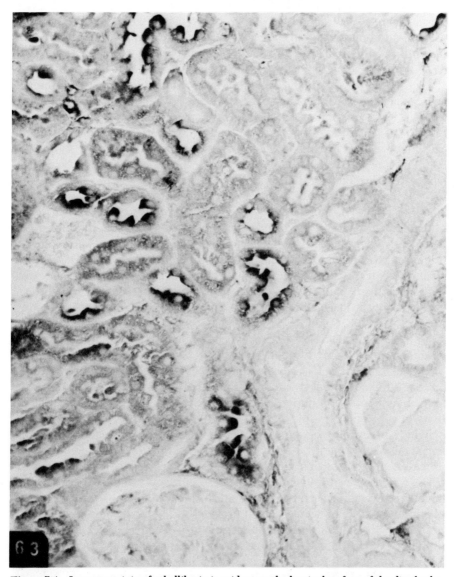

Figure 5.4 Immunostaining for kallikrein is evident on the luminal surface of the distal tubular epithelium of the rat kidney. Horseradish peroxidase bridge immunostain (X 600). (For additional detail, see Simson et al., 1979.)

munoperoxidase technique. These studies have localized renal kallikrein to the segment of distal tubule reaching from the juxtaglomerular apparatus to, or through, the collecting duct (Fig. 5.4). Both studies observed an intense luminal rim of immunoreactive kallikrein, which is similar to kallikrein localization in some salivary ducts (Ørstavik et al., 1975). Data supportive of these histochemical efforts has been obtained by Ward et al. (1975), who biochemically fractionated renal cortex and found that kallikrein was enriched in a plasma membrane fraction, which probably originated from distal tubular cells. In addition, studies of intact rat renal cortical cells in suspension have shown that kallikrein is predominantly a membrane-bound ectoenzyme with its active sites facing the external environment (Chao and Margolius, 1978a).

There is controversy about kallikrein localization in other parts of the kidney. Some studies (Mann, Geiger, and Werle, 1976) have found kallikrein activity in isolated glomeruli, while others (Scicli et al., 1976) have concluded that no enzyme is present in this or associated structures. Immunohistochemical efforts have not disclosed kallikrein in the glomeruli. Nevertheless, it would be premature to rule out the possible presence of kallikrein in some component of the juxtaglomerular apparatus since the data are inconclusive, and such a localization could begin to explain the relations being observed amongst kallikrein, renin, renal perfusion pressure, etc. To summarize, all available evidence at present indicates that renal kallikrein is localized predominantly in or upon the luminal cells of the distal nephron. It gains access to urine from this site. How the enzyme might reach renal lymph (DeBono and Mills, 1974) or the renal venous effluent (Roblero et al., 1976) is unclear. Additional unanswered questions remain, many of which relate to how little is known about the localization of other components of the renal kallikrein-kinin system.

An inhibitor that may be important in regulating the activity of renal kallikrein has been isolated from a preparation of rat renal tubules (Geiger and Mann, 1976). The localization of this low molecular weight (4,700 daltons) protein is unknown, but it can inhibit both plasma and various glandular kallikreins and may be an important regulator of renal and urinary kallikrein activity in situ.

Urine contains microgram quantities of three kinins of renal origin, bradykinin, kallidin, and met-lys-bradykinin (Hial et al., 1976). Kinins appear in the urine stream at the level of the distal nephron (Scicli, Gandolfi, and Carretero, 1978), which seems to suggest that they are products formed by the action of membrane-bound or secreted kallikrein in this locale. However, kidney kallikrein forms kallidin, as mentioned previously. The bradykinin is probably a product of the action of an aminopeptidase present in urine upon kallidin (Brandi et al., 1976), and data have recently been gathered to show that met-lys-bradykinin is formed by a uropepsin, another urinary serine proteinase active at an acid pH. Since urinary kinin collections are made into 0.1 N hydrochloric acid, this kinin is being formed in vitro and is of little significance except in artifactually altering measured levels of urinary kinin. The function of kinin formed in the distal nephron is unclear, although there is no longer a lack of hypotheses or data concerning possible roles.

Kininase II is present in kidney in high concentration (Erdös and Yang, 1976) and has been localized immunohistochemically in glomeruli, along the proximal tubule and the vascular endothelium (Caldwell et al., 1976). Brush border preparations from proximal convoluted tubular cells are rich in kininase II (Ward et al., 1976), and this localization probably accounts for the lack of appearance of arterially infused kinins in urine (Nasjletti, Colina-Chourio, and McGiff, 1975), or the similar disappearance of kinins microperfused into the proximal convoluted tubule (Carone et al., 1976).

Less is known about the origin and localization of the substrate kininogen(s) within the kidney than other components of the renal kallikrein-kinin system. Hial and colleagues (1976) and Pisano, Yates, and Pierce (1978) have detected an antigen in human urine which cross-reacted with an antibody made against plasma low molecular weight kininogen. However, this urokininogen, while a substrate for uropepsin and able to release kinin after tryptic digestion, seems not to be a good substrate for urinary kallikrein. Therefore, another area of perplexity and insufficient knowledge concerns the nature of the substrate for renal and urinary kallikrein. Whether it is produced in another organ (plasma kininogens seem to be of hepatic origin) and is filtered to gain access to renal tubular kallikrein, or is secreted into the tubular lumen upstream (or in conjunction with kallikrein) are matters of conjecture.

THE ROLE OF KALLIKREIN AND KININS IN RENAL FUNCTION

Renal hemodynamics

Studies in normal human subjects (Gill et al., 1965), anesthetized dogs (Webster and Gilmore, 1964), or isolated perfused kidneys (McGiff, Itskovitz, and Terragno, 1975) have established that either intravenously or intra-arterially administered bradykinin or kallidin cause renal arteriolar vasodilatation. However, the fact that pharmacologic doses of kinin produce vasodilatation does not prove that the renal kallikrein-kinin system performs this function in situ. As stated by Nasjletti and Colina-Chourio (1976):

Inference of physiological roles on the basis of the aforementioned observations [results of infusions of kinins intravenously or into the renal artery] should be regarded with caution, since probably no route of administration of kinins reproduces the effects evoked by release of kinins intrarenally, in terms of either concentrations achieved at their sites of action, localization of activity, or the sequence of vascular elements affected.

When one keeps this proviso in mind, along with the evidence available thus far on the localization of components of the renal kallikrein-kinin system already discussed, plus the presence of inhibitory or destructive limits upon kinin viability in plasma, it becomes difficult to conclude a priori that kinins produced in kidney have major effects upon renal vascular resistance. On the other hand, some data have been generated which are consistent with that possibility.

Hilton and Lewis (Hilton, 1970) first proposed that the function of kinins formed in salivary glands was to produce local vasodilation, by showing that kininogen consumption, kallikrein release, and kinin formation accompanied glandular vasodilation in response to parasympathetic nerve stimulation. This perspective was challenged by Schacter et al. (1970) because vasodilation could be produced by other maneuvers without demonstrable changes in levels of components of the kallikrein-kinin system. This recently dormant controversy is being reawakened by the data and points of view of Nustad and colleagues (1978) who claim that ^{125}I-labelled kallikrein infused back into salivary ducts finds its way into venous blood. Earlier work had shown that labelled pancreatic kallikrein reached the mesenteric circulation after intragut application (Moriwaki, Yamaguchi, and Moriya, 1974b). Further, using a radioimmunoassay for rat submandibular gland kallikrein, an antigen immunologically similar to this enzyme has been found in rat plasma. This antigen may be an inhibitor-complexed glandular kallikrein, but it is clearly not free glandular kallikrein (Nustad et al., 1978). Since renal distal tubules are in close association with the postglomerular capillary network, an analogous situation may exist resulting in local alterations in blood flow after glandular kallikrein liberation into blood. Because no one has yet repeated the Hilton and Lewis studies in the kidney and other available data are not conclusive, a reiteration of the following statement is warranted; Definitive evidence for liberation of glandular (i.e., renal) kallikrein into plasma, which then affects blood flow, is lacking.

However, there are other pieces of evidence to support a direct correlation between the activity of the kallikrein-kinin system and renal blood flow. Nasjletti and Colina-Chourio (1976) showed that parenteral SQ20881 significantly increased renal blood flow in dogs, concomitant with increased urinary kinin excretion and renal venous kinin concentrations. The likelihood that diminished angiotensin II formation intrarenally contributed to the observed change in blood flow was considered slight because previous studies (Freeman et al., 1973) had shown that an angiotensin II receptor antagonist did not alter renal blood flow in dogs. This may be correct, but correlations between increased endogenous kinin activity and blood flow may not indicate causality in experiments where both the kallikrein-kinin and renin-angiotensin systems might be altered by a single drug. However, confirmatory data has been obtained in conscious, sodium-deficient dogs in which continuous infusions of SQ20881 produced significant increases in effective renal plasma flow and blood kinins, as well as a somewhat unexpected decrease in kallikrein excretion (McCaa, Hall, and McCaa, 1978). These studies do not differentiate between the possible effects of delayed destruction of blood kinins formed by the action of circulating, activated plasma prekallikrein or those effects possibly induced by kinins produced by the action of renal kallikrein. In other words, whether the resultant increase in blood flow occurs because of *plasma-generated* or *renally generated* kinin is uncertain. More specific kallikrein inhibitors or kinin receptor blockers will help clarify the basis for these observations, when they become available.

Other data support a direct correlation between the system and renal blood flow. Acute renal artery constriction decreases urinary kallikrein (Bevan,

MacFarlane, and Mills, 1974). In conscious dogs, previously operated to chronically narrow a renal artery and with bilateral ureterostomies, there was an excellent correlation between the decrease in renal blood flow produced by tightening the ligature and the decrease in kallikrein excretion (Keiser et al., 1976a). In both the acute and chronic studies, changes in renal blood flow were due to the constriction. Therefore, the changes noted in kallikrein excretion were most probably secondary rather than causally related to reduced blood flow. In a study of normal and hypertensive men, Levy et al. (1977) showed a direct correlation between urinary kallikrein esterase activity and renal blood flow in almost all groups of subjects. Again, whether these data reflect a contribution by the renal kallikrein-kinin system to the regulation of renal vascular resistance and blood flow still remains to be determined.

Renal excretory function

Whether the renal kallikrein-kinin system participates directly in the control of electrolyte and water excretion and if so, as a natriuretic/diuretic or an antinatriuretic/antidiuretic influence is uncertain. Injected kinins increase sodium and water excretion (Gill et al., 1965; Webster and Gilmore, 1964), even in the face of ADH infusions (Barraclough and Mills, 1965). Increased sodium excretion produced by bradykinin infusions was shown to be secondary to increased renal blood flow by Willis et al. (1969), and Stein et al. (1972) found that although renal arterial bradykinin infusions did not affect sodium reabsorption in micropunctured superficial nephron proximal tubules, sodium excretion was increased by the peptide. They suggested that blood flow redistribution occurred and was accompanied by a decrease in sodium reabsorption in deeper nephrons. There is no convincing evidence available showing that bradykinin has *direct* inhibitory or stimulatory actions on tubular electrolyte or water transport, although Capelo and Alzamora (1977) have shown that intra-arterial infusions of bradykinin seemed to reduce proximal reabsorption of sodium and water and decreased PAH secretion during periods of stop-flow in the dog. Bradykinin can inhibit reversibly the ADH-induced increase in water permeability in the toad bladder (Furtado, 1971).

In the isolated, blood-perfused kidney, intra-arterial bradykinin increased free water clearance without increasing sodium excretion (McGiff et al., 1975). In this study, there was actually a fall in urinary sodium excretion, although these changes were considered insignificant. Interestingly, the subsequent administration of indomethacin augmented fractional sodium excretion after bradykinin. McGiff et al. (1975) and McGiff and Wong (1979) have suggested that a prostaglandin mediates the diuretic action of bradykinin and simultaneously attenuates the actions of kinins upon renal sodium excretion.

In the previously mentioned studies of the effects of SQ20881 in anesthetized dogs (Nasjletti and Colina-Chourio, 1976), there were significant increases in urine flow and sodium excretion, which were positively correlated with increased levels of kinins in blood and urine, and in renal blood flow.

Marin-Grez (1974) measured sodium, potassium, and water excretion in rats receiving saline infusions before and after treatment with an antibradykinin serum. This rabbit antiserum reduced sodium and water excretion while normal rabbit serum did not. PAH or inulin clearance were not different. The effect of this maneuver on renal venous or urinary kinin levels was not determined, but the inference to be gathered from these studies is that endogenous kinin activity augments sodium and water excretion. Again, whether this means intravascular or renal tubular kinin activity is unknown.

Mills and coworkers have shown direct correlations between sodium and kallikrein excretion in man (Adetuyibi and Mills, 1972), as well as rabbits and rats on free salt and water intake, but not in rabbits when dietary sodium intake was constant and either high or low (Mills and Ward, 1975). Both plasma kinins and urinary kallikrein were increased in dogs after oral saline but not water loading. Finally, a positive correlation between urinary kallikrein and volume has been noted in normal man (Adetuyibi and Mills, 1972).

All of the above pharmacologic studies and measurements of kallikrein or kinin activity suggest that the system is associated with natriuretic and diuretic processes.

However, a body of data has been gathered which appears inconsistent with the notion that the endogenous renal kallikrein-kinin system promotes natriuresis and diuresis. These studies (Geller et al., 1972; Margolius et al., 1974a; Abe et al., 1977; Johnston et al., 1976; Lawton and Fitz, 1977; Vinci et al., 1977; Mimran et al., 1977; Levy et al., 1978) have shown that the urinary excretion of kallikrein is increased by low dietary sodium intake in humans and in the rat. In addition, increased potassium intake (Horwitz, Margolius, and Keiser, 1978), administration of fludrocortisone to human subjects, or desoxycorticosterone or aldosterone to rats or dogs (Adetuyibi and Mills, 1972; Geller et al., 1972; Marin-Grez, Oza, and Carretero, 1973; Margolius et al., 1972, 1974a; Nasjletti, McGiff, and Colina-Chourio, 1978) also increases urinary kallikrein excretion. Furthermore, normal subjects whose kallikrein excretion had been increased by a low sodium diet showed a marked decrease in kallikrein during treatment with the specific aldosterone antagonist, spironolactone (Margolius et al., 1974a). Similar relations between kallikrein production or levels and sodium-retaining steroids and antagonists have been observed in isolated renal cortical cells in suspension (Kaizu and Margolius, 1975) or in whole kidney homogenates (Nasjletti et al., 1978). It has been suggested that kallikrein excretion is determined, at least in part, by the effective level of circulating sodium-retaining steroid hormone, presumably as a consequence of some action of steroids on renal cells (Margolius et al., 1974a; Margolius, Chao, and Kaizu, 1976).

In clinical studies of a large population of normal adults, Margolius et al. (1974a) were unable to confirm earlier data (Adetuyibi and Mills, 1972) showing a direct correlation between urinary sodium and kallikrein excretion. Neither Greco et al. (1974) nor Seino et al. (1975) saw such a relation in hypertensive adults. Over a five-year period, repeated studies of urinary kallikrein in relation to urinary electrolytes in over 600 normal children did not disclose any positive correlation between urinary sodium and kallikrein (Zinner et al., 1976, 1978). On the contrary, a repeatedly detectable significant negative correlation existed between these variables, whereas a strongly positive correlation between urinary kallikrein and potassium was observed.

Other indirect evidence suggesting relations between the kallikrein-kinin system and sodium homeostasis comes from the demonstration of decreased plasma kinin levels with saline infusions into normal human subjects (Wong et al., 1975), a result opposite to that seen by Marin-Grez, Cottone, and Carretero (1972) in dogs. Recent studies of human subjects (Vinci et al., 1977) add further perplexity to what is known of connections amongst the renal kallikrein-kinin system, electrolyte homeostasis, and sodium-retaining steroid activity. The positive relation of urinary kallikrein excretion to adrenal sodium-retaining steroid activity is confirmed in these studies. In addition, plasma kinins are increased significantly as was shown previously by Wong et al. (1975). However, urinary kinin excretion, presumptively a product of renal and urinary kinin activity, is unchanged by either prolonged periods of low dietary sodium intake (Vinci et al., 1978), administration of fludrocortisone, or of ACTH, all of which increase significantly the excretion of urinary kallikrein. Thus at least a few paradoxes are apparent. The first is the known natriuretic/diuretic effects of exogenously administered, and possibly endogenously produced, kinins and the repeatedly observed increase in kallikrein excretion under conditions in which little sodium is being excreted. Another paradox is why increased urinary kallikrein with decreased sodium intake is not reflected by increased urinary kinins (Vinci et al., 1977), which they seem optimally localized to produce, but is, instead, accompanied by increased plasma kinins.

The positive correlation between urine volume and kallikrein excretion noted by Adetuyibi and Mills (1972) has not been confirmed in other studies of human subjects (Margolius et al., 1974a). However, Levy et al., (1978) have seen significant increases in kallikrein excretion in normal men produced by intravenous water loading during prolonged sodium restriction, but not during periods of normal sodium intake. Whether increased kallikrein excretion with increased urine flow represents an inconsistently observed and passive washout phenomenon, a variably present finding owing to methodologic differences, or a physiologically meaningful observation, is still unclear.

It is obvious that, at present, the role of the renal kallikrein-kinin system in water or electrolyte homeostasis is unclear. Nevertheless, the recent and impressive findings on the localization of components of the system along the nephron; the availability of improving methodology to measure substrate, enzyme, products, and inhibitors in both renal tissue and urine; the long observed effects of kinin peptides on renal vascular and excretory function; and the relations between kallikrein and aldosterone, suggest more intensified investigation of the system in relation to water and electrolyte homeostasis. Exploration of these relations will be important not only because of the presence of system components at renal sites where electrolyte and water transport are primary functions but also because of discovered relations between the kallikrein-kinin system and hypertensive and other diseases related to renal dysfunction.

THE SYSTEM IN HYPERTENSIVE AND RENAL DISEASES

Hypertensive animal models

Components of the kallikrein-kinin system have been measured predominantly in the hypertensive rat. The models used include the Okamoto-Kyoto, New Zealand, and Bianchi strains of spontaneously hypertensive rats (SHR); the Dahl salt-sensitive and salt-resistant animals; a diabetic-hypertensive rat model; renovascular hypertensive rats with either partial renal artery occlusion or aortic coarctation; and desoxycorticosterone-salt hypertensive rats.

In the first study of kallikrein excretion in a spontaneously hypertensive rat, the Okamoto-Kyoto SHR was found to excrete more kallikrein than NIH-Wistar rats used as normotensive controls (Margolius et al., 1972). However, when the study was repeated using the newly available Wistar-Kyoto normotensive rat, urinary kallikrein excretion was found to be lower in the spontaneously hypertensive than in the normotensive animals (Geller et al., 1975)—representing yet another example of the importance of appropriate control strains for rat studies. Similarly reduced kallikrein excretion has been noted in the hypertensive Wistar strain of Bianchi (Porcelli, Bianchi, and Croxatto, 1975) and, perhaps, in the New Zealand genetically hypertensive animal (Carretero et al., 1977). The salt-sensitive rats of Dahl excrete significantly less kallilkrein than salt-resistant animals (Rapp, Tan and Margolius, 1978; Carretero et al., 1978). Parenthetically, the latter study has set a new standard for kallikrein measurement in urine by using three separate methods of assay, including a direct radioimmunoassay, a measure of kinin-generating activity, and an esterolytic assay (Fig. 5.5). Although significant quantitative differences existed, all methods detected reduced kallikrein in salt-sensitive animals.

When hypertension was induced in rats drinking 1 percent saline, via subcutaneous implantation of DOCA pellets, there was a marked increase in urinary kallikrein excretion in the hypertensive animals compared with control groups drinking either 1 percent saline or water (Margolius et al., 1972). However, it was later observed that DOCA alone increased kallikrein excretion in the absence of elevated systemic arterial pressure (Geller et al., 1972).

Urinary kallikrein excretion has almost universally been observed to be reduced in renal hypertensive rats (Croxatto and San Martin, 1970; Margolius et al., 1972; Jenner and Croxatto, 1973; Carretero et al., 1974). However, in one study, increased kallikrein excretion in the two-kidney model and no change in the one-kidney animal was reported (Johnston, Matthews, and Dax, 1976). This study used a radioimmunoassay of generated kinins for measurement of kallikrein and may be revealing some additional insight into urinary kallikrein activity in these rats. In conscious dogs with chronic unilateral renal artery

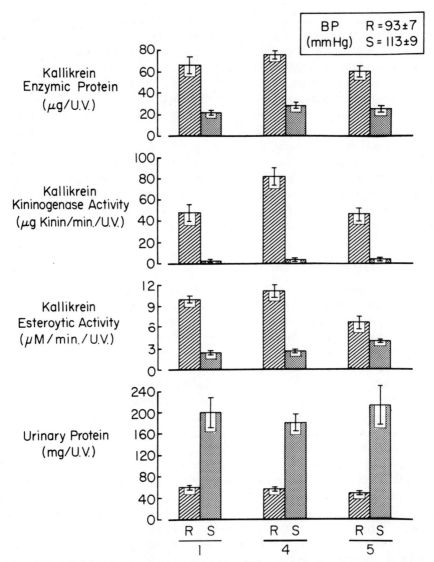

Figure 5.5   Kallikrein excretion measured by three different methods and urinary protein excretion in Dahl salt-resistant (R) and salt-sensitive (S) rats. Number under R S indicates date of urine collection. (From Carretero et al., 1978, by permission of the American Heart Association, Inc., and the author)

stenosis, Keiser et al. (1976a) found markedly reduced kallikrein excretion rates in the ureter from the compromised versus the normally perfused kidney, results that correlated well with the measured and reduced renal blood flow produced by the ligature.

Tissue kallikrein levels have been measured in the kidneys of Bianchi-Milan spontaneously hypertensive rats (Favaro et al., 1975) and in renal hypertensive rats (Croxatto et al., 1974; Carretero et al., 1974). In both models, renal kallikrein activity was significantly lower than in normotensive controls. Plasma kininogen levels have been measured in a single study in renal hypertensive rats and found to be significantly increased (Albertini et al., 1974).

These studies represent almost all of the experience gathered by measuring components of the kallikrein-kinin system in hypertensive animal models. They do not show that an abnormality in the renal kallikrein-kinin system plays any role in the pathogenesis of the hypertensive diseases associated with these models. None of the studies precedes 1970 or includes measurements of multiple components of the renal kallikrein-kinin system. However, these efforts collectively have shown convincing alterations in at least one system component in hypertensive animal models. Because similar abnormalities are present in humans, they have served to provoke an increased interest in the renal kallikrein-kinin system.

Human hypertension

The first study of the kallikrein-kinin system in human hypertension was that of Elliot and Nuzum (1934). Using large groups of normotensive and hypertensive subjects without demonstrable renal impairment, they showed the latter had significantly lower kallikrein excretion rates than the former. This finding was quickly confirmed, but further investigation was not forthcoming until 1971 when their result was reconfirmed (Margolius et al., 1971) (Fig. 5.6). Several additional studies have shown that kallikrein excretion is lower than normal in patients with essential hypertension (Greco et al., 1974; Miyashita, 1971; Shkhvatsabaia et al., 1973; Levy et al., 1977; Seino et al., 1975; Mitas et al., 1978) but predictably, some recent efforts suggest that this conclusion is not applicable to all patients. A study designed to measure urinary kallikrein excretion in normal and hypertensive white or black men during periods of normal sodium intake showed that excretion rates were decreased significantly in white hypertensive compared with white normotensive men but that black men, regardless of their level of blood pressure, had uniformly low levels (Levy et al., 1977). However, another study of kallikrein excretion in white hypertensive men with normal plasma renin activities compared with age-matched white normotensives did not find lower kallikrein excretion in this setting (Lawton and Fitz, 1977).

The relations among sodium intake, aldosterone, and kallikrein excretion in patients with moderate but sustained hypertension have been examined (Margolius et al., 1974b). This study showed that when sodium intake was changed from ad libitum to 9 mEq/day, kallikrein excretion increased in some of the hypertensive patients, but significantly less than in normal subjects, whereas aldosterone excretion was similarly increased in both groups. Thus, the lowered kallikrein excretion seen during periods of normal or low sodium intake in hypertensive patients was not due to differences in sodium intake nor the result of differences in sodium-retaining steroid activity. However, the same group (Horowitz et al., 1978) was unable to detect differences between

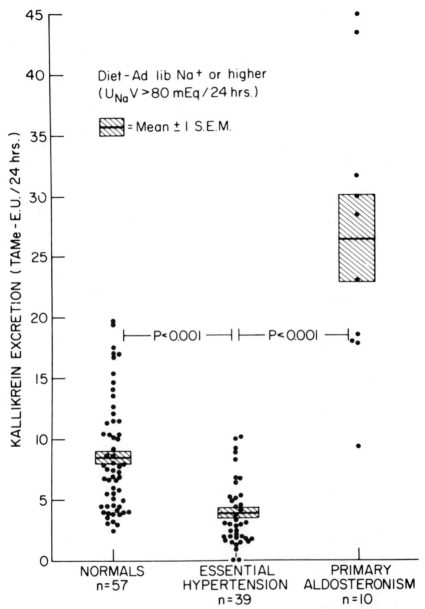

Figure 5.6   Kallikrein excretion in normal subjects, essential hypertension and primary aldosteronism. (From Margolius et al., 1974b, by permission of the American Heart Association, Inc.)

hypertensive and normotensive subjects in response to altered dietary potassium intake. Although a daily potassium intake of 185 mEq increased urinary kallikrein excretion significantly, there was no clear-cut difference between the responses of hypertensive and normotensive subjects. Levy et al. (1977) evaluated the change in kallikrein excretion with low sodium diet in hypertensive and normotensive men separately by race and found that black hypertensive men did not show increased excretion.

In summary, it is clear that low basal or stimulated kallikrein excretion is not uniformly present in all patients with essential hypertension, but the preponderance of evidence indicates lowered kallikrein excretion in patients with this disorder, at least in larger groups of Caucasian or Oriental subjects. The meaning of this alteration is uncertain, although data are beginning to be gathered which measures other system components that might be more likely to clarify the observations. For example, Shimamoto et al. (1978) have shown that a small group of Japanese patients with essential hypertension seem to be excreting less urinary kinin than normal.

A different approach to possible relations between the kallikrein-kinin system and hypertensive disease was taken in a large-scale, long-term epidemiologic study (Zinner et al., 1976; 1978). Urinary kallikrein concentration and excretion rates were measured in an initial population of over 600 normal children and their mothers in 163 families. Blood pressures, urinary electrolytes and other variables were also evaluated on two separate occasions 3 to 4 years apart. Urinary kallikrein was found to be familially aggregated amongst the children. Several variables correlated positively with kallikrein, with the highest direct correlation between it and urinary potassium. There was no direct relation between urinary kallikrein and urinary sodium concentrations by single regression analysis, but an inverse correlation existed after the effects of other variables were removed in multiple regression analyses. Normotensive black children repeatedly had markedly lower urinary kallikrein levels than did normotensive white children (Table 5.1). This was also the case when timed kallikrein excretion rates were measured. The relation observed between urinary kallikrein and blood pressure in these normal children was of interest. As all recorded blood pressures were within normal limits, those families of children with the highest 10 percent or 20 percent of mean family kallikrein levels were selected and their blood pressure scores (in standard deviation units, see Zinner et al., 1978) compared with those of families with the lowest 10 percent or 20 percent of mean family kallikrein levels. Table 5.2 shows that either systolic or diastolic blood pressure scores for the "low kallikrein" families were significantly higher than for the "high kallikrein" families. The reverse procedure, that is, selecting children with the highest or lowest diastolic pressures showed significant inverse correlations between

Table 5.1 Urinary kallikrein concentration by race

	N	Log E.U.[a] /ml ± SD
Black children	243	3.835 ± 0.75
White children	146	4.372 ± 0.74[b]

[a] E.U. = Esterase Units
[b] $P < 0.001$
(From Zimmer et al., 1978, by permission of the American Heart Association, Inc., and the author.)

Table 5.2 Mean blood pressure scores (in standard deviation units) at extremes of population for log urinary kallikrein/creatinine concentrations

White families	Mean log kall/creat	
	Lowest 10%	Highest 10%
Systolic blood pressure	0.344 ± 0.064	-1.465 ± 0.61
No. families	5	5
No. children	14	20
	$P < 0.002$	

Black families	Mean log kall/creat	
	Lowest 20%	Highest 20%
Diastolic (K4) blood pressure	0.635 ± 0.99	-0.210 ± 1.03
No. families	14	14
No. children	49	59
	$P < 0.05$	

(From Zinner et al., 1978, by permission of the American Heart Association, Inc., and the author.)

blood pressure and urinary kallikrein. This long-term study confirms the earlier finding of blood pressure tracking in childhood (Zinner et al., 1975), and establishes in a free-living population of normal children what appear to be stable relations between the activity of urinary kallikrein and blood pressure. In addition, the striking difference in levels relative to race is providing fuel for new hypothesis formulation concerning the kallikrein-kinin system and hypertensive diseases. These data do not necessarily demonstrate a relation between the activity of the renal kallikrein-kinin system and processes involved in the pathogenesis of human hypertensive diseases. Nor do they predict that children with low urinary kallikrein levels and/or high blood pressures (for their age or sex groups) will be at risk for developing hypertensive diseases in later life. However, they do demonstrate the feasibility and reinforce the necessity of examination of any variables thought to be related to the pathogenesis of hypertension in populations considered to be at risk for the development of the disease, namely, normal children.

Elevated kallikrein excretion is present in patients with primary aldosteronism (Margolius et al., 1971, 1974b; Miyashita, 1971). It was this observation that led to delineation of the relation between urinary kallikrein excretion and sodium-retaining steroid hormone activity noted above. The meaning of this finding, in terms of what other system alterations exist in this disorder and of what relations, if any, may exist to any renal abnormalities associated with the disease, is unknown. It has been suggested that the localizing of glandular kallikrein at sites where aldosterone is known to act (renal distal tubule, salivary ducts, sweat glands, colonic mucosa) and the increasing of enzyme activity in urine and renal cell suspensions (Kaizu and Margolius, 1975) by aldosterone but the decreasing of enzyme activity by spironolactone may mean that kallikrein is one of the induced proteins involved in aldosterone-mediated sodium translocation across these cell membranes (Margolius et al., 1976). In any event, the data in patients with primary aldosteronism are consistent with that in rats treated with desoxycorticosterone and suggest that measurement of urinary kallikrein excretion may be useful in evaluating adrenal-renal interactions in hypertensive patients. However, the effects of most other steroid hormones on the activity of components of the system are as yet unknown.

Patients with renovascular hypertension excrete low to undetectable amounts of kallikrein in urine (Keiser et al., 1976b). This is consistent with the data in rats with induced renovascular disease but studies of other system components have not yet been carried out. In a single patient with a renin-secreting juxtaglomerular cell tumor and severe hypertension, urinary kallikrein excretion was abnormally elevated but fell after tumor removal (Mimran et al., 1978). In this case, high kallikrein was interpreted as being secondary to increased aldosterone production.

Kallikrein excretion has been measured in several patients with pheochromocytoma (Margolius et al., 1971). Excretion was high and, in the single case studied, fell after tumor removal. The finding has been confirmed in two other cases (Wingfield et al., unpublished results). Since it has been shown that certain catecholamines are potent releasers of kallikrein from salivary glands (Nustad et al., 1978), it is possible that further insight into the regulation of the renal system will be gained by studies of sympathetic nervous system kallikrein-kinin interactions.

Bartter's syndrome and other renal diseases

Patients with Bartter's syndrome excrete more kallikrein than normal subjects (Lechi et al., 1976; Halushka et al., 1977; Vinci et al., 1978). In addition, plasma bradykinin is elevated without increased plasma prekallikrein activity and, surprisingly, urinary kinins are significantly decreased. These alterations are accompanied by increased urinary immunoreactive prostaglandin E excretion. Indomethacin, a prostaglandin synthetase inhibitor, decreased urinary prostaglandin excretion as well as urinary kallikrein and plasma bradykinin levels, but increased urinary kinin excretion (Fig. 5.7). The available data suggested to Vinci et al. (1978) that prostaglandins somehow mediate the low kinin excretion and high plasma kinin levels and that the aldosterone-dependent increase in urinary kallikrein excretion returns to normal after indomethacin, in concert with reduced plasma renin and aldosterone activity. What should be left with the reader is that clear-cut evidence for abnormal activity of the renal kallikrein-kinin system in Bartter's syndrome has been gathered but its significance is not yet clear.

On the contrary, other examples of renal pathology have generally been found to be accompanied by low urinary kallikrein excretion. Mitas et al. (1978) found that subjects with renal parenchymal diseases such as chronic glomerulonephritis or polycystic disease had extremely low kallikrein excretion. Glasser and Michael (1976) showed that two types of experimentally in-

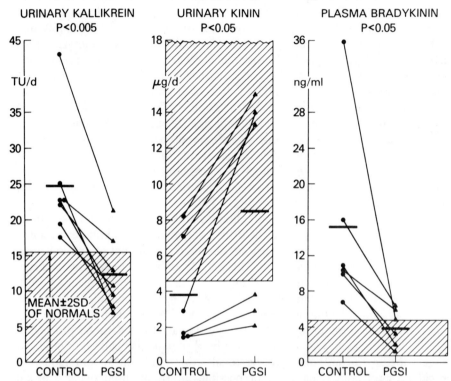

EFFECTS OF PROSTAGLANDIN SYNTHETASE INHIBITION ON THE KALLIKREIN-KININ SYSTEM IN BARTTER'S SYNDROME

Figure 5.7 Effect of prostaglandin synthetase inhibition (PGSI) on urinary kallikrein, urinary kinin, and plasma bradykinin in patients with Bartter's syndrome. (From Vinci et al., 1978, with permission of the publisher and author)

duced renal disease in rats, antiglomerular basement membrane nephritis and aminonucleoside nephrosis, each cause a prompt reduction in kallikrein excretion not consistently related to a generalized proteinuria or the presence of urinary kallikrein inhibitors. Boscolo et al. (1978) carried out an interesting study of lead workers in a car battery factory after showing that hospitalized lead-intoxicated patients excrete less kallikrein than normal. In factory workers aged 34 to 52, there was significantly reduced kallikrein excretion compared with matched controls, but younger workers (22–32 years) did not show reduced kallikrein excretion compared with matched control population. Blood pressure measurements were not reported.

DRUGS AND OTHER AGENTS WHICH AFFECT THE SYSTEM

Spironolactone, the aldosterone antagonist and distally active diuretic, decreases urinary kallikrein excretion in normal subjects and patients with primary aldosteronism (Margolius et al., 1975a & b) and kallikrein production by renal cortical cells in suspension (Kaizu and Margolius, 1975). Furosemide increases urinary kallikrein excretion in the rat (Croxatto et al., 1973) and in normal man (Abe et al., 1978). In the latter study, the short-lasting (30 min.) kallikrein increase was accompanied by an equally evanescent increase in urinary kinins and prostaglandin E. Another study in man has not confirmed these findings (Halushka et al., 1979) and thus the matter is presently in dispute. Other diuretics have also seemingly increased kallikrein excretion in rats. These include acetazolamide (Croxatto et al., 1975), bumetanide (Olsen and Ahnfelt-Rønne, 1976), and benzoflumethazide (Nielsen and Arrigoni-Martelli, 1977). It has been suggested that the observed changes may relate to renal blood flow increases produced by these agents under the experimental circumstances of their usage (Nielsen and Arrigoni-Martelli, 1977). However, preliminary evidence indicates that the diuretic drug, amiloride, may inhibit kallikrein directly (Chao and Margolius, 1978b).

The effects of indomethacin on kallikrein and kinins in Bartter's syndrome were mentioned previously, but the drug also decreases kallikrein excretion in normal volunteers on a low dietary sodium intake while not affecting urinary kinin excretion (Vinci et al., 1978). This may be an indirect effect secondary to aldosterone suppression after the drug.

Chronic subcutaneous aprotinin administration to rats significantly reduces urinary and renal kallikrein activity as well as blunting the increases in each seen after sodium-retaining steroids (Nasjletti et al., 1978). Urinary prostaglandin E-like substance was also decreased by this glandular kallikrein inhibitor, suggesting to the authors that the renal kallikrein-kinin system modulates renal prostaglandin release. Other possible interrelations between the kallikrein-kinin system and prostaglandins in the kidney have been reviewed recently by McGiff and Wong (1979).

The effects of converting enzyme inhibitors (SQ20881, SQ14255, etc.) have been mentioned previously, and more published data is likely to be forthcoming in the near future.

SUMMARY

In this chapter we have reviewed what has been discovered about the renal kallikrein-kinin system. Even though there is much uncertainty about the meaning or significance of various bits of data, the reader should appreciate that there has been accelerating interest in this system over the last decade. A perusal of the reference list should disclose that most of the work available for citation has been carried out since 1970. In their comprehensive review of the kallikrein-kinin system as of 1968, Kellemeyer and Graham (1968) questioned whether kinins had any notable action in the regulation of normal renal function. Although at this point the reader may be of a similar mind, the possibility that kallikrein and kinins play some part in kidney function in health and disease has been enhanced by data that localize and characterize system components, that indicate their pharmacologic effects and responses to various maneuvers and drugs, and that observe system abnormalities in hypertensive diseases or renal pathology.

ACKNOWLEDGMENT

Some of the work cited was supported by NIH grants HL 17705 and GM 20387. Harry S. Margolius is a Burroughs Wellcome Scholar in Clinical Pharmacology. The secretarial assistance of Marie Truesdell is appreciated.

REFERENCES

Abe, K., Irokawa, N., Yasujima, M., Seino, M., Chiba, S., Sakurai, Y., Yoshinaga, K. & Saito, T. (1978). The kallikrein-kinin system and prostaglandins in the kidney. Their relation to furosemide-induced diuresis and to the renin-angiotensin-aldosterone system in man. *Circulation Research*, **43**, 254.

Abe, K., Seino, M., Yasujima, M., Chiba, S., Sakurai, Y., Irokawa, N., Miyazaki, S., Saito, K., Ito, T., Otsuka, Y. & Yoshinaga, K. (1977). Studies in renomedullary prostaglandin and renal kallikrein-kinin system in hypertension. *Japanese Circulation Journal*, **41**, 873.

Adetuyibi, A. & Mills, I. H. (1972). Relation between urinary kallikrein and renal function, hypertension, and excretion of sodium and water in man. *Lancet*, **2**, 203.

Albertini, R., Roblero, J., Corthorn, J. & Croxatto, H. R. (1974). Blood kininogen in uninephrectomized and hypertensive rats. *Acta Physiologica Latinoamericana*, **24**, 443.

Barraclough, M. A. & Mills, I. H. (1965). Effect of bradykinin on renal function. *Clinical Science*, **28**, 69.

Beaven, V., Pierce, J. V. & Pisano, J. J. (1970). A sensitive isotopic procedure for the assay of esterase activity: Measurement of human urinary kallikrein. *Clinica Chimica Acta*, **32**, 67.

Bevan, D. R., MacFarlane, N. A. A. & Mills, I. H. (1974). The dependence of urinary kallikrein excretion on renal artery pressure. *Journal of Physiology* (London), **241**, 34P.

Boscolo, P., Porcelli, G., Cecchetti, G., Salimei, E. & Iannaccone, A. (1978). Urinary kallikrein activity of workers exposed to lead. *British Journal of Industrial Medicine*, **35**, 226.

Brandi, C. M. W., Prado, E. S., Prado, M. J. & Prado, J. L. (1976). Kinin-converting aminopeptidase from human urine: Partial purification and properties. *International Journal of Biochemistry*, **7**, 335.

Brandtzaeg, P., Gautvik, K. M., Nustad, K. & Pierce, J. V. (1976). Rat submandibular gland kallikreins: Purification and cellular localization. *British Journal of Pharmacology*, **56**, 155.

Caldwell, P. R. B., Seegal, B. C., Hsu, K. C., Das, M. & Soffer, R. L. (1976). Angiotensin-converting enzyme: Vascular endothelial localization. *Science*, **191**, 1050.

Capelo, L. R. & Alzamora, F. (1977). A stop flow analysis of the effects of intrarenal infusion of bradykinin. *Archives Internationales de Pharmacodynamie et de Therapie*, **230**, 156.

Carone, F. A., Pullman, T. N., Oparil, S. & Nakamura, S. (1976). Micropuncture evidence of rapid hydrolysis of bradykinin by rat proximal tubule. *American Journal of Physiology*, **230**, 1976.

Carretero, O. A., Amin, V. A., Ocholik, T., Scicli, A. G. & Koch, J. (1978). Urinary kallikrein in rats bred for their susceptibility and resistance to the hypertensive effect of salt. *Circulation Research*, **42**, 727.

Carretero, O. A., Oza, N. B., Piwonska, A., Ocholik, T. & Scicli, A. G. (1976). Measurement of urinary kallikrein activity by kinin radioimmunoassay. *Biochemical Pharmacology*, **25**, 2265.

Carretero, O. A., Oza, N. B., Scicli, A. G. & Schork, A. (1974). Renal tissue kallikrein, plasma renin, and plasma aldosterone in renal hypertension. *Acta Physiologica Latinoamericana*, **24**, 448.

Carretero, O. A., Scicli, A. G., Pivonska, A. & Koch, J. (1977). Urinary kallikrein in rats bred for susceptibility and resistance to the hypertensive effect of salt and in New Zealand genetically hypertensive rats. *Mayo Clinic Proceedings*, **52**, 465.

Chao, J. & Margolius, H. S. (1978a). Identification of kallikrein on external cell surfaces. *Federation Proceedings, Federation of American Societies for Experimental Biology*, **37**, 657A.

Chao, J. & Margolius, H. S. (1978b). Identification of kallikrein in toad urinary bladder and skin and its inhibition by amiloride. *Clinical Research*, **26**, 63A.

Chao, J. & Margolius, H. S. (1979). Isozymes of rat urinary kallikrein. *Biochemical Pharmacology*, in press.

Cheung, H. S. & Cushman, D. W. (1973). Inhibition of homogeneous angiotensin-converting enzyme of rabbit lung by synthetic venom peptides of *Bothrops jararaca*. *Biochimica et Biophysica Acta*, **293**, 451.

Coleman, R. (1974). Formation of human plasma kinin. *New England Journal of Medicine*, **291**, 509.

Collier, J. G., Robinson, B. F. & Vane, J. R. (1973). Reduction of pressor effects of angiotensin I in man by synthetic nonapeptide (BPP$_{9a}$ or SQ20,881) which inhibits converting enzyme. *Lancet*, **1**, 72.

Corthorn, J., Imanari, T., Yoshida, H., Kaizu, T., Pierce, J. V. & Pisano, J. J. (1977). Inactive kallikrein in human urine. *Federation Proceedings, Federation of American Societies for Experimental Biology*, **36**, 893.

Croxatto, H. R., Albertini, R., Roblero, J. & Corthorn, J. (1974). Renal kallikrein (kininogenase activity) in hypertensive rats. *Acta Physiologica Latinoamericana*, **24**, 439.

Croxatto, H. R., Huidobro, F., Rojas, M., Roblero, J. & Albertini, R. (1975). The effect of water, sodium overloading and diuretics upon urinary kallikrein. In *Advances in Experimental Medicine and Biology. Kinins: Pharmacodynamics and Biologic Roles*, eds. Sicuteri, F., Back, N. & Haberland, G. L. Vol. 70, p. 361, New York: Plenum.

Croxatto, H. R., Roblero, J., Garcia, R., Corthorn, J. & San Martin, M. (1973). Urinary kallikrein under furosemide and plasma kininogen levels in normal and hypertensive rats. *Acta Physiologica Latinoamericana*, **23**, 556.

Croxatto, H. R. & San Martin, M. (1970). Kallikrein-like activity in the urine of renal hypertensive rats. *Experientia*, **26**, 1216.

DeBono, E. & Mills, I. H. (1974). Simultaneous increases in kallikrein in renal lymph and urine during saline infusion. *Journal of Physiology* (London), **241**, 127P.

Elliot, A. H. & Nuzum, F. R. (1934). Urinary excretion of a depressor substance (kallikrein of Frey and Kraut) in arterial hypertension. *Endocrinology*, **18**, 462.

Erdös, E. G. (1975). Angiotensin I converting enzyme. *Circulation Research*, **36**, 247.

Erdös, E. G. (1976). The kinins. A status report. *Biochemical Pharmacology*, **25**, 1563.

Erdös, E. G. (1979). *Handbook of Experimental Pharmacology, Bradykinin, Kallidin and Kallikrein*. Vol. 25 (Suppl.). New York: Springer.

Erdös, E. G. & Yang, H. Y. T. (1976). An enzyme in microsomal fractions of kidney that inactivates bradykinin. *Life Sciences*, **6**, 569.

Favaro, S., Baggio, B., Antonello, A., Zen, A., Connella, G., Todesco, S. & Borsatti, A. (1975). Renal kallikrein content of spontaneously hypertensive rats. *Clinical Science and Molecular Medicine*, **49**, 69.

Ferreira, S. H. (1965). A bradykinin-potentiating factor (BPF) present in the venom of *Bothrops jararaca*. *British Journal of Pharmacology*, **24**, 163.

Fiedler, F. (1976). Pig pancreatic kallikreins A and B. In *Methods in Enzymology-Proteolytic Enzymes*, ed. Lorand, L. Vol. 45, p. 289, New York: Academic Press.

Fränki, J. E., Jansén, C. T. & Hopsu-Havu, V. K. (1970). Human sweat kallikrein. *Acta Dermato-Venereologica*, **50**, 321.

Freeman, R. H., Davis, J. O., Vitale, S. J. & Johnson, J. A. (1973). Intrarenal role of angiotensin I. *Circulation Research*, **32**, 692.

Frey, E. K., Kraut, H., Werle, E., Vogel, R., Zickgraf-Rüdel, G. & Trautschold, I. (1968). *Das Kallikrein-Kinin System und seine Inhibitoren*. Stuttgart: Ferdinand Enke.

Fujimoto, Y., Moriya, H. & Moriwaki, C. (1973). Studies on human salivary kallikrein—I. Isolation of human salivary kallikrein. *Journal of Biochemistry* (Tokyo), **74**, 239.

Furtado, M. (1971). Inhibition of the permeability response to vasopressin and oxytocin in the toad bladder: Effects of bradykinin, kallidin, eledoisin and physalaemin. *Journal of Membrane Biology*, **4**, 165.

Gravras, H. Brunner, H. R., Turini, G. A., Kershaw, G. R., Tifft, C. D., Cuttelod, S., Garvas, I., Vukovich, R. A. & McKinstry, D. N. (1978). Antihypertensive effect of the oral angiotensin-converting enzyme inhibitor SQ14225 in man. *New England Journal of Medicine*, **298**, 991.

Geiger, R. & Mann, K. (1976). A kallikrein-specific inhibitor in rat kidney tubules. *Hoppe-Seyler's Zeitschrift für Physioligsche Chemie*, **357**, 553.

Geller, R. G., Margolius, H. S., Pisano, J. J. & Keiser, H. R. (1975). Urinary kallikrein in spontaneously hypertensive rats. *Circulation Research*, **36/37**, Suppl. I, 103.

Geller, R. G., Margolius, H. S., Pisano, J. J. & Keiser, H. R. (1972). Effects of mineralocorticoids, altered sodium intake and adrenalectomy on urinary kallikrein in rats. *Circulation Research*, **31**, 857.

Gill, J. R., Jr., Melmon, K. L., Gillespie, L., Jr., & Bartter, F. C. (1965). Bradykinin and renal function in normal man: Effects of adrenergic blockade. *American Journal of Physiology*, **209**, 844.

Glasser, R. J. & Michael, A. F. (1976). Urinary kallikrein in experimental renal disease. *Laboratory Investigation*, **34**, 616.

Greco, A. V., Porcelli, G., Croxatto, H. R., Fedeli, G. & Ghirlanda, G. (1974). Ipertensione arteriosa e callicreina urinaria. *Minerva Medica*, **65**, 3058.

Halushka, P. V., Margolius, H. S., Allen, H. & Conradi, E. C. (1979). Urinary excretion of prostaglandin E-like material and kallikrein: Effects of furosemide. *Prostaglandins*, in press.

Halushka, P. V., Wohltmann, H., Privitera, P. J., Hurwitz, G. & Margolius, H. S. (1977). Bartter's syndrome: Urinary prostaglandin E-like material and kallikrein; indomethacin effects. *Annals of Internal Medicine*, **87**, 281.

Hial, V., Diniz, C. R. & Mares-Guia, M. (1974). Purification and properties of a human urinary kallikrein (kininogenase). *Biochemistry*, **13**, 4311.

Hial, V., Keiser, H. R. & Pisano, J. J. (1976). Origin and content of methionyl-lysyl-bradykinin, lysyl-bradykinin and bradykinin in human urine. *Biochemical Pharmacology*, **25**, 2499.

Hilton, S. M. (1970). The physiological role of glandular kallikreins. In *Handbook of Experimental Pharmacology, Bradykinin, Kallidin and Kallikreins*, ed. Erdös, E. G. Vol. 25, p. 389, New York: Springer.

Horwitz, D., Margolius, H. S. & Keiser, H. R. (1978). Effects of dietary potassium and race on urinary excretion of kallikrein and aldosterone in man. *Journal of Clinical Endocrinology and Metabolism*, **47**, 296.

Jenner, S. & Croxatto, H. R. (1973). Urinary kallikrein from normal and hypertensive rats. *Experientia*, **29**, 1359.

Johnston, C. I., Matthews, P. G. & Dax, E. (1976). Effects of dietary sodium, diuretics and hypertension on renin and kallikrein. In *Systemic Effects of Antihypertensive Agents*, ed. Sambhi, M. P. P. 328, New York: Stratton Intercontinental.

Kaizu, T. & Margolius, H. S. (1975). Studies on rat renal cortical cell kallikrein. I. Separation and measurement. *Biochimica et Biophysica Acta*, **411**, 305.

Keiser, H. R., Andrews, M. J., Jr., Guyton, R. A., Margolius, H. S. & Pisano, J. J. (1976a). Urinary kallikrein in dogs with constriction of one renal artery. *Proceedings of the Society for Experimental Biology and Medicine*, **151**, 53.

Keiser, H. R., Margolius, H. S., Brown, R., Rhamey, R. & Foster, J. (1976b). Urinary kallikrein in patients with renovascular hypertension. In *Chemistry and Biology of the Kallikrein-Kinin System in Health and Disease*, ed. Pisano, J. J. & Austen, K. F. P. 423. Fogarty International Center Proceedings, No. 27. Washington: U.S. Government Printing Office.

Kellermeyer, R. W. and Graham, R. C., Jr. (1968). Kinins—possible physiologic and pathologic roles in man. *New England Journal of Medicine*, **279**, 754.

Lawton, W. J. & Fitz, A. E. (1977). Urinary kallikrein in normal renin essential hypertension. *Circulation*, **56**, 856.

Lechi, A., Covi, G., Lechi, C., Mantero, F. & Scuro, L. A. (1976). Urinary kallikrein excretion in Bartter's syndrome. *Journal of Clinical Endocrinology and Metabolism*, **43**, 1175.

Levy, S. B., Frigon, R. P. & Stone, R. A. (1978). The relationship of urinary kallikrein activity to renal salt and water excretion. *Clinical Science and Molecular Medicine*, **54**, 39.

Levy, S. B., Lilley, J. J., Frigon, R. P. & Stone, R. A. (1977). Urinary kallikrein and plasma renin activity as determinants of renal blood flow. *Journal of Clinical Investigation*, **60**, 129.

Mann, K., Geiger, R. & Werle, E. (1976). A sensitive kinin-liberating assay for kininogenase in rat urine, isolated glomeruli and tubules of rat kidney. *Advances in Experimental Biology and Medicine, Kinins, Pharmacodynamics and Biological Roles*, eds. Sicuteri, F., Back, N. & Haberland, G. L. P. 65. New York: Plenum Press.

Margolius, H. S., Chao, J. & Kaizu, T. (1976). The effects of aldosterone and spironolactone on renal kallikrein. *Clinical Science and Molecular Medicine*, **51**, Suppl. 3, 279S.

Margolius, H. S., Geller, R. G., deJong, W., Pisano, J. J. & Sjoerdsma, A. (1972). Altered urinary kallikrein excretion in rats with hypertension. *Circulation Research*, **30**, 358.

Margolius, H. S., Geller, R., Pisano, J. J. & Sjoerdsma, A. (1971). Altered urinary kallikrein excretion in human hypertension. *Lancet*, **2**, 1063.

Margolius, H. S., Horwitz, D., Geller, R. G., Alexander, R. W., Gill, J. R., Jr., Pisano, J. J. & Keiser, H. R. (1974a). Urinary kallikrein excretion in normal man. Relationships to sodium intake and sodium-retaining steroids. *Circulation Research*, **35**, 812.

Margolius, H. S., Horwitz, D., Pisano, J. J. & Keiser, H. R. (1974b). Urinary kallikrein in hypertension: Relationship to sodium intake and sodium-retaining steroids. *Circulation Research*, **35**, 820.

Marin-Grez, M. (1974). The influence of antibodies against bradykinin on isotonic saline diuresis in the rat. *Pflügers Archiv*, **350**, 231.

Marin-Grez, M., Cottone, P. & Carretero, O. A. (1972). Evidence for an involvement of kinins in regulation of sodium excretion. *American Journal of Physiology*, **223**, 794.

Marin-Grez, M., Oza, N. B. & Carretero, O. A. (1973). The involvement of urinary kallikrein in the renal escape from the sodium retaining effect of mineralocorticoids. *Henry Ford Hospital Medical Journal*, **21**, 85.

Matsuda, Y., Miyazaki, K., Moriza, H., Fujimoto, Y., Hojima, Y. & Moriwaki, C. (1976). Studies on urinary kallikreins—I. Purification and characterization of human urinary kallikreins. *Journal of Biochemistry* (Tokyo), **80**, 671.

McCaa, R. E., Hall, J. E. & McCaa, C. S. (1978). The effects of angiotensin I-converting enzyme inhibitors on arterial blood pressure and urinary sodium excretion. Role of the renin-angiotensin and kallikrein-kinin systems. *Circulation Research*, **43**, Supp. I, I–32.

McGiff, J. C. (1976). Kinins, renal function and blood pressure regulation. *Federation Proceedings, Federation of American Societies for Experimental Biology*, **35**, 172.

McGiff, J. C., Itskovitz, H. D. & Terragno, N. A. (1975). The actions of bradykinin and eledoisin in the canine isolated kidney: Relationships to prostaglandins. *Clinical Science and Molecular Medicine*, **49**, 125.

McGiff, J. C. & Wong, P. Y-K. (1979). Compartmentalization of prostaglandins and prostacyclin within the kidney: Implications for renal function. *Federation Proceedings, Federation of American Societies for Experimental Biology*, **38**, 89.

Miller, E. D., Samuels, A. I., Haber, E. & Barger, A. C. (1972). Inhibition of angiotensin conversion in experimental renovascular hypertension. *Science*, **177**, 1108.

Mills, I. H. & Ward, P. E. (1975). The relationship between kallikrein and water excretion and the conditional relationship between kallikrein and sodium excretion. *Journal of Physiology* (London), **246**, 695.

Mimran, A., Baudin, G., Casellas, D. & Soulas, D. (1977). Urinary kallikrein and changes in endogenous aldosterone in the rat. *European Journal of Clinical Investigation*, **7**, 497.

Mimran, A., Leckie, B. J., Fourcade, J. C., Baldet, P., Navratil, H. & Barjon, P. (1978). Blood pressure, renin-angiotensin system and urinary kallikrein in a case of juxtaglomerular cell tumor. *American Journal of Medicine*, **65**, 527.

Mitas, J. A., Levy, S. B., Holle, R., Frigon, R. D. & Stone, R. A. (1978). Urinary kallikrein activity in the hypertension of renal parenchymal disease. *New England Journal of Medicine*, **299**, 162.

Miyashita, A. (1971). Urinary kallikrein determination and its physiological role in human kidney. *Japanese Journal of Urology*, **62**, 507.

Moriwaki, C., Miyazaki, K., Matsuda, Y., Moriya, H., Fujimoto, Y. & Ueki, H. (1976). Dog renal kallikrein: Purification and some properties. *Journal of Biochemistry* (Tokyo), **80**, 1277.

Moriwaki, C., Watanuki, N., Fujimoto, Y. & Moriya, H. (1974a). Further purification and properties of kininogenase from the guinea-pig's coagulating gland. *Chemical and Pharmaceutical Bulletin*, **22**, 628.

Moriwaki, C., Yamaguchi, K. & Moriya, H. (1974b). Studies on kallikreins—III. Intra-intestinal administration of hog pancreatic kallikrein and its appearance in the perfusate from the mesenteric vein. *Chemical and Pharmaceutical Bulletin*, **22**, 1975.

Nasjletti, A. & Colina-Chourio, J. (1976). Interaction of mineralocorticoids, renal prostaglandins, and the renal kallikrein-kinin system. *Federation Proceedings, Federation of American Societies for Experimental Biology*, **35**, 189.

Nasjletti, A., Colina-Chourio, J. & McGiff, J. C. (1975). Disappearance of bradykinin in the renal circulation of dogs. Effects of kininase inhibition. *Circulation Research, 37*, 59.

Nasjletti, A., McGiff, J. C. & Colina-Chourio, J. (1978). Interrelations of the renal kallikrein-kinin system and renal prostaglandins in the conscious rat. Influence of mineralocorticoids. *Circulation Research, 43*, 799.

Nielsen, K. & Arrigoni-Martelli, E. (1977). Effects on rat urinary kallikrein excretion of bumetanide, benzoflumethazide, and hydralazine. *Acta Pharmacologica Toxicologica, 40*, 267.

Nustad, K., Gautvik, K. M. & Pierce, J. V. (1976). Glandular kallikreins: Purification, characterization and biosynthesis. In *Chemistry and Biology of the Kallikrein-Kinin System in Health and Disease*, ed. Pisano, J. J. & Austen, K. F. P. 77. Fogarty International Center Proceedings, No. 27. Washington: U.S. Government Printing Office.

Nustad, K., Ørstavik, T. B., Gautvik, K. M. & Pierce, J. V. (1978). Glandular kallikreins. *General Pharmacology, 9*, 1.

Nustad, K. & Pierce, J. V. (1974). Purification of rat urinary kallikreins and their specific antibody. *Biochemistry, 13*, 2312.

Nustad, K., Vaaje, K. & Pierce, J. V. (1975). Synthesis of kallikreins by rat kidney slices. *British Journal of Pharmacology, 53*, 229.

Obika, L. F. O. (1978). Recent developments in urinary kallikrein research. *Life Sciences, 23*, 765.

Odya, C. E. & Goodfriend, T. L. (1977). Bradykinin receptors. *Clinical Research, 25*, 364A.

Ole-Moi Yoi, O., Austen, K. F. & Spragg, J. (1977). Kinin-generating and esterolytic activity of purified human urinary kallikrein (urokallikrein). *Biochemical Pharmacology, 26*, 1893.

Olsen, U. B. & Ahnfelt-Rønne, J. (1976). Bumetanide-induced increase of renal blood flow in conscious dogs and its relation to local renal hormones (PGE, kallikrein and renin). *Acta Pharmacologica Toxicologica, 38*, 219.

Ondetti, M. A., Rubin, B. & Cushman, D. W. (1977). Design of specific inhibitors of angiotensin-converting enzyme: New class of orally active antihypertensive agents. *Science, 196*, 441.

Ørstavik, T. B., Brandtzaeg, P., Nustad, K. & Halvorsen, K. M. (1975). Cellular localization of kallikreins in rat submandibular and sublingual salivary glands. Immunofluorescence tracing related to histological characteristics. *Acta histochemica, 54*, 183.

Ørstavik, T. B., Nustad, K., Brandtzaeg, P. & Pierce, J. V. (1976). Cellular origin of urinary kallikreins. *Journal of Histochemistry and Cytochemistry, 24*, 1037.

Oza, N. B. (1977). A direct assay for urinary kallikrein. *Biochemical Journal, 167*, 305.

Oza, N. B., Amin, V. M., McGregor, R. K., Scicli, A. G., & Carretero, O. A. (1976). Isolation of rat urinary kallikrein and properties of its antibodies. *Biochemical Pharmacology, 25*, 1607.

Pierce, J. V. (1968). Structural features of plasma kinins and kininogens. *Federation Proceedings, 27*, 52.

Pierce, J. V. & Guimarães, J. A. (1976). Further characterization of highly purified human plasma kininogens. In *Chemistry and Biology of the Kallikrein-Kinin System in Health and Disease*, ed. Pisano, J. J. & Austen, K. F. P. 121. Fogarty International Center Proceedings, No. 27. Washington: U.S. Government Printing Office.

Pierce, J. V. & Webster, M. E. (1961). Human plasma kallidins: Isolation and chemical studies. *Biochemical and Biophysical Research Communications, 5*, 353.

Pisano, J. J. (1975). Chemistry and biology of the kallikrein-kinin system. In *Proteases and Biological Control*, ed. Reich, E., Rifkin, D. B. & Shaw, E. P. 199. Cold Spring Harbor, N.Y.: Cold Spring Harbor Laboratory.

Pisano, J. J., Yates, K. & Pierce, J. V. (1978). Kininogen in human urine. *Agents and Actions, 8*, 153.

Porcelli, G., Bianchi, G. & Croxatto, H. (1975). Urinary kallikrein in a spontaneously hypertensive strain of rats. *Proceedings of the Society for Experimental Biology and Medicine, 149*, 983.

Porcelli, G., Marini-Bettolo, G. B., Croxatto, H. R. & Di Iorio, M. (1974). Purification and chemical studies on rabbit urinary kallikrein. *Italian Journal of Biochemistry, 23*, 154.

Prado, E. S., Prado, J. L. & Brandi, C. M. W. (1962). Further purification and some properties of horse urinary kallikrein. *Archives Internationales de Pharmacodynamie et de Therapie, 137*, 358.

Rapp, J. P., Tan, S. Y. & Margolius, H. S. (1978). Plasma mineralocorticoids, plasma renin and urinary kallikrein in salt-sensitive and salt-resistant rats. *Endocrine Research Communications*, **5**, 35.

Roblero, J., Croxatto, H., Garcia, R., Corthorn, J. & DeVito, E. (1976). Kallikrein-like activity in perfusates and urine of isolated rat kidneys. *American Journal of Physiology*, **231**, 1383.

Schachter, M. (1970). Vasodilatation in the submaxillary gland of the cat, rabbit and sheep. In *Handbook of Experimental Pharmacology, Bradykinin, Kallidin and Kallikrein*, ed. Erdös, E. G. Vol. 25, p. 400. New York: Springer.

Scicli, A. G., Carretero, O. A., Hampton, A., Cortes, P. & Oza, N. B. (1976). Site of kininogenase secretion in the dog nephron. *American Journal of Physiology*, **230**, 533.

Scicli, A. G., Gandolfi, R. & Carretero, O. A. (1978). Site of formation of kinins in the dog nephron. *American Journal of Physiology*, **234**, F36.

Sealey, J. E., Atlas, S. A., Laragh, J. H., Oza, N. B. & Ryan, J. W. (1978). Human urinary kallikrein converts inactive to active renin and is a possible physiological activator of renin. *Nature* (London), **275**, 144.

Seino, J., Abe, K., Otsuka, Y., Saito, T., Irokawa, N., Yasujima, M., Ciba, S. & Yoshinaga, K. (1975). Urinary kallikrein excretion and sodium metabolism in hypertensive patients. *Tohoku Journal of Experimental Medicine*, **116**, 359.

Shimamoto, K., Ando, T., Nakao, T., Tanaka, S., Sakuma, M. & Miyabara, M. (1978). A sensitive radioimmunoassay for urinary kinins in man. *Journal of Laboratory and Clinical Medicine*, **91**, 721.

Shimamoto, K., Tanaka, S., Nakao, T., Ando, T., Nakahashi, Y., Sakuma, M. & Miyahara, M. (1979a). Measurement of urinary kallikrein activity by kinin radioimmunoassay. *Japanese Circulation Journal*, **43**, in press.

Shimamoto, K., Margolius, H. S., Chao, J., & Croswell, A. F. (1979b). A direct radioimmunoassay of rat urinary kallikrein and comparison with other measures of urinary kallikrein activity. *Journal of Laboratory and Clinical Medicine*, in press.

Shkhvatsabaia, I. K., Nekrasova, A. A., Chernova, N. A. & Khukharev, V. V. (1973). Kinin system of the kidneys in the pathogenesis of hypertensive disease. *Terapevticheskii Arkhiv*, **10**, 71.

Simson, J. A. V., Spicer, S. S., Chao, J., Grimm, L. & Margolius, H. S. (1979). Kallikrein localization in rodent salivary glands and kidney with the immune-peroxidase bridge technique. *Journal of Histochemistry and Cytochemistry*, in press.

Stein, J. H., Congbaloy, R. C., Karsh, D. L., Osgood, R. W. & Ferris, T. F. (1972). The effect of bradykinin on proximal tubular sodium reabsorption in the dog: Evidence for functional nephron heterogeneity. *Journal of Clinical Investigation*, **51**, 1709.

Tschesche, H., Mair, G., Förg-Brey, B. & Fritz, H. (1976). Isolation of porcine urinary kallikrein. In *Advances in Experimental Medicine and Biology, Kinins, Pharmacodynamics and Biological Roles*, eds. Sicuteri, F., Back, N. & Haberland, G. L. Vol. 70, p. 119. New York: Plenum Press.

Vahatera, E. & Hamburg, V. (1976). Absence of binding of pancreatic and urinary kallikreins to α_2-macroglobulin. *Biochemical Journal*, **157**, 521.

Vinci, J. M., Gill, J. R., Jr., Bowden, R. E., Pisano, J. J., Izzo, J. L., Jr., Radfar, N., Taylor, A. A., Zusman, R. M., Bartter, F. C. & Keiser, H. R. (1978). The kallikrein-kinin system in Bartter's syndrome and its response to prostaglandin synthetase inhibition. *Journal of Clinical Investigation*, **61**, 1671.

Vinci, J., Zusman, R., Bowden, R., Horwitz, D. & Keiser, H. (1977). Relationship of urinary and plasma kinins to sodium-retaining steroids and plasma renin activity. *Clinical Research*, **25**, 450A.

Ward, P. E., Erdös, E. G., Gedney, C. D., Dowben, R. M. & Reynolds, R. C. (1976). Isolation of membrane-bound renal enzymes that metabolize kinins and angiotensins. *Biochemical Journal*, **157**, 643.

Ward, P. E., Gedney, C., Dowben, R. M. & Erdös, E. G. (1975). Isolation of membrane-bound renal kallikrein and kininase. *Biochemical Journal*, **151**, 755.

Ward, P. E. & Margolius, H. S. (1979). Renal and urinary kallikreins. In *Handbook of Experimental Pharmacology, Bradykinin, Kallidin and Kallikrein*, ed. Erdös, E. G. Vol. 25, Supplement, New York: Springer. In press.

Webster, M. E. & Gilmore, J. P. (1964). Influences of kallidin-10 on renal function. *American Journal of Physiology*, **206**, 714.

Webster, M. E., Mares-Guia, M. & Diniz, C. R. (1970). Kallikreins in glandular tissues. In

Handbook of Experimental Pharmacology. Bradykinin, Kallidin and Kallikrein, ed. Erdös, E. G. Vol. 25, p. 131. New York: Springer.

Webster, M. E. & Pierce, J. V. (1961). Action of kallikreins on synthetic ester substrates. *Proceedings of the Society for Experimental Biology and Medicine,* **107,** 186.

Willis, L. R., Ludens, J. H., Hook, J. B. & Williamson, H. E. (1969). Mechanism of natriuretic action of bradykinin. *American Journal of Physiology,* **217,** 1.

Wong, P. Y., Talamo, R. C., Williams, G. H. & Coleman, R. W. (1975). Response of the kallikrein-kinin and renin-angiotensin systems to saline infusion and upright posture. *Journal of Clinical Investigation,* **55,** 691.

Zinner, S. H., Margolius, H. S., Rosner, B. & Kass, E. H. (1978). Stability of blood pressure rank and urinary kallikrein concentration in childhood: an eight-year follow-up. *Circulation,* **58,** 908.

Zinner, S. H., Margolius, H. S., Rosner, B., Keiser, H. R. & Kass, E. H. (1976). Familial aggregation of urinary kallikrein concentration in childhood. *American Journal of Epidemiology,* **104,** 124.

Zinner, S. H., Martin, L. F., Sacko, F., Rosner, B. & Kass, E. H. (1975). A longitudinal study of blood pressure in children. *American Journal of Epidemiology,* **100,** 437.

6

Factors regulating the secretion and metabolism of arginine vasopressin (antidiuretic hormone)

RICHARD E. WEITZMAN

INTRODUCTION

Arginine vasopressin (AVP) has been shown to have a number of distinct physiological effects on renal and extrarenal tissues other than its antidiuretic action on the collecting duct and its pressor effects on vascular smooth muscle. AVP produces dose-dependent inhibition of renal renin release (Shade et al., 1973; Khokhär et al., 1976; Hesse and Nielsen, 1977), stimulation of renal medullary prostaglandin synthesis (Zusman and Keiser, 1977), and stimulation of pituitary secretion of ACTH (Yates et al., 1971). It also influences several central nervous system functions, namely, morphine tolerance (VanRee and De Wied, 1977) and memory (DeWied, 1971). It is, therefore, not surprising that AVP secretion is regulated by a large number of osmolar and nonosmolar stimuli, all of which interact to determine the net secretion rate of AVP (Fig. 6.1). To fur-

REGULATION OF AVP SECRETION AND THIRST

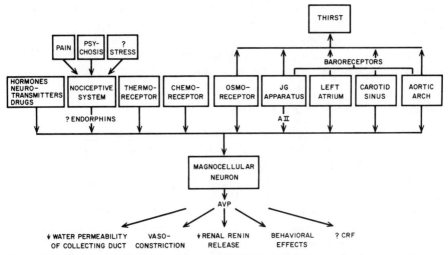

Figure 6.1 Regulation of AVP secretion and thirst. Osmoreceptors and volume sensitive receptors (carotid sinus, aortic arch, left atrium, and renal juxtaglomerular apparatus) influence both AVP secretion and thirst while chemoreceptors, hormones, nociceptive influences, and thermoreceptors influence mainly AVP. Magnocellular neurons in the supraoptic and paraventricular nuclei synthesize AVP and package it into neurosecretory granules for transport down the pituitary stalk to the neural lobe where it is released into the circulation. Circulating AVP influences not only renal water permeability and vascular tone but also memory, corticotrophin release and renal release of renin.

ther complicate matters, plasma concentrations of AVP only indirectly reflect secretion rate; the metabolic clearance and distribution of AVP must be taken into account to assess minute-to-minute AVP secretion from serial measurements of plasma AVP levels. This review covers new developments in regulation of AVP secretion and metabolism, many of which were made possible by the development of sensitive and specific AVP radioimmunoassays. Several comprehensive reviews, which cover earlier work in the field, are recommended (Lauson, 1974; Moses and Miller, 1974; Gauer and Henry, 1976; Share, 1976; Robertson, 1977).

OSMOTIC REGULATION

Verney Hypothesis

Verney (1947) first demonstrated that extracellular fluid osmolality influences AVP secretion; he observed a marked reduction in urine flow after intracarotid injections of hypertonic saline. This antidiuresis is qualitatively similar to that produced by intravenous injection of pituitary extract, and Verney (1947) pointed out that a similar antidiuresis can be produced by intracarotid injections of dextrose or fructose, suggesting that the effect of sodium chloride is a reflection of its osmotic activity and not intrinsically related to the sodium ion itself. However, in Verney's studies the response to dextrose was somewhat less than that which was anticipated on the basis of osmolality; moreover, a similar rise in osmolality produced by intracarotid injection of urea had no antidiuretic effects. Verney (1947) concluded that the effectiveness of any substance in inducing an antidiuretic response is a function of both its osmotic activity and its membrane permeability.

Periventricular sodium hypothesis

There have been several challenges to the osmoreceptor hypothesis in recent years. A number of Scandinavian workers observed that sodium chloride is uniquely effective in producing an antidiuresis after injection into the cerebral ventricles whereas injections of saccharide solutions actually inhibit antidiuresis (Andersson and Olsson, 1977). It was felt that these studies demonstrated the existence of a specific periventricular sodium receptor for control of AVP release and that the inhibition of antidiuresis which occurred after injection of saccharide solutions was merely a reflection of the dilution of ventricular sodium concentration by the injected solutions. According to this hypothesis, injection of hyperosmotic substances into the carotid artery serves to induce a water shift across the blood-brain barrier, producing a rise in the cerebrospinal fluid sodium concentration and stimulation of AVP secretion. In other studies the sodium receptor appeared to act synergistically with a periventricular receptor for angiotensin, since injection of subthreshold quantities of angiotensin II greatly potentiates the effects of intraventricular NaCl (Andersson and Westbye, 1970). The effect of sodium upon AVP release is inhibited by intracerebroventricular injections of either glycerol or deuterium, both of which are effective inhibitors of $Na+-K+-ATP$-ase activity, suggesting that such activity mediates the response to saline (Andersson and Olsson, 1977).

In vitro studies

Recently, studies have been conducted to determine the osmotic reactivity of the hypothalamic neurohypophyseal system in vitro by measurement of AVP release from cultured hypothalamic-neural lobe explants (Sladek and Knigge, 1977). Such explants respond to subtle variations in the osmolality of the culture medium ($\pm$ 15–20 mOsm) with significant alterations in AVP release into the bathing medium (Fig. 6.2a). AVP release occurs when osmolality is increased with either sodium or mannitol but not with glucose or urea (Fig. 6.2b). These in vitro studies appear to confirm the in vivo studies of Verney (1947) but do not exclude the concurrent existence of the periventricular sodium receptors described above. Robertson, Shelton, and Athar (1976) have demonstrated differential effectiveness of equi-osmolar doses of saline, mannitol, urea, and glucose on the stimulation of immunoreactive AVP release in humans. Their studies are in essential agreement with those cited above except that in their hands infusions of glucose have actually inhibited AVP release.

These observations raise the question of whether the polyuria seen in hyper-glycemic states represents both an osmotic and a water diuresis.

Relationship between plasma osmolality and plasma AVP

The interaction between plasma osmolality and plasma concentrations of AVP has been the subject of considerable interest for many years. Verney (1947) attempted to quantify AVP release in dogs from the quantity of pitui-tary extract required to produce a similar pattern of antidiuresis to that occur-ring after intracarotid injection of hypertonic saline. He found that there is a sigmoid relationship between the dose of injected solute and the antidiuretic response. O'Connor (1962) pursued these investigations using the same animal model and reported that the antidiuretic response increases very sharply with higher plasma osmotic pressures. He attributed this type of response curve to sequential recruitment of secretory units with randomly distributed stimula-tion thresholds. Robertson and coworkers have directly determined plasma AVP and osmolality in paired samples from large numbers of either normal human subjects or from rats over wide ranges of hydration. They have pro-posed that a linear relationship exists between plasma AVP and osmolality (Robertson and Athar, 1976; Dunn et al., 1973). This relationship appears to be remarkably consistent in a given individual over time, but may vary substan-tially among normal subjects (Robertson, 1977). Robertson and colleagues have reported that the x intercept of this relationship (which they have designated the osmotic threshold) can be shifted to the left or to the right by the presence of hypovolemia or hypervolemia while the slope of the relationship remains unchanged (Fig. 6.3; Robertson et al., 1976). These observations suggest that volume changes do not override osmolar control of AVP secretion, but merely raise or lower the level of plasma osmolality required to initiate AVP secretion without changing the subsequent responsiveness to changes in osmolality (gain).

Weitzman and Fisher (1977) analysed the relationship between "integrated plasma AVP concentration" and plasma osmolality in sheep. Results of earlier studies of AVP determinations collected serially at three-minute intervals dur-ing osmotic stimulation reveal a peak-and-valley pattern suggestive of episodic secretion (Weitzman et al., 1977b). They attempted to minimize this variation by determining "integrated" plasma AVP concentrations (measured as the mean of ten samples collected over a 30-minute period under various condi-tions of hydration). They found that IpAVP varied as an exponential function of plasma osmolality such that $\log \mathrm{IpAVP} = \lambda \mathrm{pOsm} + b$ where λ is the re-sponse slope and b is the y intercept. The log linear model predicted that IpAVP would increase by a constant log quantity (fold change above baseline) for any given increment in plasma osmolality irrespective of the baseline values. Furthermore, this model provides an alternative to the critical osmolal-ity (or threshold) concept for AVP secretion since a progressive logarithmic increase in IpAVP with increasing osmolality would have the appearance of a

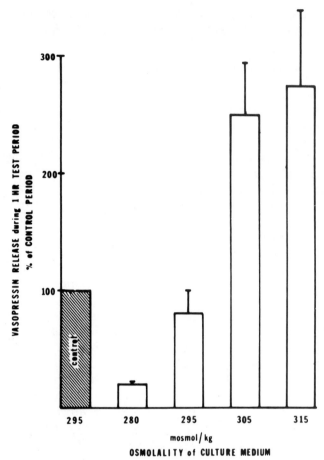

Figure 6.2   A. Effect of alterations in bath osmolality on AVP release from organ cultured rat hypothalamic-neurohypophyseal units. Hypoosmolality significantly depresses and hyperosmolality significantly increases AVP release.

threshold when viewed in the conventional manner. The data presented by these authors, however, was insufficient to determine with certainty whether or not such a threshold exists. Subsequent studies by these authors showed that infusion of hypertonic saline to both randomly hydrated and water-loaded sheep produces differing increments in the absolute concentrations of IpAVP while the log IpAVP responses are not significantly different, further supporting the log linear model (Weitzman and Fisher, 1977).

Leake et al. (1978) have extended these studies to newborn lambs and have found that the osmotic responsiveness (defined by the stimulus response ratio, Δ log plasma AVP/Δ plasma osmolality) to either infusion of hypertonic saline or hypotonic dextrose in water is remarkably similar to that in adults. Similar studies by Weitzman et al. (1978a) employing osmotic stimulation in fetal sheep have shown that the stimulus response ratio is actually enhanced relative to the response ratios of newborn or adult sheep. The explanation for this enhanced fetal AVP responsiveness is not clear. It is possible that either rela-

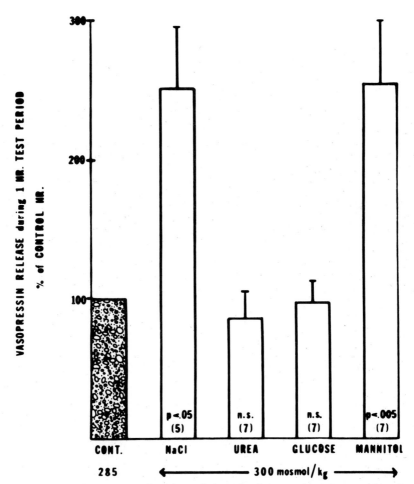

Figure 6.2 (*continued*)   B. Equimolar solutions of NaCl and mannitol have comparable effects on AVP release while urea and glucose do not stimulate AVP release. (From Sladek and Knigge, 1978, reproduced with permission.)

tive fetal hypovolemia or the elevated fetal angiotensin II levels may alter osmotic responsiveness. These studies suggested that the hypothalamic-neurohypophyseal system is functionally mature by at least the last third of gestation.

In summary, alterations in plasma tonicity have a major effect on AVP secretion. Most evidence is consistent with Verney's original hypothesis that extracellular fluid osmolality directly influences hypothalamic neurohypophysial synthesis and release of AVP.

VOLUME REGULATION

Roll of left atrial and carotid sinus baroreceptors

The basic mechanisms for volume regulation of AVP secretion have been extensively reviewed by Share (1974). Removal of blood or a reduction in blood

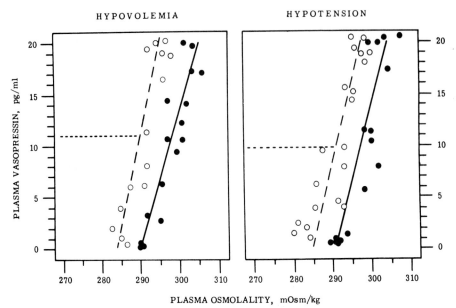

Figure 6.3 Effect of hypovolemia or hypotension on AVP release in rats. Both a decrease in blood volume or blood pressure shift the plasma AVP-plasma osmolality relationship to the left such that there is increased AVP release at any given level of plasma osmolality. The slope or gain of the relationship is unchanged. (From Robertson, Athar, and Shelton, 1976, reproduced with permission.)

pressure both result in an exponential rise in plasma levels of AVP (Robertson, 1977; Dunn et al., 1973). There is considerable evidence to suggest that two distinct baroreceptor systems mediate AVP release; low pressure stretch receptors in the left atrium responding to changes in central blood volume and high pressure baroreceptors in the carotid sinus and aortic arch responding to changes in arterial blood pressure (Share, 1967; Share, 1976; Zehr, Johnson and Moore, 1969; Claybaugh and Share, 1973). Gauer and Henry (1976) have proposed that the cardiac stretch receptors, particularly those in the left atrium, play an important role in the day-to-day regulation of extracellular fluid volume. Decreases in blood volume cause decreased stretch in these receptors (without any changes in systemic pressure) and result in stimulation of AVP secretion. The subsequent water retention then tends to restore blood volume to normal. In an extensive critique of the low pressure baroreceptor hypothesis, Goetz, Bond, and Smith (1974) have found it unconvincing. They argue that most stimuli which are supposed to influence left atrial pressure selectively also have substantial effects on systemic hemodynamics and may thus have multiple sites of action. Furthermore, they point out that the demonstration of an inverse correlation between left atrial pressure and plasma AVP levels does not prove the existence of a cause and effect relationship for AVP secretion. They pointed to the failure of plasma AVP to increase after upright posture or phlebotomy in human subjects as evidence against the view that such receptors play an important role in day-to-day regulation of volume status.

There are several recent studies in dogs employing radioimmunoassay determinations of AVP levels in plasma to assess the response of left atrial stretch receptors. These studies suggest a dissociation of low and high pressure baroreceptors in control of AVP release. DeTorrente and coworkers (1975) measured plasma AVP levels, left atrial pressure, systemic pressure, and free water clearance before and after left atrial balloon inflation. They observed a significant fall in plasma AVP levels associated with a rise in left atrial pressure but with a fall in arterial pressure. The fall in plasma AVP coincided with an increase in free water clearance. Conversely, Yaron and Bennett (1978) demonstrated that inflation of a balloon in the pulmonary artery decreases left atrial pressure and elevated plasma AVP while systemic pressure increases. Taken together, these studies demonstrate that during experimental conditions of opposing left atrial and systemic pressures, left atrial pressures appear to dominate in the effect on plasma AVP levels. However, it remains to be shown that the changes in left atrial pressure occurring under day-to-day conditions play an important role in the regulation of AVP release.

Volume regulation of AVP secretion in primates

Arnauld and associates (1977) have studied plasma AVP responses to hemorrhage in trained, conscious monkeys. In contrast to earlier studies in dogs in which nonhypotensive hemorrhage produced AVP release, these investigators found that hemorrhage stimulates AVP release only if there is an associated fall in systolic pressure. They interpreted their data as suggesting that the arterial baroreceptors rather than atrial stretch receptors are responsible for AVP release in primates. A recent report by Gilmore and Zucker (1978) provides support for the viewpoint that the low pressure baroreceptors are relatively unimportant in regulation of AVP secretion in primates. They studied the effects of balloon distension of the left atrium in monkeys and were unable to detect significant changes in salt or water excretion after balloon inflation. Their studies were carried out in anesthetized monkeys who had undergone extensive surgical preparation and changes in AVP secretion were inferred from changes in free water clearance. Nonetheless, their data and those of Arnauld et al. (1977) raise important questions about the applicability of the Gauer-Henry hypothesis to humans. There is relatively little direct data regarding volume control of AVP release in humans. Goetz et al. (1974) reported that phlebotomy of a unit of blood has no consistent effect on plasma levels of AVP or renin in normal human subjects. The failure of a 9 to 10 percent fall in blood volume to stimulate AVP release in human subjects was taken as evidence against a sensitive low-pressure baroreceptor system. There is considerable dispute as to whether upright posture, a potent stimulus to renin secretion, has any significant effect on plasma AVP. Most observers have failed to see any consistent effect of upright posture on plasma AVP in randomly hydrated subjects, although some workers have reported a significant postural elevation in dehydrated subjects (Share et al., 1972; Kimura et al., 1976; Robertson and Athar, 1976; Baylis and Heath, 1977). Segar and Moore (1968) have reported a substantial rise in plasma AVP in normal subjects with upright posture. However, subjects in their study were propped passively against a stool instead of ambulating quietly or standing still. Under such conditions pooling of blood in the lower extremities would result in a larger apparent volume deficit.

Davies, Forsling, and Slater (1977) utilized the principle of passive upright tilting as a provocative test for AVP release. They observed a significant rise in plasma AVP and renin after an 85 degree head-up tilt. It is pertinent that the peak rise in plasma AVP occurred between 30 to 45 minutes after tilting in the absence of any significant change in systolic pressure. The mechanism for AVP release under these conditions remains to be defined.

Volume factors have potent effects on AVP secretion. There is evidence supporting a role in quadripeds for cardiac stretch receptors that mediate changes in AVP secretion after small changes in blood volume but recent data suggest that in primates the effects of alterations in body fluid volume on AVP are mediated by high pressure baroreceptors in the carotid sinus and aortic arch.

INTERACTION OF OSMOLAR AND VOLUME STIMULI

Early articles on regulation of AVP secretion have contained lengthy discussions on the relative dominance of osmolar and volume factors on AVP secretion. Arndt (1965) studied the effect of a subthreshold hemorrhage (6 percent of blood volume) on the water diuresis produced by intracarotid infusion of distilled water. He found that minimal hemorrhage inhibited the water diuresis even though it had no effect on either arterial pressure or heart rate. These results were interpreted as supporting the hypothesis that the inhibitory effects of hypoosmolality on AVP secretion can be overcome by a hypovolemic stimulus. Johnson, Zehr, and Moore (1970) studied the effects of various combinations of osmolar and volume stimuli on AVP secretion, left atrial pressure, and systemic pressure in conscious sheep. They found that independent alterations in either blood volume or osmolality were capable of appropriately modifying plasma AVP levels. Concomittant alterations in osmolality and volume produced additive effects and opposing osmolar and volume stimuli had no net effect on AVP secretion. The authors concluded that neither system appeared to predominate over the other. It must be pointed out, however, that the opposing stimuli were not of equal magnitude; a 1.2 percent fall in osmolality was able to counterbalance a 10 percent fall in blood volume, suggesting greater sensitivity of the osmocontrol system.

Significant insights into the interaction of osmolar and volume stimuli were provided by the studies of Dunn et al. (1973) and Robertson and Athar (1976). The results suggested that hypovolemia sensitizes the osmoregulatory mechanism for AVP release rather than merely having an additive effect on AVP secretion. Such an interaction would permit a wide range of AVP responses to circumstances with variable degrees of opposing osmolar and volume stimuli. It is pertinent that approximately equal and opposite perturbations of osmolality and volume produce a net change in secretion dictated by the change in osmolality, whereas larger perturbations in volume can either equalize or overwhelm the opposing osmolar force (Arndt, 1965; Johnson et al., 1970; Kimura et al., 1976). Salt depletion appears to represent a physiologic circumstance in which opposing osmolar and volume forces are present. Losses of body stores of sodium produce depletion of extracellular fluid volume and, eventually, dilution of extracellular fluid tonicity (McCance, 1936). It is notable, therefore, that the relatively substantial changes in body fluid volumes seen in experimental salt depletion in humans have not been shown to elevate plasma AVP although they do produce significant increases in plasma renin activity (Share et al., 1972; Brennan and Malvin, 1977; Weitzman et al., 1977a). It was felt that this reflects the dominance of osmolar over volume homeostasis for AVP secretion; increased AVP secretion would impair water excretion and produce further dilution of extracellular fluids.

In addition to the effect of alterations of blood volume on osmotically stimulated AVP release, a recent preliminary report suggests that alterations of plasma osmolality can similarly modify AVP release occurring after hemorrhage (Weitzman et al., 1978b). Water loading, dehydration, or infusion of hypertonic saline significantly alters baseline values for plasma AVP relative to randomly hydrated controls but does not modify the increase in log AVP (i.e., fold increase from control) per unit volume of blood removed. These observations suggest that osmolar and volume factors mutually interact on AVP secretion with no one system "dominant" over the other. Osmolality may appear at times to be the predominant factor, but this is merely a reflection of the steeper relative response curve for this system. A 1 to 2 percent change in osmolality has a comparable effect on AVP secretion as that of an 8 to 10 percent change in volume (Dunn et al., 1973) (Fig. 6.4).

RENIN-ANGIOTENSIN-AVP INTERACTIONS

Renin or angiotensin have repeatedly been shown to stimulate AVP secretion after cerebroventricular administration (Mouw et al., 1971; Keil, Summy-Long and Severs, 1975; Malayan and Reid, 1976). Intravenous administration of angiotensin II has been shown to elevate plasma AVP concentrations in both humans and experimental animals, although some groups have been unable to reproduce these results (Bonjour and Malvin, 1970; Uhlich et al., 1975; Claybaugh, 1976; Ramsay et al., 1978; Cadnapaphornchai et al., 1975; Shimizu, Share, and Claybaugh, 1973). Part of the explanation for the discrepant results may lie in the observation by Claybaugh (1976) that dehydration enhances the AVP response to infusions of renin. Thus, prior water loading may have abolished or obscured the response (Cadnapaphornchai et al., 1975). Furthermore, the pressor action of angiotensin in intact animals may inhibit AVP secretion via an effect on the arterial baroreceptors (Cadnapaphornchai et al., 1975). Angiotensin does not appear to stimulate AVP secretion directly but rather augments osmotically stimulated AVP release (Shimizu et al., 1973). This augmentation is specific for osmolality and does not occur for AVP re-

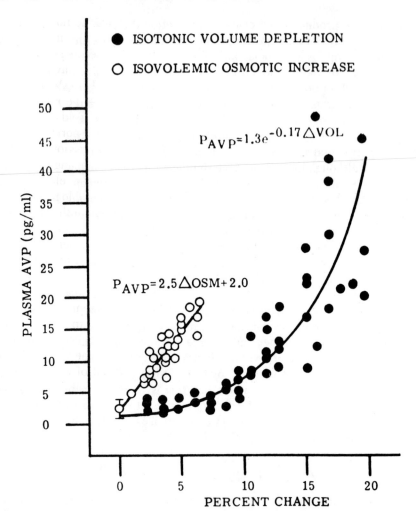

Figure 6.4   Dose response curve for changes in blood volume or osmolality upon AVP release in rats. Changes in plasma volume are considerably more potent than changes in osmolality in influencing AVP secretion. (From Dunn et al., 1973)

lease stimulated by hypovolemia or hypotension (Claybaugh and Share, 1972; Morton et al., 1977).

The physiological significance of the angiotensin effect on AVP secretion is controversial. Brennan and Malvin (1977) have proposed that elevations of plasma renin activity acting in concert with baroreceptors serve to counterbalance osmotic influences and maintain AVP secretion under conditions of sodium restriction. On the contrary, Share et al. (1972) have pointed out that both sodium depletion and upright posture are potent stimuli to renin secretion but have no consistent effect on AVP; such a dissociation argues against the renin angiotensin system playing a significant role in AVP release. Davies et al. (1977) have demonstrated that passive upright tilting is a reproducible stimulus to both AVP and renin secretion in humans. Since no significant changes in arterial blood pressure were observed after tilting, the authors speculated that the rise in plasma renin activity may play a role in mediating the rise in plasma AVP. They tested this hypothesis by means of intravenous infusions of propranolol, which abolished the renin response. The AVP response was unaffected by the propranolol infusion, suggesting that the renin-angiotensin system is not a necessary mediator for AVP release. Padfield and Morton (1977) have determined plasma AVP and angiotensin levels in normal subjects after fluid deprivation, water loading, upright posture, and angiotensin infusion and in a group of patients with pathological elevations of angiotensin II. They found that angiotensin II infusions do produce definite elevations in plasma AVP levels but only with doses that produce supraphysiological plasma levels of angiotensin II. Furthermore, no consistent relationship between plasma levels of AVP and angiotensin II could be detected in either the normal volunteers or the patients. The authors also concluded that there is no evidence to suggest that angiotensin II plays a significant role in vasopressin regulation in humans.

While there is considerable controversy regarding the significance of angiotensin in modifying AVP release, there is substantial agreement that infusions of AVP inhibit renal secretion of renin in both humans and experimental animals (Tagawa et al., 1971; Shade et al., 1973; Khokhär et al., 1976; Hesse and Nielsen, 1977). The effect on renin secretion appears to be mediated by a direct action of AVP upon the macula densa similar to that of angiotensin II (Shade et al., 1973). This observation may be of considerable clinical utility in the differential diagnosis of hyponatremic states. Patients with hyponatremia owing to salt depletion or with hyponatremia owing to cirrhosis, nephrosis, or heart failure would all be expected to have elevated levels of plasma renin activity while those with SIADH would have suppressed renin activity. (Share et al., 1972; Brennan and Malvin, 1977; Weitzman et al., 1977a; Chonko et al., 1977; Fichman, Michelakis, and Horton, 1974). This, indeed, seems to be the case. Fichman et al. (1974) have found low or undetectable levels of plasma renin activity in both patients with SIADH and in normal subjects treated with pitressin tannate in oil.

THE EFFECT OF HYPOXIA OR HYPERCAPNIA ON AVP RELEASE

Abnormalities in renal diluting ability have been observed in patients with chronic obstructive pulmonary disease, suggesting the possibility that either hypoxia or hypercapnia may influence AVP secretion (White and Woodings, 1971). A possible afferent limb for such secretion may involve the carotid chemoreceptors. Share and Levy (1966) perfused isolated carotid chemoreceptors with deoxygenated blood and demonstrated a significant rise in plasma AVP concentrations in a group of dogs that had been previously vagotomized and artificially ventilated. A similar response did not occur in another group of dogs who had been similarly perfused but were breathing spontaneously. The authors postulated that the reflex changes in ventilation and blood pressure in the latter group of animals served to counter the impulses from the perfused chemoreceptor blocking the stimulation of AVP release. They concluded that the chemoreceptors had only a weak effect upon AVP release.

Forsling and Rees (1975) studied the effect of hypoxia produced by breathing 13 percent oxygen in nitrogen and hypercapnia produced by breathing 5 percent carbon dioxide in oxygen in spontaneously ventilating anesthetized cats. They found that hypoxia produced a consistent rise in plasma AVP but hypercapnia stimulated AVP release only in those animals that experienced an increase in respiratory rate of greater than 15 percent. Berns et al. (1978) also studied the effects of hypercapnia using anesthetized dogs. They found that hypercapnic acidosis resulted in an antidiuresis associated with a significant fall in mean arterial blood pressure and a rise in plasma AVP concentration. The rise in plasma AVP levels could not be prevented when the fall in blood pressure was abolished using an intravenous infusion of norepinephrine. This suggested that baroreceptors did not mediate the response. Attempts to transpose these experiments to humans have been less successful in identifying an effect of altered ventilation on AVP release. Both Forsling and Milledge (1977) and Baylis, Stockley, and Heath (1977) failed to observe a consistent effect of hypoxia on plasma levels of AVP in normal volunteers breathing 9 to 10 percent oxygen. Farber et al. (1975, 1977) studied water handling and AVP release in hypoxic patients who had chronic obstructive lung disease and who were either normocapnic or hypercapnic. They found that the hypercapnic patients had significant impairment in their ability to excrete a water load but that this appeared to be related to enhanced renal reabsorption of bicarbonate or reduced renal blood flow rather than to abnormal elevations of plasma AVP (Farber et al., 1975). Indeed, careful studies using water loading or hypertonic saline infusion to alter plasma osmolality failed to identify any subtle disturbances in the osmotic reactivity of the two groups of patients compared to normal controls (Farber et al., 1977). Taken together, these studies do not suggest any clinically significant effects of either hypoxia or hypercapnia on neurohypophyseal function.

NOCICEPTIVE INFLUENCES ON AVP SECRETION

In 1859 Claude Bernard reported that a decrease in urine flow occurs in patients undergoing surgery. This phenomenon was investigated by Rydin and Verney (1938) who used weak faradic currents to induce pain and emotional stress in dogs. They concluded that the diminution in urine flow is most likely owing to the release of a posterior pituitary antidiuretic substance. Support for this view was provided by Hayward and Jennings (1973) who found that noxious stimuli accelerate the firing rate of neurosecretory neurons of the supraoptic nucleus, a response similar to that achieved after injection of hypertonic saline. Moreover, there is direct evidence that pain is a potent stimulus for AVP release. Moran et al. (1964) found that surgical incisions produce AVP release in patients who receive general anesthesia and are presumably not subject to emotional stress. Abdominal traction had a particularly strong effect on AVP release (Moran et al., 1964). The effect of skin incision appears to be mediated by afferents in somatic nerves while the effect of visceral manipulation is mediated by afferents in the vagus nerve. Pain of a lesser degree than general surgery can also stimulate AVP release in humans. Kendler, Weitzman, and Fisher (1978) observed a twofold elevation in plasma AVP levels in conscious patients complaining of pain in an emergency room compared to controls.

The effect of stress other than pain on AVP secretion is less certain. Brennan, Shelton, and Robertson (1975) studied the effects of three stressful situations in rats on plasma levels of AVP and corticosterone. They were unable to demonstrate any significant effects of ether stress, water immersion, or pain produced by intraperitoneal injections of isotonic saline upon plasma AVP, although all three stimuli had potent effects on plasma corticosterone. These findings were confirmed by Keil and Severs (1977) who subjected rats to both ether stress and acceleration stress (centrifugation at 4.1 × G). They found that both stresses were without effect on plasma AVP in randomly hydrated animals and actually reduced pAVP in dehydrated animals. In contrast, plasma corticosterone rose markedly after both stimuli. The dissociation between corticosterone and AVP release suggested that in rats stress sufficient to activate the hypothalamic-pituitary-adrenal axis does not provoke AVP release.

There is considerable evidence in humans, however, that severe emotional disturbances may be associated with alterations of thirst and AVP secretion. (Dubovsky et al., 1973; Raskind, Orenstein and Christopher, 1975). In a prospective study Raskind and coworkers (1978) found significantly elevated plasma AVP levels in a series of eight psychotic patients compared to either normal controls or patients with acute anxiety.

A possible explanation for the AVP release observed with psychosis and pain may be that both circumstances are associated with elevated levels of beta-endorphin, a central nervous system peptide hormone with opiate activity. Guillemin et al. (1977) have found elevated levels of beta-endorphin in the blood of rats subjected to fracture of the tibia-fibula and intracerebroventricular injection of beta-endorphin is known to produce a catatonic state in experimental animals (Bloom et al., 1976). It is therefore conceivable that elevations of endogenous beta-endorphin in either pain or psychosis may act to mediate AVP release since intravenous infusion of beta-endorphin has been shown to stimulate AVP secretion in vivo (Weitzman et al., 1977c). On the other hand, other forms of stress that produce adrenal steroid and catecholamine release may not necessarily affect AVP.

EMESIS-INDUCED AVP SECRETION

Nausea and vomiting have been known for some time to inhibit a water diuresis in experimental animals (Andersson and Larsson, 1954). Robertson

(1977) has described a paradoxical increase in plasma AVP after water loading that occurred in patients who became nauseated after ingestion of water. In subsequent studies it was found that injections of apomorphine, a potent emetic causes significant elevations of plasma AVP in humans (Shelton, Kinney, and Robertson, 1976). However, the drug has only minimal effects on AVP in rats, a species lacking an emetic reflex. These results suggest that the effect of apomorphine is mediated by afferents to the neurohypophysis from the emetic center. Hayward and Pavasuthipaisit (1976) examined the antidiuretic action of nicotine in monkeys. They found that nicotine infusion results in significant increases in plasma AVP accompanied by restlessness and retching. Pretreatment with either intravenous promethazine or diphenhydramine significantly reduces both the AVP release and the behavioral changes. The authors suggested that the action of nicotine on AVP release is likely mediated by activation of intra-abdominal vagal receptors or by a direct effect on the chemoreceptor trigger zone and that these effects can be attenuated by drugs with antiemetic activity. Taken together, these studies suggest the presence of important regulatory pathways for AVP release with afferents in the gastrointestinal tract. It should be recalled that visceral manipulation has a uniquely potent effect on AVP release during major surgery. It is possible that stimulation of these pathways may be the explanation for neurohypophyseal hormone release in some patients found to have "idiopathic" SIADH (Robertson, 1977).

THERMOREGULATION

Exposure to cold ambient temperatures characteristically produces an increase in urine volume and decrease in urine specific gravity that has been designated cold diuresis. In man this response is observed not only in adults but also in newborn infants who are cooled to ambient temperatures from the warmer environment of the uterus (Fisher, 1967). Segar and Moore (1968) determined plasma levels of AVP by bioassay in normal subjects exposed to either cold or heated environments. Sixty minutes of exposure to a temperature of 13° C produced a fall in plasma AVP from a control value of 2.2 ± 0.6 μU/ml at 26° C to 1.3 ± 0.4 μU/ml. Increased ambient temperature (50° C) for 2 hours resulted in a significant rise in plasma AVP from 1.6 ± 0.4 μU/ml to 5.2 ± 0.7 μU/ml. Neither heating nor cooling had any significant effects on plasma osmolality. The authors proposed that the effects on AVP secretion are mediated by the left atrial baroreceptors which respond to changes in central blood volume caused by peripheral vasoconstriction after cold exposure or vasodilation after heating.

Andersson and Larsson (1961) demonstrated the presence of thermosensitive areas in the anterior hypothalamus with the finding that local heating of the preoptic area in conscious goats produces enhanced water intake. Subsequently, Hayward and Baker (1968) were able to produce a typical cold diuresis in monkeys by selective chilling of the midpreoptic region of the hypothalamus and could abolish this response by infusion of vasopressin. The mechanism for this effect was not clear. The authors proposed that redistribution of blood flow occurs as the consequence of the thermoregulatory response but a direct action on the hypothalamic neurons regulating AVP secretion can not be excluded. The former hypothesis (baroreceptor mediation) needs to be reevaluated in light of the recent studies of Gilmore and Zucker (1978), which raises questions about the validity of the Gauer-Henry reflex in primates. It is therefore unlikely that changes in blood distribution after thermal stimulation will affect AVP release in primates unless there are also significant changes in systemic pressure.

Subsequent reports using environmental or localized temperature changes in other species have revealed inconsistent and occasionally contradictory results (Sadowski, Nazar, and Szczepánska-Sadowska, 1972; Szczepánska-Sadowska, 1974; Forsling, Ingram, and Stanier, 1976; Simon-Oppermann and Jessen, 1977; Sadowski, Kruk, and Chwalbínska-Moneta, 1977). From the available evidence it seems likely that alterations in body core temperature can influence AVP release, but the precise mechanism by which it does so remains to be defined.

HORMONAL INFLUENCES OF AVP SECRETION

Many hormones and neurotransmitters have been found to have substantial excitatory or inhibitory effects on AVP secretion, the details of which are described in several comprehensive reviews (Schrier and Berl, 1975; Schrier et al., 1976; McDonald et al., 1976). Many of these effects do not appear to represent unique regulatory pathways for AVP secretion and will not be discussed in this section. For example, most studies support the view that isoproterenol stimulation and norepinephrine inhibition of AVP secretion are indirect effects mediated by changes in blood pressure perceived by the baroreceptor control system (Schrier and Berl, 1975; Schrier et al., 1976). On the other hand, there is evidence that some hormones may have a direct influence on hypothalamic-posterior lobe neurosecretion similar to that described for angiotensin II. Hormone deficiency states, notably myxedema and adrenal insufficiency have been associated with elevated plasma levels of AVP (Seif et al., 1975; Seif et al., 1977; Skowsky and Fisher, 1977; Boykin et al., 1976; Mandell et al., 1977). The pathogenesis of the enhanced AVP secretion in myxedema has not been fully elucidated. Possible mechanisms include a direct effect of thyroid hormone deficiency on the supraoptic and paraventricular nuclei or baroreceptor stimulation from decreased cardiac output. The explanation for the increased plasma AVP levels in the adrenal insufficient state may be more complicated. Boykin et al. (1976) have proposed that baroreceptor stimulation owing to functional hypovolemia could result in nonosmolar stimulation of AVP. However, Mandell et al. (1977) recently reported that volume loading with a high salt diet and deoxycorticosterone acetate fails to restore defective water excretion to normal in adrenalectomized rats. Furthermore, there is evidence that glucocorticoid hormones may have a direct influence on neurosecretion. Aubrey et al. (1965) have shown that administration of cortisol increases the apparent osmotic threshold for AVP release (as detected by a fall in free water clearance) in normal subjects. Recently Stillman et al. (1977) have described increased staining of vasopressin and its neurophysin in the zona externa of the median eminence of adrenalectomized rats. This pattern of staining was inhibited by treatment with glucocorticoids and was not observed in a control group of rats subjected to water deprivation for 5 days. These observations suggest that glucocorticoids regulate the content of vasopressin in a specific neurosecretory pathway extending from the neurosecretory nuclei to the origin of the hypothalamo-hypophyseal portal system. Since it has previously been shown that high concentrations of AVP are present in portal blood and AVP is known to influence ACTH (Zimmerman et al., 1973; Yates et al., 1971) secretion, it is reasonable to speculate that a negative feedback loop exists such that a fall in plasma cortisol causes increased AVP secretion into the hypothalamo-hypophyseal portal system, which in turn enhances the secretion of ACTH.

Many drugs are also known to influence AVP secretion, but there is relatively limited information about their specific site of action (Miller and Moses, 1976). There is no evidence at the present time to suggest the existence of additional regulatory pathways to mediate these effects.

DISTRIBUTION AND METABOLISM

After being released by the neural lobe, or after intravenous injection, AVP is rapidly distributed into a volume that is larger than plasma volume (Forsling et al., 1973; Wilson, Weitzman, and Fisher, 1978). The pattern of disappearance follows a biexponential pattern with a half-life ranging from 6 to 9 minutes in humans (Skowsky, Rosenbloom, and Fisher, 1974; Beardwell et al., 1975; Morton, Padfield, and Forsling, 1975). There is evidence that AVP is not bound to plasma proteins; rather it appears to be rapidly bound to an extravascular pool that may consist, in part, of the biological receptors for the hormone (Brook and Share, 1966; Shimamoto et al., 1977; Weitzman and Fisher, 1978). AVP is also detected in lymph and cerebrospinal fluid, but the latter is due to neurosecretory pathways terminating in the third ventricle (Brook and Share, 1966; Dogterom, van Wimersma Greidanus and Swaab, 1978).

AVP is metabolized in roughly equal fractions by the liver and kidneys (Lauson, 1974; Share, Shade and Rabkin, 1978). The renal clearance persists after ureteral ligation and appears to be in large measure independent of glomerular filtration (Share et al., 1978). Both renal and total body removal of AVP are saturable with diminished clearance observed with higher plasma levels. These and other data suggest that the clearance of the hormone may be, in part, related to its biological action (Levi, Rosenfield and Kleeman, 1974; Weitzman and Fisher, 1978).

A circulating enzyme, cystine aminopeptidase, is present in the plasma of pregnant primates and is capable of rapidly inactivating vasopressin (and oxytocin) in vitro (Rosenbloom, Sack, and Fisher, 1975). Its impact on overall hormone turnover in intact animals is not known but increased vasopressin requirements are occasionally noted during pregnancy in patients with diabetes insipidus (Phelan, Guay, and Newman, 1978). The plasma of orders other than primates also is capable of degrading AVP but at a considerably slower rate (Wilson et al., 1978). The direct plasma degradation of AVP in nonpregnant primates does not significantly contribute to total hormone turnover, but it does warrant special handling of plasma samples for either bio- or immunoassay.

The rapid half-life and extensive distribution of AVP limit the ability to infer very much about moment-to-moment secretion rates from a single plasma sample, particularly after acute stimulation. Serial determinations of plasma AVP concentrations can be collected and the mean value determined to better approximate neurosecretion.

SUMMARY

Neurohypophyseal secretion of arginine vasopressin represents the algebraic sum of multiple influences, the most potent being the osmosensitive cells of the hypothalamus. Body fluids also play a major role through their effects on central blood volume sensed by left atrial stretch receptors and arterial blood pressure sensed by baroreceptors in the aortic arch and carotid sinus. Recent evidence has led to reservations about the importance of the left atrial stretch receptors as a mechanism for regulation of water balance in primates. Volume factors appear to interact with osmolar factors in regulating AVP secretion. The renin-angiotensin system has been shown to have significant effects upon neurohypophyseal hormone release, but the physiological significance of this pathway has been questioned. Hypoxia and hypercapnia can also influence AVP secretion partially through effects on carotid chemoreceptors, but these effects are relatively mild and are clinically insignificant. Noxious stimuli and emesis may stimulate AVP release, but stress apparently does not, at least in rats. There is some evidence that thermosensitive cells in the hypothalamus can initiate AVP release but such an effect cannot be dissociated from temperature-induced changes in central blood volume. Finally, several hormones, notably cortisol, may have direct effects on the hypothalamic neurohypophyseal system to influence AVP release. AVP is cleared rapidly from blood and is metabolized largely in the liver.

ACKNOWLEDGMENT

Supported by grants MG 2472 from the American Heart Association and HD 09690 from NICHD.

Dr. Delbert Fisher and Dr. Richard Glassock graciously reviewed the manuscript. Mrs. Rita Kemp provided expert secretarial assistance.

REFERENCES

Andersson, B. & Larsson, S. (1954). Inhibitory effects of emesis on water diuresis in the dog. *Acta Physiologica Scandinavica*, **32**, 19–27.
Andersson, B. & Larsson, B. (1961). Influence of local temperature changes in the preoptic area and rostral hypothalamus on the regulation of food and water intake. *Acta Physiologica Scandinavica*, **52**, 75–89.

Andersson, B. & Olsson, K. (1977). Evidence for periventricular sodium-sensitive receptors of importance in the regulation of ADH secretion. In *Neurohypophysis*, ed. Moses, A.M. & Share, L. Pp. 118–127. Basel: S. Karger.

Andersson, B. & Westbye, O. (1970). Syntergistic action of sodium and angiotensin on brain mechanisms controlling fluid balance. *Life Sciences*, 9, 601–608.

Arnauld, E., Czernichow, P., Fumoux, F. & Vincent, J. D. (1977). The effects of hypotension and hypovolemia on the liberation of vasopressin during hemorrhage in the unanesthetized monkey. *Pflügers Archiv* 371, 193–200.

Arndt, J. O. (1965). Diuresis induced by water infusion into the carotid loop and its inhibition by small hemorrhage. *Pflügers Archiv* 282, 313–322.

Aubrey, R. H., Nankin, H. R., Moses, A. M. & Streeten, D. H. P. (1965). Measurement of the osmotic threshold for vasopressin release in human subjects and its modification by cortisol. *Journal of Clinical Endocrinology and Metabolism*, 25, 1481–1492.

Baylis, P. H. & Heath, D. A. (1977). Influence of presyncope and postural change upon plasma arginine vasopressin concentrations in hydrated and dehydrated man. *Clinical Endocrinology*, 7, 79–83.

Baylis, P. H., Stockley, R. A. & Heath, D. A. (1977). Effects of acute hypoxaemia on plasma arginine vasopressin in conscious man. *Clinical Science and Molecular Medicine*, 53, 401–404.

Beardwell, C. G., Geelen, G., Palmer, H. M., Roberts, D. & Salmanson, L. (1975). Radioimmunoassay of plasma vasopressin in physiological and pathological states in man. *Journal of Endocrinology*, 67, 189–202.

Bernard, C. (1859). Lecons sur les propriétés physiologiques et les altérations pathologiques des liquides de l'organisme. *Paris: J.B. Ballière et fils*, pp. 297–298.

Berns, A. S., Arnold, P. E., McDonald, K. M. & Anderson, R. J. (1978). Effect of hypercapnic acidosis on renal water excretion. *Clinical Research*, 26, 138A.

Bloom, F., Segal, D., Ling, N. & Guillemin, R. (1976). Endorphins: Profound behavioral effects in rats suggest new etiological factors in mental illness. *Science*, 194, 630–632.

Bonjour, J. P. & Malvin, R. L. (1970). Stimulation of ADH by the renin angiotensin system. *American Journal of Physiology*, 218, 1555–1559.

Boykin, J., McCool, A., McDonald, K., Robertson, G. & Schrier, R. W. (1976). Mechanism of effect of glucocorticoid deficiency on renal water excretion in the conscious dog. *Clinical Research*, 24, 269A.

Brennan, L. A. & Malvin, R. L. (1977). Concentrations of antidiuretic hormone in plasma during human sodium restriction. *Nephron*, 19, 284–287.

Brennan, T. C., Shelton, R. L. & Robertson, G. L. (1975). Effect of stress on plasma vasopressin and corticosterone in rats. *Clinical Research*, 23, 234A.

Brook, A. H. & Share, L. (1966). On the question of protein binding and the diffusibility of circulating antidiuretic hormone in the dog. *Journal of Clinical Endocrinology and Metabolism*, 78, 779–785.

Cadnapaphornchai, P., Boykin, P., Harbottle, J. A., McDonald, K. M. & Schrier, R. W. (1975). Effect of angiotensin II on renal water excretion. *American Journal of Physiology*, 228, 155–159.

Chonko, A. M., Bay, W. H., Stein, J. H. & Fenis, T. F. (1977). The role of renin and aldosterone in the salt retention of edema. *American Journal of Medicine*, 63, 881–889.

Claybaugh, J. R. (1976). Effect of dehydration on stimulation of ADH release by heterologous renin infusions in conscious dogs. *American Journal of Physiology*, 231, 655–660.

Claybaugh, J. R. & Share, L. (1972). Role of the renin angiotensin system in the vasopressin response to hemorrhage. *Endocrinology*, 90, 453–460.

Claybaugh, J. R. & Share, L. (1973). Vasopressin, renin, and cardiovascular responses to continuous slow hemorrhage. *American Journal of Physiology*, 224, 519–523.

Davies, R., Forsling, M. L. & Slater, J. D. H. (1977). The interrelationship between the release of renin and vasopressin as defined by orthostasis and propranalol. *Journal of Clinical Investigation*, 60, 1438–1441.

DeTorrente, A., Robertson, G. L., McDonald, K. M. & Schrier, R. W. (1975). Mechanism of diuretic response to increased left atrial pressure in the anesthetized dog. **Kidney International**, 8, 355–361.

DeWied, D. (1971). Long term effect of vasopressin on the maintenance of a conditioned avoidance response in rats. *Nature* (London), 232, 58.

Dogterom, J., van Wimersma Greidanus, Tj. B. & Swaab, D. F. (1977). Evidence for the release of vasopressin and oxytocin into cerebrospinal fluid measurements in plasma and CSF of intact and hypophysectomized rats. *Neuroendocrinology,* **24**(2), 108–118.

Dubovsky, S. L., Grabon, S., Berl, T. & Schrier, R. W. (1973). Syndrome of inappropriate secretion of antidiuretic hormone with exacerbated psychosis. *Annals of Internal Medicine,* **79**, 551–554.

Dunn, F. L., Brennan, T. J., Nelson, A. E. & Robertson, G. L. (1973). The role of blood osmolality and volume in regulating vasopressin in the rat. *Journal of Clinical Investigation,* **52**, 3212–3219.

Farber, M. O., Bright, T. P., Strawbridge, R. A., Robertson, G. L. & Manfredi, F. (1975). Impaired water handling in chronic obstructive lung disease. *Journal of Laboratory and Clinical Medicine,* **85**, 41–49.

Farber, M. O., Kiblawi, S. S. O., Strawbridge, R. A., Robertson, G. L., Weinberger, M. H. & Manfredi, F. (1977). Studies on plasma vasopressin and the renin-angiotensin-aldosterone system in chronic obstructive lung disease. *Journal of Laboratory and Clinical Medicine,* **90**, 373–380.

Fichman, M. P., Michelakis, A. M. & Horton, R. (1974). Regulation of aldosterone in the syndrome of inappropriate antidiuretic hormone secretion (SIADH). *Journal of Clinical Endocrinology and Metabolism,* **39**, 136–144.

Fisher, D. A. (1967). Cold diuresis in the newborn. *Pediatrics,* **40**, 636–641.

Forsling, M. L., Ingram, D. I. & Stanier, M. W. (1976). Effects of various ambient temperatures and of heating and cooling the hypothalamus and cervical spinal cord on antidiuretic hormone secretion and urinary osmolality in pigs. *Journal of Physiology,* **257**, 673–686.

Forsling, M. L., Martin, M. J., Sturdy, J. C. & Burton, A. M. (1973). Observations on the release and clearance of neurophysin and the neurohypophyseal hormones in the rat. *Journal of Endocrinology,* **57**, 307–315.

Forsling, M. L. & Milledge, J. S. (1977). Effect of hypoxia on vasopressin release in man. *Journal of Physiology,* **247**, 22P–23P.

Forsling, M. L. & Rees, M. (1975). Effects of hypoxia and hypercapnia on plasma vasopressin concentration. *Journal of Endocrinology,* **63**, 579–580.

Gauer, O. H. & Henry, J. P. (1976). Neurohormonal control of plasma volume. In *International Review of Physiology, Cardiovascular Physiology II,* ed. Guyton, A. C. & Cowley, A. W., Vol. 9, pp. 145–191, Baltimore: University Park Press.

Gilmore, J. P. & Zucker, I. H. (1978). Failure of left atrial distention to alter renal function in the nonhuman primate. *Circulation Research,* **42**, 267–270.

Goetz, K. L., Bond, G. C. & Bloxam, D. D. (1975). Atrial receptors and renal function. *Physiological Reviews,* **55**, 157–205.

Goetz, K. L., Bond, G. C. & Smith, W. E. (1974). Effect of moderate hemorrhage in humans on plasma ADH and renin. *Proceedings of the Society for Experimental Biology and Medicine,* **145**, 277–280.

Guillemin, R., Vargo, T., Rossier, J., Minick, S., Ling, N., Rivier, C., Vale, W. & Bloom, F. (1977). β-endorphin and adrenocorticotropin are secreted concomittantly by the pituitary gland. *Science,* **197**, 1367–1369.

Hayward, J. N. & Baker, M. A. (1968). Diuretic and thermoregulatory responses to preoptic cooling in the monkey. *American Journal of Physiology,* **214**, 843–850.

Hayward, J. N. & Jennings, D. P. (1973). Influenced sleepwalking and nociceptor induced behavior on the activity of supraoptic neurons in the hypothalamus of the monkey. *Brain Research,* **57**, 461–466.

Hayward, J. N. & Pavasuthipaisit, K. (1976). Vasopressin released by nicotine in the monkey. *Neuroendocrinology,* **21**, 120–129.

Hesse, B. & Nielsen, J. (1977). Suppression of plasma renin activity by intravenous infusion of antidiuretic hormone in man. *Clinical Science and Molecular Medicine,* **52**, 357–360.

Johnson, A., Zehr, J. E. & Moore, W. W. (1970). Effects of separate and concurrent osmotic and volume stimuli on plasma ADH in sheep. *American Journal of Physiology,* **218**, 1273–1280.

Keil, L. C. & Severs, W. B. (1977). Reduction in plasma vasopressin levels of dehydrated rats following acute stress. *Endocrinology,* **100**, 30–38.

Keil, L. C., Summy-Long, J. & Severs, W. B. (1975). Release of vasopressin by angiotensin II. *Endocrinology,* **96**, 1063–1064.

Kendler, K. L., Weitzman, R. E. & Fisher, D. A. (1978). The effect of pain on plasma arginine vasopressin concentrations in man. *Clinical Endocrinology*, **8**, 89–94.

Khokhär, A. M., Slater, J. D. H., Forsling, M. L. & Payne, N. N. (1976). Effect of vasopressin on plasma volume and renin release in man. *Clinical Science and Molecular Medicine*, **50**, 415–424.

Kimura, T., Minai, K., Matsui, K., Mouri, T., Sata, T., Yoshinaga, K. & Hoshi, T. (1976). Effect of various states of hydration on plasma ADH and renin in man. *Journal of Clinical Endocrinology and Metabolism*, **42**, 79–87.

Lauson, H. D. (1974). Metabolism of the neurohypophyseal hormones. In *Handbook of Physiology*, Section 7: Endocrinology, Vol. 4, Part I, The Pituitary Gland and Its Neuroendocrine Control, ed. Knobil, E. & Sawyer, W. H., pp. 287–393. Washington, D.C.: American Physiological Society.

Leake, R. L., Weitzman, R. E., Weinberg, J. A. & Fisher, D. A. (1979). Control of vasopressin secretion in the newborn lamb. *Pediatric Research*, **13**, 257–260.

Levi, J., Rosenfield, S. & Kleeman, C. R. (1974). Inactivation of arginine vasopressin by the isolated perfused rabbit kidney. *Journal of Endocrinology*, **62**, 1–10.

Malayan, S. A. & Reid, I. A. (1976). Antidiuresis produced by injection of renin into the third cerebral ventricle of the dog. *Endocrinology*, **98**, 329–335.

Mandell, I., DeFronzo, R., Robertson, G. & Forrest, J. N. (1977). Incomplete suppression of plasma arginine vasopressin during water diuresis. In *Glucocorticoid Deficiency Program* of The Annual Meeting of the American Society of Nephrology, pp. 114A.

McCance, R. A. (1936). Experimental sodium chloride deficiency in man. *Proceedings of the Royal Society of London, Section B*, **119**, 245–268.

McDonald, K. M., Miller, P. D., Anderson, R. J., Berl, T. & Schrier, R. (1976). Hormonal control of renal water excretion. *Kidney International*, **10**, 38–45.

Miller, M. & Moses, A. M. (1976). Drug-induced states of impaired water excretion. *Kidney International*, **10**, 96–103.

Moran, W. H., Jr., Miltenberger, F. W., Shuáyb, W. A. & Zimmerman, B. (1964). Relationship of antidiuretic hormone secretion to surgical stress. *Surgery*, **56**, 99–108.

Morton, J. J., Padfield, P. L. & Forsling, M. L. (1975). A radioimmunoassay for plasma arginine vasopressin in man and dog, applications to physiological and pathological states. *Journal of Endocrinology*, **65**, 411–424.

Morton, J. J., Semple, P. F., Ledingham, I. McA., Stuart, B., Tehrani, M. A., Garcia, A. R. & McGarrity, G. (1977). Effect of angiotensin-converting enzyme inhibitor (SQ20881) on the plasma concentration of angiotensin I, angiotensin II and arginine vasopressin in the dog during hemorrhagic shock. *Circulation Research*, **41**, 301–308.

Moses, A. M. & Miller, M. (1974). Osmotic influences on the release of vasopressin. In *Handbook of Physiology*, Section 7: Endocrinology, Vol. 4, Part I, The Pituitary Gland and Its Neuroendocrine Control, ed. Knobil, E. & Sawyer, W. H. Pp. 225–242. Washington, D.C., American Physiological Society.

Mouw, D., Bonjour, J. P., Malvin, R. L. & Vander, A. (1971). Central action of angiotensin in stimulating ADH release. *American Journal of Physiology*, **220**, 239–242.

O'Connor, W. J. (1962). Release of antidiuretic hormone from the neurohypophysis. In *Renal Function*. P. 59. London: Arnold.

Padfield, P. L. & Morton, J. J. (1977). Effects of angiotensin II on arginine-vasopressin in physiological and pathological situations in man. *Journal of Endocrinology*, **74**, 251–259.

Phelan, J. P., Guay, A. T. & Newman, C. (1978). Diabetes insipidus. In *Pregnancy, A Case Review. American Journal of Obstetrics and Gynecology*, **130**, 365–366.

Ramsay, D. J., Keil, L. C., Sharpe, M. C. & Shinsako, J. (1978). Angiotensin II infusion increases vasopressin ACTH and II-hydroxycorticosteroid secretion. *American Journal of Physiology*, **234**, R66–R71.

Raskind, M. A., Orenstein, H. & Christopher, T. G. (1975). Acute psychosis, increased water ingestion and inappropriate antidiuretic hormone secretion. *American Journal of Psychiatry*, **132**, 907–910.

Raskind, M. A., Weitzman, R. E., Orenstein, H., Fisher, D. A. & Courtney, N. (1978). Antidiuretic hormone is elevated in psychosis. *Biological Psychiatry*, **13**, 385–390.

Robertson, G. L. (1977). The regulation of vasopressin function in health and disease. *Recent Progress in Hormone Research*, **33**, 333–385.

Robertson, G. L. & Athar, S. (1976). The interaction of blood osmolality and blood volume in regulating plasma vasopressin in man. *Journal of Clinical Endocrinology and Metabolism*, **42**, 613–620.

Robertson, G. L., Athar, S. & Shelton, R. L. (1976). The osmoregulation of vasopressin. *Kidney International*, **10**, 25–37.

Rosenbloom, A. A., Sack, J. & Fisher, D. A. (1975). The circulating vasopressinase of pregnancy: Species comparison with radioimmunoassay. *American Journal of Obstetrics and Gynecology*, **121**, 316–320.

Rydin, H. & Verney, E. G. (1938). The inhibition of water diuresis by emotional stress and by muscular exercise. *Quarterly Journal of Experimental Physiology and Cognate Medical Sciences*, **27**, 343–374.

Sadowski, J., Kruk, B. & Chwalbínska-Moneta (1977). Renal function changes during preoptic-anterior hypothalamic heating in the rabbit. *Pflügers Archiv*, **370**, 51–57.

Sadowski, J., Nazar, K. & Szczepánska-Sadowska, E. (1972). Reduced urine concentration in dogs exposed to cold; Relation to plasma ADH and 17-OHCS. *American Journal of Physiology*, **222**, 607–610.

Schrier, R. W. & Berl, T. (1975). Nonosmolar factors affecting renal water excretion. *New England Journal of Medicine*, **292**, 81–88, 141–145.

Schrier, R. W., Berl, T., Anderson, R. J. & McDonald, K. M. (1976). Humoral, neural and hemodynamic influences on renal water excretion. In *International Conference on the Neurohypophysis*, ed. Moses, A. M. & Share, L. Pp. 144–152. Basel: S. Karger.

Segar, W. E. & Moore, W. W. (1968). The regulation of antidiuretic hormone release in man. I. Effects of change in position and ambient temperature on blood ADH levels. *Journal of Clinical Investigation*, **47**, 2143–2151.

Seif, S. M., Huellmantel, A. B., Stillman, M., Recht, L. & Robinson, A. G. (1975). Neurophysin and vasopressin in the plasma and hypothalamus of adrenalectomized and normal rats. *Program of the 57th Annual Meeting of the Endocrine Society*, pp. 186.

Seif, S. M., Zenser, T. V., Huellmantel, A. B., & Davis, B. B. (1977). Elevated plasma vasopressin and impaired renal cyclic nucleotide generation in myxedematous rats. *Endocrinology (Supplement)*, **100**, 243.

Shade, R. E., Davis, J. O., Johnson, J. A., Gotshall, R. W. & Spielman, W. S. (1973). Mechanism of action of angiotensin II and antidiuretic hormone on renin secretion. *American Journal of Physiology*, **224**, 926–929.

Share, L. (1967). Role of peripheral receptors in the increased release of vasopressin in response to hemorrhage. *Endocrinology*, **81**, 1140–1146.

Share, L. (1974). Blood pressure, blood volume, and the release of vasopressin. In Handbook of Physiology, Section 7: Endocrinology, Vol. IV, Part I, *The Pituitary Gland and Its Neuroendocrine Control*, ed. Knobil, E. & Sawyer, W. H. Pp. 243–255. Washington, D.C. American Physiological Society.

Share, L. (1976). Role of cardiovascular receptors in the control of ADH release. *Cardiology* (Supplement), **61**, 51–64.

Share, L., Claybaugh, J. R., Hatch, F. E., Johnson, J. G., Lee, S., Muirhead, E. E. & Shaw, P. (1972). Effects of change in posture and of sodium depletion on plasma levels of vasopressin and renin in normal human subjects. *Journal of Clinical Endocrinology and Metabolism*, **35**, 171–174.

Share, L. & Levy, M. (1966). Effect of carotid chemoreceptor stimulation on plasma antidiuretic hormone titer. *American Journal of Physiology*, **210**, 157–161.

Share, L., Shade, R. E. & Rabkin, R. (1978). Studies on the metabolism of vasopressin with emphasis on the role of the kidney. In *Neurohypophysis*, ed. Moses, A. M. and Share, L. Basel: S. Karger.

Shelton, R. L., Kinney, R. M. & Robertson, G. L. (1976). Emesis: A species-specific stimulus for vasopressin (AVP) release. *Clinical Research*, **24**, 531A.

Shimamoto, K., Ando, T., Nakao, T., Watorai, I. & Miyahara, M. (1977). Permeability of antidiuretic hormone and other hormones through the dialysis membranes in patients undergoing hemodialysis. *Journal of Clinical Endocrinology and Metabolism*, **45**, 818–820.

Shimizu, K., Share, L. & Claybaugh, J. R. (1973). Potentiation by angiotensin II of the vasopressin response to an increasing plasma osmolality. *Endocrinology*, **93**, 42–50.

Simon-Oppermann, C. & Jessen, C. (1977). Antidiuretic responses to thermal stimulation of hypothalamus spinal cord in the conscious goat. *Pflügers Archiv*, **368**, 33–37.

Skowsky, W. R. & Fisher, D. A. (1977). Arginine vasopressin secretion in thyroidectomized sheep. *Endocrinology*, **100**, 1022–1026.

Skowsky, W. R., Rosenbloom, A. A. & Fisher, D. A. (1974). Radioimmunoassay measurement of arginine vasopressin in serum, development and application. *Journal of Clinical Endocrinology and Metabolism*, **38**, 278–287.

Sladek, C. D. & Knigge, K. M. (1977). Osmotic control of vasopressin release by rat hypo-thalamo-neurohypophyseal explants in organ culture. *Endocrinology*, **101**, 1834–1838.

Stillman, M. A., Recht, L. D., Rosario, S. L., Seif, S. M., Robinson, A. G. & Zimmerman, E. A. (1977). The effects of adrenalectomy and glucocorticoid replacement on vasopressin and vasopressin neurophysin in the zona externa of the median eminence of the rat. *Endocrinology*, **101**, 42–49.

Szczepánska-Sadowska, E. (1974). Plasma ADH increase and thirst suppression elicited by preoptic heating in the dog. *American Journal of Physiology*, **226**, 155–161.

Tagawa, H., Vander, A. J., Bonjour, J. P. & Malvin, R. L. (1971). Inhibition of renin secretion by vasopressin secretion in unanesthetized sodium-deprived dogs. *American Journal of Physiology*, **220**, 949–951.

Uhlich, E., Weber, P., Eigler, J. & Gröshel-Stewart, U. (1975). Angiotensin stimulated AVP-release in humans. *Klinische Wochenschrift*, **53**, 177–180.

VanRee, J. M. & DeWied, D. (1977). Effect of neurohypophyseal hormones on morphine de-pendence. *Psychoneuroendocrinology*, **2**, 35–41.

Verney, E. B. (1947). Croonian lecture: The antidiuretic hormone and the factors which de-termine its release. *Proceedings, Royal Society of London*, **135**, 25–105.

Weitzman, R. E., Farnsworth, L., MacPhee, R., Wang, C. & Bennett, C. M. (1977a). The ef-fect of opposing osmolar and volume factors on plasma arginine vasopressin in man. *Mineral Electrolyte Metabolism*, **1**, 43–47.

Weitzman, R. E. & Fisher, D. A. (1977). Log linear relationship between plasma arginine vasopressin and plasma osmolality. *American Journal of Physiology*, **233**, E37–E40.

Weitzman, R. E. & Fisher, D. A. (1978). Arginine vasopressin metabolism in dogs. I. Evi-dence for receptor mediated mechanism. *American Journal of Physiology*, **235**, E591–E597.

Weitzman, R. E., Fisher, D. A., DiStefano, J. J. & Bennett, C. M. (1977b). Episodic secretion of arginine vasopressin. *American Journal of Physiology*, **233**, E32–E36.

Weitzman, R. E., Fisher, D. A., Minick, S., Ling, N. & Guillemin, R. (1977c). β-endorphin stimulates secretion of arginine vasopressin *in vivo*. *Endocrinology*, **101**, 1643–1646.

Weitzman, R. E., Fisher, D. A., Robillard, J., Erenberg, A., Kennedy, R. & Smith, F. (1978a). Arginine vasopressin response to an osmotic stimulus in the fetal sheep. *Pediatric Research*, **12**, 35–38.

Weitzman, R. E., Reviczky, A., Oddie, T. H. & Fisher, D. A. (1978b). The effect of blood pressure and plasma osmolality on arginine vasopressin release following hemorrhage. *Clinical Research*, **26**, 314A.

White, R. J. & Woodings, D. F. (1971). Impaired water handling in chronic obstructive air-way disease. *British Medical Journal*, **2**, 561–563.

Wilson, K. L., Weitzman, R. E. & Fisher, D. A. (1978). Arginine vasopressin metabolism in dogs: II, modeling and system analysis. *American Journal of Physiology*, **235**, E598–E605.

Yaron, M., Bennett, C. M. (1978). Mechanism of impaired water excretion in acute right ventricular failure in conscious dogs. *Circulation Research*, **42**(6), 801–805.

Yates, F. E., Russell, S. M., Dallman, M. F., Hedge, G. A., McCann, S. M. & Dhariwal, A. P. (1971). Potentiation by vasopressin of corticotropin release induced by corticotropin re-leasing factor. *Endocrinology*, **88**, 3–11.

Zehr, J. E., Johnson, J. A. & Moore, W. W. (1969). Left atrial pressure, plasma osmolality and ADH levels in the unanesthetized ewe. *American Journal of Physiology*, **217**, 1672–1680.

Zimmerman, E. A., Carmel, P. W., Husain, M. K., Ferin, M., Tannerbaum, M., Frantz, A. G. & Robinson, A. G. (1973). Vasopressin and neurophysin, high concentrations in monkey hypophyseal portal blood. *Science*, **182**, 925–927.

Zusman, R. M. & Keiser, H. R. (1977). Prostaglandin E_2 biosynthesis by rabbit renomedul-lary interstitial cells in tissue culture; Mechanisms of stimulation by angiotensin II, brady-kinin, and arginine vasopressin. *Journal of Biological Chemistry*, **151**, 2069–2071.

7

Physiologic and metabolic effects of parathyroid hormone

EDUARDO SLATOPOLSKY
KEITH HRUSKA
KEVIN MARTIN
JEFFREY FREITAG

INTRODUCTION

Parathyroid hormone (PTH), in conjunction with vitamin D, is responsible for the maintenance of calcium homeostasis in living organisms. Perturbations of parathyroid gland function may produce severe changes in plasma calcium that may be fatal in some circumstances. Major advances in our understanding of the synthesis, biochemistry, and metabolism of parathyroid hormone have been made in the past decade. With the development of radioimmunoassays for parathyroid hormone, specific for certain regions of the PTH molecule, the fate of the circulating PTH in blood has been partially clarified. Recent evidence suggests that the kidney, liver, and skeleton are the major sites of PTH degradation.

Glandular production of PTH and its precursors

Recently (Cohn et al., 1972; Habener et al., 1972 and Hamilton et al., 1974) it has been shown that parathyroid hormone, a single-chain polypeptide containing 84 amino acids, is synthesized within the parathyroid gland from a biosynthetic precursor, a prohormone known as pro-PTH. Pro-PTH has an extra six amino acids added to the NH_2-terminus of the PTH 1–84 molecule. The sequence of the hexapeptide has been determined by the automated degradation procedure of Edman and Begg (1967). The prohormone is heavily basic, four of the six additional amino acids are positively charged (3 lysine, 1 arginine). The content of pro-PTH within the bovine parathyroid gland has been established to be less than 10 percent of that of PTH and its biological activity in a bioassay system is greatly reduced when compared with the potency of PTH (Cohn et al., 1972). Pro-PTH is synthesized in the rough endoplasmic reticulum (RER) of the chief cells in the parathyroid glands. Pro-PTH is converted to PTH by proteolytic cleavage in approximately 20 min. (Kemper et al., 1972; Habener et al., 1974) in the Golgi apparatus. So far there is no good evidence that pro-PTH is present in circulating blood; however, pathological conditions such as adenomas may be responsible for the secretion of pro-PTH along with the hormone. Martin, Greenbert, and Michelangeli (1973) suggested that pro-PTH was secreted in the media of culture cells derived from human PTH adenoma. The storage form of PTH 1–84 is packaged in secretory granules that take several hours to mature. There is evidence to suggest that a portion of the newly synthesized PTH may be secreted without equilibration in the pool of secretory granules (MacGregor, Hamilton, and Cohn, 1975). It would seem that the transfer of the prohormone from the RER to the Golgi region is independent of the synthesis of the prohormone and its conversion to the hormone. The translocation process requires metabolic energy and appears to be mediated by microtubules. Kemper et al. (1975) have studied PTH biosynthesis in bovine gland slices incubated in vitro in the presence of either colchicine or vinblastine, drugs that disrupt the microtubules. Although conversion of pro-PTH to PTH is delayed in the presence of colchicine or vinblastine, this effect was only partial and can be overcome with prolonged incubations. Studies performed in our laboratory in the rat (Chanard et al., 1977), using pharmacological doses of colchicine or vinblastine, clearly indicate that disruption of the microtubules does not impair the release of PTH in response to a hypocalcemic stimulus. Thus, at least in the rat, the absence of microtubules does not prevent the release of PTH.

Recently, a precursor of pro-PTH called pre-pro-PTH consisting of a 25 amino acid sequence covalently linked to the amino-terminal portion of pro-PTH has been demonstrated (Kemper et al., 1976; Habener et al., 1976). Thus, pre-pro-PTH has 115 amino acids, pro-PTH 90, and PTH 84.

The role of calcium and magnesium in the synthesis and release of PTH

Although calcium plays a key role in the secretion of PTH and changes as small as 0.1 mg/100 ml in ionized calcium are important stimuli for the release of PTH (Blum et al., 1974), it seems that the biosynthesis of pro-PTH is modified only slightly by the extracellular calcium. However, it would seem that the efficiency of conversion of pro-PTH to PTH will increase in conditions characterized by hypocalcemia. Chu et al. (1973) studied rats maintained on a low calcium diet for a period of 13 days. His studies suggest that the parathyroid glands of the rat may adapt to diets low in calcium by increasing the efficiency of conversion of pro-PTH to PTH. On the other hand, magnesium does not affect either the synthesis or the conversion of proparathyroid hormone (Hamilton et al., 1971; Habener and Potts, 1976). Magnesium has an important role in the release of parathyroid hormone. Hypermagnesemia suppresses and hypomagnesemia enhances the release of parathyroid hormone. However, severe magnesium depletion decreases the release of parathyroid hormone (Anast et al., 1972).

Biochemistry of PTH

The role of the parathyroid glands in prevention of tetany has been known since the late 19th century (MacCallum and Voegtlin, 1909). However, it was not until 1959 when Aurbach (1959) introduced important modifications to preliminary methods that high yields of active PTH were obtained. Subsequently, the extraction of PTH from parathyroid tissue was further modified by homogenization with 8 M urea HCl (Rasmussen, Sze and Young, 1964) followed by gel filtration and ion exchange chromatography on carboxymethlycellulose (CMC) (Keutman et al., 1971; Hamilton et al., 1971). Moreover, with the use of CMC columns PTH was separated from pro-PTH. Parathyroid hormone is characterized by a single-chain polypeptide devoid of cysteine with a free amino group at the amino-terminus (Potts et al., 1971). In addition, the sequence of the first 34 amino acid residues of human PTH has recently been determined in separate laboratories (Brewer et al., 1972; Niall et al., 1974). However, the sequence of human PTH 1–34 from the two laboratories differs in the amino acid residues found in positions 22, 28, and 30. Brewer et al. (1972) have found that amino acids in the positions 22, 28, and 30 are composed of glutamine, lysine, and leucine, respectively. On the other hand, Niall et al. (1974) have found glutamic acid in position 22, leucine in position 28, and asparagine in position 30. The basis for these discrepancies remains to be clarified as does the sequence of the remaining portion of the human PTH molecule. The importance of determining the correct sequence of amino acids of human PTH 1–34 is crucial for the development of antibodies to this fragment. Unfortunately, since there is a discrepancy at the present time in three of the first 34 amino acids, antibodies produced with either antigen may have varying specificities for the amino-terminal portion of the native human PTH molecule and therefore may give misleading results using RIA in humans.

Biological activity

Recently studies have shown that the interpretation of biological activity should be cautious since it depends on the method used to determine the potency of the peptide (Marcus and Aurbach, 1969; Parsons, Reit and Robinson, 1973). It seems that different results may be obtained if biological activity is measured by using the rat renal cortical adenyl cyclase system in vitro or the chick hypercalcemic response in vivo. In the chicken, the activity of the 1–34 fragment is greater on the molar basis than the native hormone. If a few amino acids are removed and the 1–28 peptide is used, it is still slightly active in the rat renal cortical adenyl cyclase system but is inactive in the chick hypercalcemic assay. On the other hand, deletion of the first amino acid (2–34 peptide) is still active in the chicken and inactive in the cyclase system. It would seem from these studies that the carboxyl two-thirds of the molecule does not have biological activity. However, because PTH has other actions that may influence immunological responses, carbohydrate metabolism, lipid metabolism, marrow fibrosis, sexual potency, erythropoiesis, etc., it is not known if some of the carboxyl fragments that do not have biological activity in the two systems mentioned above may have some role in pathological processes such as seen in patients with far advanced renal failure.

Heterogeneity of PTH

One of the most controversial aspects in the understanding of the metabolism of parathyroid hormone has been the elucidation and interpretation of the appearance of parathyroid hormone fragments in peripheral blood. Early studies (Berson and Yalow, 1966; Reiss and Canterbury, 1968) with radioimmunoassay gave different results in patients with primary hyperparathyroidism. It was thought that the radioimmunoassay for parathyroid hormone was measuring in blood the peptide secreted by the parathyroid glands. However, Berson and Yalow described (1968) that parathyroid hormone in plasma of humans was heterogeneous and differed immunologically from the hormone extracted from human glands. Using different antisera, they clearly demonstrated the presence of fragments with very short half-lives, which became undetectable after parathyroidectomy, and of other fragments with prolonged half-lives in the circulation. They also demonstrated that the half-life of immunoreactive PTH was markedly prolonged in patients with uremia. It was clear from studies performed in several laboratories that the predominant circulating species of i-PTH had a smaller molecular weight (approximately 7,000) compared to the native hormone (M.W. 9,500). Moreover, Canterbury, Levey, and Reiss (1973), employing gel filtration of concentrated serum samples from patients with hyperparathyroidism, demonstrated three peaks. Peak 1 was consistent with the native parathyroid hormone; Peak 2, which was the main component, was found to be biologically inactive, therefore representing a carboxyl portion of the molecule; and Peak 3, with a molecular weight around 4,000, demonstrated to have biological activity in the adenyl cyclase system using rat renal cortical membranes. Controversy persists as to the origin of PTH fragments. There is evidence to suggest that PTH fragments are made in the peripheral circulation particularly by liver and kidney (Canterbury et al., 1975; Hruska et al., 1977; and Martin et al., 1976). Habener et al. (1971) demonstrated in patients with hyperparathyroidism that blood obtained from the thyroid veins had mainly the intact hormone similar to the one obtained from the parathyroid adenomas. On the other hand, when blood was obtained from a peripheral vein, smaller molecular fragments were present, indicating that most of the fragments were made in the periphery and were not being directly secreted by the parathyroid glands. More recently, it has been demonstrated that in patients with primary hyperparathyroidism, samples obtained in the thyroid venous effluent demonstrated the presence of carboxyl-terminal fragments (Flueck et al., 1977). On the other hand, there is considerable evidence that the PTH fragments present in the circulation are made by organs such as liver and kidney. Studies performed with isolated rat liver (Canterbury et al., 1975) and isolated perfused kidney (Hruska et al., 1977) show that both organs have the capability of degrading the hormone, and the appearance of amino and carboxyl-terminal fragments was demonstrated in the blood leaving these organs.

Peripheral metabolism of parathyroid hormone

Hruska et al. (1975) demonstrated in vivo that the kidney plays a key role in the metabolism of parathyroid hormone. After the injection of bovine parathyroid hormone 1–84 in dogs, the kidneys account for approximately 60 percent of the total metabolic clearance rate of carboxyl-terminal immunoreactive parathyroid hormone. The remaining 40 percent, therefore, is due to PTH uptake at extrarenal sites. Further studies were performed to characterize the role of the peritubular uptake and glomerular filtration rate in the renal handling of parathyroid hormone. Martin et al. (1977) demonstrated that both glomerular filtration rate and peritubular uptake are important mechanisms for the renal PTH uptake. The degradation of carboxyl-terminal fragments of PTH is dependent exclusively upon glomerular filtration and tubular reabsorption, whereas peritubular uptake can only be demonstrated for biologically active intact 1–84 or its biologically active fragment syn b-PTH 1–34 (Figure 7.1).

As we mentioned before, the liver also plays a critical role in the degradation of parathyroid hormone. Studies in our laboratory in the dog (Martin et al., 1976) indicate that the hepatic uptake of immunoreactive PTH is selective for intact hormone, and this organ does not remove either carboxyl-terminal or amino-terminal fragments from the circulation. Two minutes after a bolus in-

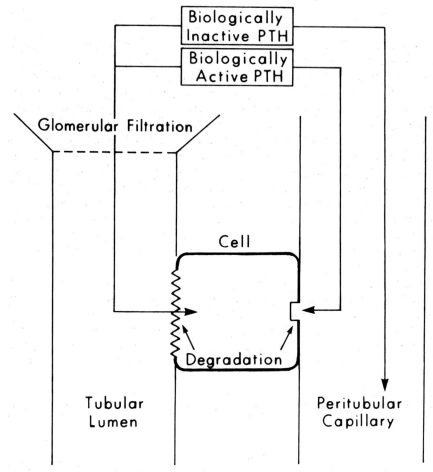

Figure 7.1   Schematic representation of the renal mechanisms of PTH uptake (Martin et al., 1977; reproduced with permission of the publisher.)

jection of intact parathyroid hormone, the liver demonstrates an A-V difference for i-PTH of roughly 35 percent. However, after 20 minutes when intact parathyroid hormone is no longer present in blood, the liver ceases to remove any fragments from the circulation. Moreover, when the synthetic 1–34 fragment has been injected in vivo into dogs, the liver again has failed to demonstrate any uptake of this fragment. Since the kidney accounts for roughly 45 percent of the metabolic clearance rate for the amino-terminal fragment of PTH, the major portion is left to be accounted for by extrarenal sites. Since bone is an important target organ for parathyroid hormone, studies were designed to examine the possibility that the skeleton may represent the extrarenal site of metabolism for the synthetic amino-terminal PTH fragments.

Using an experimental model in which the canine tibia is isolated and per-fused in vitro, Martin et al. (1978) clearly demonstrated that the isolated per-

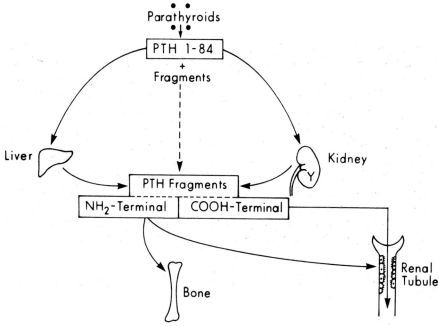

Figure 7.2 Current scheme of the peripheral metabolism of parathyroid hormone. For a complete description see text. (Martin et al., 1978; reproduced with permission of the publisher.)

fused bone has an arteriovenous difference of 35 percent for the synthetic b-PTH 1–34. However, when similar studies were performed during infusion of the native hormone (b-PTH 1–84), no significant uptake was observed. In addition, when oxidized (biologically inactive) synthetic biological 1–34 was used, no A-V difference was observed. These studies in bone suggest that in the dog the skeleton is the major site of metabolism of the amino-terminal PTH fragment synthetic bovine 1–34.

Figure 7.2 illustrates our current scheme of the metabolism of parathyroid hormone. Parathyroid hormone is secreted from the parathyroid glands predominantly in the intact form. However, there is evidence that PTH fragments also can be secreted from the glands. Intact PTH is degraded by the liver and kidney resulting in the production of amino- and carboxyl-terminal fragments. The carboxyl-terminal fragments are further metabolized by the kidney by a process of glomerular filtration and tubular reabsorption. The amino-terminal fragments, in addition to intact PTH, also act on the peritubular side of the renal tubular cells and mediate the biological effect of parathyroid hormone in the kidney. These studies suggest that the peripheral metabolism of PTH may be necessary for the biological effect of parathyroid hormone on bone. The fact that the liver removes only intact hormone and the kidney is responsible for the removal of amino- and carboxyl-terminal fragments offers an explanation for the high levels of carboxyl-terminal immunoreactive parathyroid hormone seen in patients with chronic renal failure. In primary hyper-parathyroidism the liver and the kidney degrade the hormone and the carboxyl-terminal fragments are removed by the intact kidney. In far advanced renal insufficiency, the native hormone (1–84) is degraded by the liver; however, in the absence of renal function, there is an accumulation of carboxyl-terminal fragments. Patients with advanced renal failure may have detectable levels of PTH up to two weeks after parathyroidectomy if the antibody used detects carboxyl-terminal fragments. On the other hand, 24 hours after a successful renal transplant the circulating levels of carboxyl-terminal i-PTH decreased by 80 percent (Freitag et al., 1978).

Action of parathyroid hormone

As we mentioned previously, the main role of parathyroid hormone is the maintenance of calcium homeostasis and its main target organs are the kidney and skeleton. However, in the past five years many investigators have attributed other pathological manifestations in patients with chronic renal failure to parathyroid hormone. These alterations include carbohydrate intolerance, hyperlipidemia, impotence, pruritis, anemia, etc. However, since the main target organs for parathyroid hormone are the skeleton and kidney, we will concentrate on these two systems.

Parathyroid hormone action on bone

At the cellular level the main actions of parathyroid hormone on bone are an increase in osteoclastic bone resorption and changes in the rate of bone collagen synthesis. Numerous investigators have demonstrated that an excess of parathyroid hormone in humans is characterized by an increase not only in the number but also in the activity of the osteoclasts with a characteristic osteolytic effect and increase in bone resorption. This process also is coupled to an increased remodeling phase by the osteoblasts (Rasmussen and Bordier, 1974). Thus, in conditions in which the levels of parathyroid hormone are low in blood (e.g., primary or surgical hypoparathyroidism), the remodeling process is decreased. The mechanism of action of PTH in bone is primarily mediated by activation of cyclic AMP, similar to its action on the renal cell. However, PTH stimulates bone cells by increasing cell membrane permeability to calcium with an increase in calcium influx and subsequently activation of membrane-bound adenyl cyclase. There is evidence (Parson, Near, and Potts, 1971) that after the administration of PTH, early changes are characterized by a decrease in serum calcium and increase in bone cell calcium uptake. PTH induces release of calcium from bone by at least three different mechanisms (Parfitt, 1976): (1) the osteoprogenitor cell proliferates to osteoclast; (2) the deep osteocyte mobilizes calcium from perilacunar bone; and (3) the surface osteocyte regulates calcium flux and so maintains a steady-state level of plasma calcium.

RENAL EFFECTS OF PARATHYROID HORMONE

Though much is known about the effects of PTH on the kidney, contradictions do exist in the literature. Some of the confusion is a result of species variation and the fact that the renal handling of one ion can affect that of others irrespective of PTH.

Renal function

Despite observations that exogenous administration of PTH resulted in increased glomerular filtration rate (GFR) and renal plasma flow, this phenomenon was likely due to vasoactive contaminants in the parathyroid extract (PTE) and to the relatively large amount of PTE used. In studies utilizing purified preparations of bovine PTH, no alterations of GFR or renal plasma flow were detected (Agus et al., 1973).

Phosphate

Probably the best-recognized renal effect of PTH is its ability to produce phosphaturia (Pullman et al., 1960). Parathyroidectomized animals have an increased tubular reabsorption of phosphate, which can readily be reversed with the administration of exogenous PTH (Talmage and Kraintz, 1954). PTH decreases not only proximal tubular reabsorption of phosphate, but distal reabsorption as well, thus resulting in enhanced fractional excretion of phosphate (Amiel, Kuntziger, and Richet, 1970; Knox and Lechene, 1975).

The data suggest that the inhibition of proximal tubule phosphate reabsorption is mediated via cyclic AMP (cAMP) as a result of PTH stimulated adenyl cyclase in the renal cortex (Chase and Aurbach, 1968). Studies using dibutyryl cAMP infusions were able to duplicate the PTH-induced inhibition of proximal tubular phosphate reabsorption (Agus et al., 1971). Although this effect of cAMP may extend to the loop (Kuntziger et al., 1974) and, indeed, even mediate the PTH effect on phosphate transport in the distal nephron as suggested by Goldfarb, Agus, and Goldberg (1974), recent data by Puschett and Sylk (1977) suggest that the PTH-induced inhibition of phosphate reabsorption in the distal nephron is not mediated by cAMP when "physiologic" doses of PTH are used.

PTH has also recently been shown to increase proximal tubule permeability. It is conceivable that PTH, via changes in tubule permeability, could alter proximal tubular transport by allowing increased backflow of reabsorbed substances (Lorentz, 1976).

That PTH-induced inhibition of carbonic anhydrase mediates the decreased proxmial tubule reabsorption of phosphate can be dismissed. Studies by Knox, Haas, and Lechene (1976) have shown that the increased distal phosphate delivery after acetazolamide administration was additive to that of PTH administration, thus suggesting different mechanisms of action. Furthermore, Garg

(1976) could not detect an effect of PTH or cAMP on renal carbonic anhydrase activity.

The phosphaturic response to exogenous PTH in rats is impaired in vitamin D deficiency (Forte, Nickols, and Anast, 1976), metabolic acidosis (Beck, Kim, and Kim, 1975), and phosphate depletion (Steele, 1976).

Calcium

PTH decreases the clearance of calcium by affecting both proximal and distal nephron calcium reabsorption (Sutton, Wong, and Dirks, 1976). In the proximal tubule, PTH administration results in decreased calcium reabsorption in parallel with decreased sodium reabsorption. This parallelism, however, is disrupted in the distal nephron where PTH enhances calcium reabsorption in excess of the sodium reabsorption, thereby resulting in overall decreased calcium clearance. The exact site of action of this PTH effect in the distal nephron is not known, but may be beyond the late distal tubule.

The above effects of PTH on calcium handling are, in part, mediated by cAMP. In the experiments of Agus et al. (1973) in dogs, dibutyryl cAMP administration resulted in decreased proximal tubule calcium reabsorption. Kuntziger et al. (1974), however, using rats, showed that exogenous cAMP administration caused no proximal effect, but did lower calcium absorption in the loop. Part of the conflict may be a reflection of species variation.

Magnesium

The effects of PTH on the renal handling of magnesium are not well defined and await further clarification. The bulk of data suggest that exogenous PTH administration results in an initial renal conservation of magnesium by decreasing its excretion (MacIntyre, Boss, and Troughton, 1963). This effect of PTH may be transient, as suggested by Gill, Bell, and Bartter (1967). Because increases in serum calcium with resultant increased filtered load of calcium enhance renal excretion of magnesium (Coburn, Massry, and Kleeman, 1970), interventions that themselves alter serum calcium could potentially affect renal magnesium handling by this effect alone, thus creating a potential hazard in the interpretation of results and, perhaps, accounting for some of the conflicting literature.

Exogenous administration of cAMP has been shown to increase magnesium reabsorption in the loop but not in the proximal tubule (Kuntziger et al., 1974).

Bicarbonate

Muldowney et al. (1971) observed that the systemic acidosis of hyperparathyroidism could be corrected by parathyroidectomy and postulated that the acidosis resulted from a proximal tubule defect in bicarbonate reabsorption with resultant bicarbonate loss. Subsequent studies have confirmed a decreased proximal tubule reabsorption of bicarbonate in response to PTH, though this may not always result in increased bicarbonate excretion in the urine, as the latter seems to be dependent on the amount of bicarbonate escaping proximal reabsorption (Puschett and Zurbach, 1976). Arruda et al. (1977) not only reported decreased proximal tubular bicarbonate reabsorption in response to PTH infusions in dogs but also noted decreased ammonium excretion. This occurred in the absence of an observed distal PTH effect on bicarbonate reabsorption. Bank and Aynedjian (1976), however, reported increased ammonium excretion in rats given PTH with no change in whole-kidney bicarbonate reabsorption despite decreased proximal tubule bicarbonate. These data, however, may be unique to the rat.

The proximal tubule effect of PTH on bicarbonate reabsorption does not appear to be mediated by carbonic acid inhibition (Garg, 1976). The exact mechanism of action for this PTH effect remains to be elucidated, though alterations in tubule permeability or concomitant changes in sodium and water reabsorption could be causative factors.

It has been argued that the acidosis noted by Muldowney et al. (1971) in their hyperparathyroid patients was due to factors other than a direct effect of PTH on bicarbonate reabsorption, namely, phosphate depletion. This has been shown to decrease bicarbonate reabsorption per se (Gold et al., 1973).

Sodium

In addition to decreasing proximal tubule reabsorption of calcium and phosphate, proximal tubular sodium reabsorption is also reduced by PTH (Wen, 1974). This results in only minimal natriuresis since most of the increased sodium that escapes proximal reabsorption is reabsorbed distally. As indicated above, the PTH effect on sodium absorption can be dissociated from that on phosphate and calcium.

Other

PTH has also been shown to increase T_{Mg}/GFR (Halver, 1966) as well as increase amino acid excretion in man (Short, Elsas, and Rosenberg, 1974). The mechanism of these effects remains to be elucidated.

Finally, studies have suggested that PTH enhances renal production of 1,25-dihydroxy vitamin D_3; for, in the absence of PTH, serum 1,25-dihydroxy vitamin D_3 levels were reduced (Hughes et al., 1975).

HYPERPARATHYROIDISM

Primary

Clinical features

The widespread application of multichannel automated serum testing has altered the clinical presentation of primary hyperparathyroidism. Now, the most common presentation (50–70 percent of the cases) is hypercalcemia, which is often asymptomatic (Boonstra and Jackson, 1971). This has resulted in higher estimates of the disease prevalence, which is now one per thousand of population (Potts and Deftos, 1974). The manifestations of primary hyperparathyroidism other than hypercalcemia include nephrolithiasis, osteitis fibrosa cystica, peptic ulcer disease, pancreatitis, asymptomatic abnormalities in renal function, central nervous system disturbances, neuromuscular dysfunction, ectopic calcifications, and possibly hypertension. Renal stones were the most common clinical presentation of primary hyperparathyroidism prior to the automated blood testing era. Currently, primary hyperparathyroidism accounts for 5 percent to 10 percent of patients with hypercalciuric renal stone disease (K. A. Hruska, unpublished observations). Patients with primary hyperparathyroidism have a higher incidence of calcium phosphate stones than the general population with calcium stone disease. About 20 percent of the patients have radiographically demonstrable bone involvement, with diffuse demineralization being the most prevalent feature. The radiographic and histologic features of primary hyperparathyroidism have been reviewed in depth elsewhere (Rasmussen and Bordier, 1974). Hyperparathyroidism has been described as a distinct familial disorder, and it is also a prominent feature of the multiple endocrine adenoma syndromes, both Type I and Type II.

Diagnosis

Elevation of the serum calcium is the most important criterion for the diagnosis of hyperparathyroidism. A currently debated issue is the incidence of normocalcemic primary hyperparathyroidism. In those centers with reliable determinations of ionized calcium, this entity is considered very rare. Since these patients usually present with nephrolithiasis and elevated PTH levels similar to patients with renal leak hypercalciuria, thiazide therapy is useful for detection of increased secretion of parathyroid hormone by provoking frank hypercalcemia in this instance. The other manifestations of hyperparathyroidism seen in the blood are hypophosphatemia, hyperchloremic metabolic acidosis, and elevated alkaline phosphatase.

The renal effects of hyperparathyroidism may include decreased GFR, possibly mediated by the dual effects of calcium and PTH on the renal glomerulus (Humes et al., 1978), hypercalciuria, decreased reabsorption of phosphorus, decreased hydrogen ion secretion resulting occasionally in bicarbonaturia and high urine pHs, elevated urinary hydroxyproline, and, finally, elevated urinary 3'5'-cyclic adenosine monophosphate (cAMP) (Broadus et al., 1977). When hypercalcemia is present, hyposthenuria may lead to polyuria and polydipsia.

Many of the above listed urinary findings have been utilized as indirect diagnostic tests for primary hyperparathyroidism. The tubular reabsorption of phosphorus (TRP) of less than 75 percent has been widely applied. However, for accuracy this test requires a phosphorus intake in the narrow range of 1–1.5 grams per day and performance of the test in the late morning when the diurnal variation in phosphate clearance peaks. Even then the TRP is beset with a 20 percent incidence of falsely normal results in patients with primary hyperparathyroidism. More recently, Broadus et al. (1977) have proposed the determination of nephrogenous cAMP as a test for primary hyperparathyroidism. The authors were able to point out that since PTH is the major source of renal cAMP production, expression of the clearance of cAMP as a function of glomerular filtration, or the calculation of "nephrogenous" cAMP excretion, was 91 percent effective in detecting hyperparathyroidism. In settings where sensitive PTH assays are not available, this determination appears to be a reasonable test for primary hyperparathyroidism. The source of false-positives is mainly patients with high levels of adrenergic stimulation such as pheochromocytoma.

Radioimmunoassay

The most direct method for diagnosis of hyperparathyroidism is the PTH radioimmunoassay (RIA). Over the past several years, the heterogenous nature of PTH in the circulation has been elucidated. With this knowledge, the binding specificities of the polyvalent antisera in widespread use have been characterized by the portion of the PTH molecule to which a particular antiserum is chiefly directed. Because both intact PTH and amino-terminal fragments have short half-lives in the circulation (ca. 5 min.), while carboxyl-terminal fragments have much longer half-lives, it is these peptides that comprise the bulk of the circulating hormone. In addition, recent data suggest that primary hyperparathyroidism is characterized by glandular secretion of COOH-terminal PTH fragments. Thus, antisera with binding specificities for the carboxyl-terminal portion of the molecule bind the greatest fraction of circulating PTH (intact hormone and carboxyl-terminal fragments), and these antisera display greater sensitivity in separating normal individuals from those with hyperparathyroidism. Utilizing carboxyl-terminal specific antisera, Arnaud et al. (1974) have reported several RIAs displaying abnormal PTH levels in 90 percent of patients with primary hyperparathyroidism. The experience of our laboratory with the use of carboxyl-terminal antiserum (CH9) is portrayed in Figure 7.3. Ninety-six percent of patients with surgically proven hyperparathyroidism had high PTH levels utilizing this RIA. PTH immunoassays utilizing antisera to the amino-terminal portion of the molecule generally display a 50 percent to 70 percent diagnostic ability for primary hyperparathyroidism. Since the RIA for PTH is a direct measure of parathyroid function, an assay for carboxyl-terminal immunoreactive PTH combined with serum-ionized calcium markedly diminishes the need for indirect parathyroid function tests such as nephrogenous cyclic AMP.

Recent studies have described the dependency of carboxyl-terminal fragments on glomerular filtration for their clearance from the circulation (Martin et al., 1977). Thus, in hyperparathyroid states associated with renal failure, the half-life of carboxyl-terminal fragments in the circulation is tremendously prolonged as is shown by the slow disappearance of assayable PTH from the circulation following parathyroidectomy in dialysis patients (Freitag et al., 1978). In this situation, PTH assays, utilizing antisera with amino-terminal

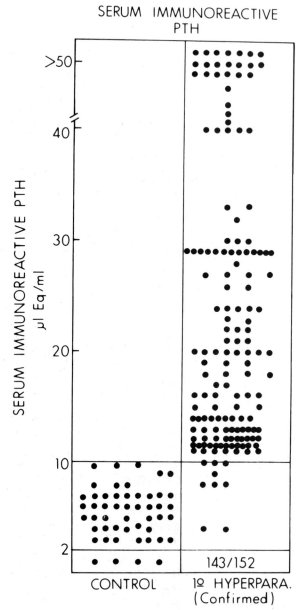

Figure 7.3 Results for serum radioimmunoassayable PTH obtained in 152 patients with surgically confirmed hyperparathyroidism. Using CH9 antibody, a predominantly C-terminal antibody, elevated levels were found in 96 percent of the patients.

binding specificities will be more useful in the acute determination of PTH secretion, for instance during a calcium infusion. However, over a longer term follow-up of weeks to months, carboxyl-terminal assays in renal failure correlate closely with the manifestations of parathyroid activity on the bone (Bordier, Marie, and Arnaud, 1975; Rutherford et al., 1977).

Treatment
The surgical management of patients with hyperparathyroidism, both primary and secondary, is difficult and controversial because of the anatomy of the parathyroids, problems with the differentiation between multiple gland hyperplasia and single-gland adenoma, and the incidence of postsurgical hyper- and hypoparathyroidism. The experience at Massachusetts General Hospital, recently reported (Wang, Potts, and Neer, 1975), is based on the observation that 80 percent of patients with primary hyperparathyroidism have single-gland adenomas. Their approach is to remove the adenoma and identify the ipsilateral gland. If this latter gland is atrophic, they do not undertake additional exploration and end the procedure. They report a very low incidence of postsurgical hypoparathyroidism and almost no recurrent hyperparathyroidism. However, in other centers the incidence of diffuse parathyroid hyperplasia has been higher, and the differentiation between diffuse hyperplasia and single adenoma has been more difficult. Thus, there has been an increasing tendency to explore all four parathyroid glands and to remove all questionably involved glands to insure adequate resection. These authors also perform 3.5 gland parathyroidectomy for all cases of diffuse hyperplasia, attempting to leave about 50 mg of tissue behind. This latter approach has become the standard treatment for the secondary hyperparathyroidism of renal disease requiring resection. Recently, Wells et al. (1976) have recommended total parathyroidectomy with autotransplantation of parathyroid tissue into the forearm's muscle, especially for secondary hyperparathyroidism in renal disease. This procedure is advocated for better control of postsurgical hyper- and hypoparathyroidism. However, it appears unnecessarily aggressive when surgeons utilizing 3.5 gland parathyroidectomies report very small rates of postsurgical hyper- or hypoparathyroidism. The latter experience has clearly been the case at Barnes Hospital, Washington University (Charles Anderson, M.D., personal communication).

The use of arteriography and venography with RIA for PTH in the thyroid venous effluent as a preoperative localizing procedure for abnormal parathyroid tissue seems to depend on the approach of the surgeon. Those who prefer limited resection and exploration utilize the procedures more than surgeons who perform complete cervical exploration and tend to perform more than single gland resections. In cases of hyperparathyroidism following prior surgery, the use of localization techniques has been shown to be of definite value, with about 80 percent effectiveness in demonstrating the abnormal parathyroid tissue and decreasing the need for mediastinal exploration. In centers where selective catheterization techniques are frequently employed, differentiation between normal subjects and those with diffuse hyperplasia has not been difficult, and significant incidences of false-positive step-ups of PTH concentrations have not been reported.

Secondary

The most common form of secondary hyperparathyroidism is that seen in patients with decreased renal function. There are several factors recently reviewed (Slatopolsky et al., 1978) that contribute to the overproduction of PTH during chronic renal disease (CRD). These include phosphate retention, calcium malabsorption, skeletal resistance to calcemic effects of PTH, and low $1,25(OH)_2D_3$ levels. Recently, the role of phosphate retention early in the course of CRD as an important stimulus to increased PTH secretion, as described by Slatopolsky et al. (1971, 1972), has been challenged (Massry, Ritz, and Verberckmoes, 1977). However, studies such as those shown in Figure 7.4 and experimental situations (Rutherford et al., 1977) clearly demonstrate that if phosphate retention is avoided secondary hyperparathyroidism does not develop. The patient portrayed in Figure 7.4 had congenital absence of one kidney, a hypernephroma in the other and was treated by nephrectomy and chronic hemodialysis. Postoperatively he was placed on phosphate binders, a controlled phosphate diet, and calcium supplementation. PTH levels remained normal or only slightly elevated for a 2-year period. Thereafter, the phosphate binders were prospectively stopped for a short period, the PTH levels rose markedly. Reinstitution of PO_4 binders decreased PTH to previous levels. Thus, although several factors are involved in the production of secondary hyperparathyroidism in CRD, phosphate retention plays an early and key role, and hyperparathyroidism does not develop when phosphate intake is controlled.

Adequate control of established secondary hyperparathyroidism in CRD is difficult when phosphate binders and calcium supplementation are the sole therapy because of the rigidity of necessary diet restrictions and poor compliance with the use of the binding agents. The potent metabolites of vitamin D are useful adjuncts for control of secondary hyperparathyroidism, and their use will be widespread in the near future. However, some patients with CRD exhibit partially autonomous secondary hyperparathyroidism; or they have such high levels of PTH with severe resorptive bone disease that subtotal parathyroidectomy has a definite role for treatment of hyperparathyroidism owing to CRD in selected patients. The surgical approach to hyperparathyroidism is discussed above under treatment of primary hyperparathyroidism.

Elevated PTH levels are seen in several other disease states on a secondary basis. These include states of malabsorption, vitamin D deficiency, renal hypercalciuria, and pseudohyperparathyroidism. The space limitations of this chapter do not permit an in-depth discussion of these disorders; however, they have been recently reviewed (Prein, Pyle, and Krane, 1976). Their pathogenesis appears to be due to factors that produce hypocalcemia either by decreasing intake, by increasing loss, or by decreasing calcemic actions of PTH.

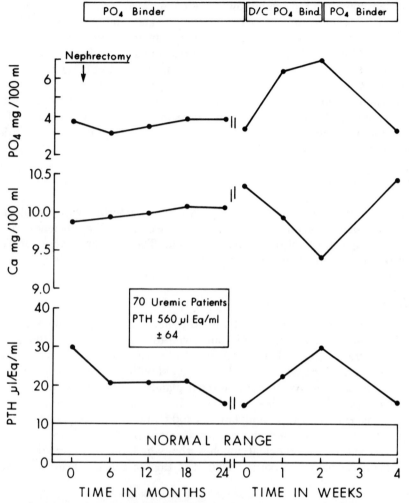

EFFECTS OF PO₄ ON SECONDARY HYPERPARATHYROIDISM IN AN ANEPHRIC PATIENT

Figure 7.4 Effects of phosphate on serum PTH in a patient with a renal cell carcinoma in a solitary kidney. Before nephrectomy the creatinine clearance was 70 ml/min. For a complete description see text. (Slatopolsky et al. 1978. *Archives of Internal Medicine,* **138,** 848–852. Copyright 1978, American Medical Association.)

Pseudohyperparathyroidism

In recent years some hypercalcemic states associated with malignancies of several types have been shown to result from ectopic production of peptides with PTH-like activity. These peptides share the gel filtration characteristics of proparathyroid hormone (Benson et al., 1974) in the instances where careful studies have been performed. Since pro-PTH is less immunoreactive than PTH 1–84 in most RIAs, this may explain why that immunoassayable PTH levels in these patients tend to be lower than they are in patients with primary hyperparathyroidism. Clinically, patients with pseudohyperparathyroidism tend to have more severe hypercalcemia. The peptides produced in pseudohyperparathyroidism tend to exhibit lower degrees of renal activity. Thus, decreased phosphate reabsorption, hypophosphatemia, and high urinary cAMP—although they are seen—are less prevalent than they are in primary hyperparathyroidism. Also, the effects of hypercalcemia override the effects of the PTH-like peptides on hydrogen ion secretion, and most of these patients have tendencies to metabolic alkalosis rather than acidosis. The hypercalcemia is responsive temporarily to conservative measures and a decrease in tumor burdon. However, hypercalcemia tends to recur with increased growth of the tumor or metastases correlating with reappearance of the PTH-like peptide in the circulation.

HYPOPARATHYROIDISM

Hypoparathyroidism is a clinical syndrome characterized by hypocalcemia, hyperphosphatemia, and tentany in the absence of renal insufficiency, rickets or osteomalacia, or intestinal malabsorption. The principal causes of hypoparathyroidism are shown in Table 7.1.

Etiology

The most common cause of hypoparathyroidism is excision or damage to the parathyroid glands at surgery. Although symptoms may develop within several days, diagnosis may be delayed for months to years. Idiopathic hypoparathyroidism is a rare disease and may be associated with hypofunction of other endocrine organs such as thyroid, adrenal glands, ovaries, particularly in the familial type (Blizzard, Chee, and Davis, 1966). Chronic mucocutaneous candidiasis may also be seen in both familial and sporadic types. Hypoparathyroidism in the DiGeorge syndrome is a consequence of failure of development of the third and fourth branchial pouches from which the parathyroids and thymus gland develop (DiGeorge, 1968). The thymic agenesis leads to a severe

Table 7.1 Principal causes of hypoparathyroidism

I. Inadequate secretion of parathyroid hormone
  A. Abnormal, damaged, or absent parathyroid glands
    1. Postoperative
      a. Thyroid surgery
      b. Parathyroid surgery
      c. Radical neck dissections
    2. Idiopathic
      a. Familial
      b. Sporadic
      c. DiGeorge syndrome
  B. Suppression of PTH secretion from normal parathyroid glands
    1. Neonatal from maternal hypercalcemia
    2. Magnesium depletion
II. Defective end-organ responsiveness to parathyroid hormone
  Pseudohypoparathyroidism Types I and II

immunodeficiency state of the cellular type. Delayed hypersensitivity reactions and allograft rejections are absent and chronic mucocutaneous candidiasis is common. Patients with this syndrome usually die in early childhood of hypocalcemia and/or severe infections.

Neonatal tetany should be watched for closely in the presence of hypercalcemia of any cause in the mother. The fetal parathyroid glands become suppressed by the maternal hypercalcemia and when the infant is stressed, for example with a phosphate load (cow's milk), tetany may result.

Although acute decreases in serum magnesium result in stimulation of PTH secretion, chronic magnesium depletion is associated with impaired secretion of PTH and is inappropriate for the associated hypocalcemia (Chase and Slatopolsky, 1974). Magnesium replenishment is associated with a rapid rise (within minutes) in circulating PTH and correction of the hypocalcemia (Anast et al., 1976).

Pseudohypoparathyroidism is a rare hereditary disorder that is characterized by symptoms and signs of hypoparathyroidism associated with distinctive skeletal and somatic defects (Albright et al., 1942). This syndrome is of considerable interest in relation to the mechanisms of the actions of parathyroid hormone and its interrelationship with vitamin D metabolism. The secretion of parathyroid hormone is increased as assessed by elevated levels of immunoreactive PTH, and thus pseudohypoparathyroidism is felt to represent endorgan unresponsiveness to parathyroid hormone. The hallmark of pseudohypoparathyroidism is an absent or subnormal response to exogenous parathyroid hormone. However, is is apparent that the severity and mechanism of the hormone resistance differs among patients with this syndrome. The hormone resistance is usually demonstrable in kidney, whereas a deficient calcemic response to exogenous PTH (skeletal resistance) may or may not be present, and several cases have been described with the skeletal changes of osteitis fibrosa (Bell, Gerard, and Bartter, 1963). The nature of the renal resistance leads to the recognition of two types of pseudohypoparathyroidism. In the classic type (Type I) there is neither a cAMP nor phosphaturic response to exogenous PTH, whereas in pseudohypoparathyroidism Type II there is no phosphaturic response while the cAMP response is normal (Drezner, Neilson, and Lebovitz, 1975). Resistance to parathyroid hormone may be restored following therapy with calcium (Rodriguez et al., 1974), vitamin D or its metabolites. Levels of 1,25-dihydroxycholecalciferol are low in this disorder, perhaps representing renal resistance to PTH stimulated 1-α-hydroxylase activity (Drezner et al., 1976).

Clinical manifestations

Carpopedal spasms (tetany) and convulsions are the most serious complications of the hypoparathyroid state. Latent tetany may be detected by tapping over the facial nerves, resulting in a contraction of the facial muscles (Chvostek's sign), or by producing carpal spasm following occlusion of arterial blood supply to the forearm (Trousseau's sign). Cataracts are common as a consequence of chronic hypocalcemia. Soft tissue calcification is not infrequent and may be related to hyperphosphatemia. In pseudohypoparathyroidism ectopic calcification may include true bone formation.

The characteristic somatic abnormalities of pseudohypoparathyroidism include short stature, round facies, short neck, and abnormalities of metacarpal and metatarsal bones. Relatives of patients with pseudohypoparathyroidism often have a similar phenotype without evidence of hypoparathyroidism (pseudo-pseudohypoparathyroidism).

Diagnosis

The diagnosis of hypoparathyroidism does not present any difficulty when tetany is accompanied by hypocalcemia and hyperphosphatemia in the absence of renal failure, rickets or osteomalacia, or intestinal malabsorption. History and physical examination usually indicate the underlying cause. A definitive diagnosis, however, particularly for pseudohypoparathyroidism, requires more detailed evaluation, including measurement of plasma i-PTH and measurement of urinary cAMP and phosphate following exogenous parathyroid hormone. Awareness of hypoparathyroidism secondary to magnesium depletion may prevent unnecessary diagnostic evaluation.

Treatment

The object of treatment of hypoparathyroidism is to raise the serum calcium towards normal to prevent symptoms of tetany and convulsions. Supplemental dietary calcium alone is relatively ineffective as intestinal calcium absorption is low in hypoparathyroidism. Thus, the use of a vitamin D preparation is usually required. Therapy with vitamin D is complicated by a narrow range between therapeutic efficacy and toxicity since large doses (50,000–100,000 units/day) are required. Hypercalciuria, which may occur even with serum calcium in the low normal range, reflects the lack of parathyroid hormone-dependent renal reabsorption of calcium and may lead to nephrolithiasis.

Recent advances in vitamin D metabolism may facilitate treatment of hypoparathyroidism. Plasma 1,25-dihydroxycholecalciferol levels are low in hypoparathyroidism reflecting the lack of PTH-stimulated 1-α-hydroxylase activity in the kidney. Accordingly, 1,25-dihydroxycholecalciferol in relatively low dosage has been shown to increase and maintain serum calcium (Neer, Holick, and DeLuca, 1975). The added advantage of this metabolite is the shorter duration of toxicity. This metabolite of vitamin D is the treatment of choice to control the hypoparathyroid state.

ACKNOWLEDGMENT

This work was supported by U.S.P.H.S. NIAMDD grants AM-09976 and AM-07126.

The authors would like to express their appreciation to Mrs. Patricia Verplancke for her assistance in the preparation of this chapter.

REFERENCES

Agus, Z. S., Puschett, J. B., Senesky, D. & Goldberg, M. (1971). Mode of action of parathyroid hormone and cyclic adenosine-3′,5′-monophosphate in renal tubular phosphate reabsorption in the dog. *Journal of Clinical Investigation*, **50**, 617–626.

Agus, Z. S., Gardner, L. B., Beck, L. H. & Goldberg, M. (1973). Effects of parathyroid hormone on renal tubular reabsorption of calcium, sodium and phosphate. *American Journal of Physiology*, **224**, 1143–1148.

Albright, F., Burnett, C. H., Smith, P. H. & Parson, W. (1942). Pseudohypoparathyroidism— an example of the Seabright-Bantam syndrome. Report of 3 cases. *Endocrinology*, **30**, 922–932.

Amiel, C., Kuntziger, H. & Richet, G. (1970). Micropuncture study of handling of phosphate by proximal and distal nephron in normal and parathyroidectomized rat. Evidence for distal reabsorption. *Pflügers Archiv*, **317**, 93–109.

Anast, C. A., Mohs, J. M., Kaplan, S. L. & Burns, T. W. (1972). Evidence for parthyroid failure in magnesium deficiency. *Science*, **177**, 606–608.

Anast, C. A., Winnacher, J. L., Forte, L. R. & Burns, T. W. (1976). Impaired release of parathyroid hormone in magnesium deficiency. *Journal of Clinical Endocrinology and Metabolism*, **42**, 707–717.

Arnaud, C. D., Goldsmith, R. S., Bordier, P. J. & Sizemore, G. W. (1974). Influence of immunoheterogeneity of circulating parathyroid hormone on results of radioimmunoassays of serum in man. *American Journal of Medicine*, **56**, 785–793.

Arruda, J. A. L., Nascimento, L., Westenfelder, C. & Kurtzman, N. A. (1977). Effect of parathyroid hormone in urinary acidification. *American Journal of Physiology*, **232**, F429–433.

Bank, N. & Ayneydjian, H. S. (1976). A micropuncture study of the effect of parathyroid hormone on renal bicarbonate reabsorption. *Journal of Clinical Investigation*, **58**, 336–344.

Beck, N., Kim, H. P. & Kim, K. S. (1975). Effect of metabolic acidosis on renal action of parathyroid hormone. *American Journal of Physiology*, **228**, 1483–1488.

Bell, N. M., Gerard, E. S. & Bartter, F. C. (1963). Pseudohypoparathyroidism with osteitis fibrosa cystica and impaired absorption of calcium. *Journal of Clinical Endocrinology and Metabolism* **23**, 759–772.

Benson, R. C., Jr., Riggs, B. L., Pickard, B. M. & Arnaud, C. E. (1974). Immunoreactive forms of circulating parathyroid hormone in primary and ectopic hyperparathyroidism. *Journal of Clinical Investigation*, **54**, 175–181.

Berson, S. A. & Yalow, R. S. (1966). Parathyroid hormone in plasma in adenomatous hyperparathyroidism, uremia and bronchogenic carcinoma. *Science*, **154**, 907–909.

Berson, S. A. & Yalow, R. S. (1968). Immunochemical heterogeneity of parathyroid hormone in plasma. *Journal of Clinical Endocrinology and Metabolism*, **28**, 1037–1047.

Blizzard, R. M., Chee, D. & Davis, W. (1966). The incidence of parathyroid and other antibodies in the sera of patients with idiopathic hypoparathyroidism. *Clinical Experimental Immunology*, **1**, 119–128.

Blum, J. W., Fischer, J. A., Schwörer, D., Hunziker, W. & Binswager, U. (1974). Acute parathyroid hormone response: Sensitivity relationship to hypocalcemia. *Endocrinology*, **95**, 753–759.

Boonstra, E. E. & Jackson, C. E. (1971). Serum Ca survey for hyperparathyroidism. *American Journal of Clinical Pathology*, **55**, 523–526.

Bordier, P., Marie, P. & Arnaud, C. D. (1975). Evolution of renal osteodystrophy: Correlation of bone histomorphometry and serum mineral and immunoreactive parathyroid hormone values before and after treatment with calcium carbonate or 25-hydroxycholecalciferol. *Kidney International*, **7**, S102–112.

Brewer, H. B., Jr., Fairwell, T., Ronan, R., Sizemore, G. W. & Arnaud, C. D. (1972). Human parathyroid hormone: Amino acid sequence of the amino-terminal residues 1–34. *Proceedings of the National Academy of Science (U.S.A.)*, **69**, 3585–3588.

Broadus, A. E., Mahaffey, J. E., Bartter, F. C. & Neer, R. M. (1977). Nephrogeneous cyclic adenosine monophosphate as a parathyroid function test. *Journal of Clinical Investigation*, **60**, 771–783.

Canterbury, J. M., Levey, G. S. & Reiss, E. (1973). Activation of renal cortical adenylate cyclase by circulating immunoreactive parathyroid fragments. *Journal of Clinical Investigation*, **52**, 524–527.

Canterbury, J. M., Bricker, L. A., Levey, G. S., Kozlovskis, P. L., Ruiz, E., Zull, J. E. &

Reiss, E. (1975). Metabolism of bovine parathyroid hormone. Immunological and biological characteristics of fragments generated by liver perfusion. *Journal of Clinical Investigation*, **55**, 1245–1253.

Chase, L. R. & Aurbach, G. D. (1968). Renal adenyl cyclase: Anatomically separate sites for parathyroid hormone and vasopressin. *Science*, **159**, 545–547.

Chase, L. R. & Slatopolsky, E. (1974). Secretion and metabolic efficacy of parathyroid hormone in patients with severe hypomagnesemia. *Journal of Clinical Endocrinology and Metabolism*, **38**, 363–371.

Chanard, J., Lewis, J., Klahr, S. & Slatopolsky, E. (1977). The effects of colchicine and vinblastine on parathyroid hormone secretion in the rat. *Endocrinology*, **101**, 1792–1800.

Chu, L. L. H., MacGregor, R. R., Anast, C. S., Hamilton, J. W. & Cohn, D. V. (1973). Studies on the biosynthesis of rat parathyroid hormone and proparathyroid hormone: Adaptation of the parathyroid gland to dietary restriction of calcium. *Endocrinology*, **93**, 915–924.

Coburn, J. W., Massry, S. G. & Kleeman, C. R. (1970). The effect of calcium infusion on renal handling of magnesium with normal and reduced GFR. *Nephron*, **7**, 131–143.

Cohn, D. V., MacGregor, R. R., Chu, L. L. H., Kimmel, J. R. & Hamilton, J. W. (1972). Calcemic fraction-A: Biosynthetic peptide precursor of parathyroid hormone. *Proceedings of the National Academy of Science* (U.S.A.), **69**, 1521–1525.

DiGeorge, A. M. (1968). Congenital absence of the thymus and its immunological consequences: Concurrence with congenital hypoparathyroidism. In *Immunological Deficiency Disease in Man*, ed. Bergsma, D. and Good, R. A. Vol. 4. Baltimore:Williams and Wilkins.

Drezner, M., Nelson, F. A. & Lebovitz, H. E. (1973). Pseudohypoparathyroidism Type II: A possible defect in the reception of the cyclic-AMP signal. *New England Journal of Medicine*, **289**, 1056–1060.

Drezner, M. K., Neelon, F. A., Haussler, M., McPherson, M. T. & Lebovitz, H. E. (1976). 1,25-dihydroxycholecalciferol deficiency: The probable cause of hypocalcemia and metabolic bone disease in pseudohypoparathyroidism. *Journal of Clinical Endocrinology and Metabolism*, **42**, 621–628.

Edman, P. & Begg, G. (1967). A protein sequenator. *European Journal of Biochemistry*, **1**, 80–91.

Flueck, J. A., DiBella, F. P., Edis, A. J., Kehrwald, J. M. & Arnaud, C. D. (1977). Immunoheterogeneity of parathyroid hormone in venous effluent serum from hyperfunctioning parathyroid glands. *Journal of Clinical Investigation*, **60**, 1367–1375.

Forte, L., Nickols, G. A. & Anast, C. S. (1976). Renal adenyl cyclase and the interrelationship between parathyroid hormone and vitamin D in the regulation of urinary phosphate and adenosine cyclic 3′,5′-monophosphate excretion. *Journal of Clinical Investigation*, **57**, 559–568.

Freitag, J., Martin, K. J., Hruska, K. A., Anderson, C., Conrades, M., Ladenson, J., Klahr, S. & Slatopolsky, E. (1978). Impaired parathyroid hormone metabolism in chronic renal failure. *New England Journal of Medicine*, **298**, 29–31.

Garg, L. C. (1975). Effect of parathyroid hormone and adenosine-3′,5′-monophosphate on renal carbonic anhydrase. *Biochemical Pharmacology*, **24**, 437–439.

Gill, J. R., Jr., Bell, N. H. & Bartter, F. (1967). Effect of parathyroid extract on magnesium excretion in man. *Journal of Applied Physiology*, **22**, 136–138.

Gold, L. J., Massry, S. G., Arieff, A. I. & Coburn, J. W. (1973). Renal bicarbonate wasting during phosphate depletion. A possible cause of altered acid-base homeostasis in hyperparathyroidism. *Journal of Clinical Investigation*, **52**, 2556–2562.

Goldfarb, S., Agus, Z. S. & Goldberg, M. (1974). Tubular sites of action of dibutyryl cyclic AMP (DBC-AMP) on renal phosphate reabsorption. *Kidney International*, **6**, 47A.

Habener, J. F., Powell, D., Murray, T. M. & Potts, J. T., Jr. (1971). Parathyroid hormone: Secretion and metabolism in vivo. *Proceedings of the National Academy of Science* (U.S.A.), **68**, 2986–2991.

Habener, J. F., Kemper, B., Potts, J. T. & Rich, A. (1972). Proparathyroid hormone: Biosynthesis by human parathyroid adenomas. *Science*, **178**, 630–633.

Habener, J. F., Kemper, B., Potts, J. T., Jr., & Rich, A. (1975). Pre-proparathyroid hormone identified by cell-free translation of messenger RNA from hyperplastic human parathyroid tissue. *Journal of Clinical Investigation*, **56**, 1328–1333.

Habener, J. F., Potts, J. T., Jr., & Rich, A. (1976). Pre-proparathyroid hormone. *Journal of Biological Chemistry*, **251**, 3893–3899.

Habener, J. F. & Potts, J. T., Jr. (1976). Relative effectiveness of magnesium and calcium on the secretion and biosynthesis of parathyroid hormone in vitro. *Endocrinology*, **98**, 197–202.

Halver, B. (1966). The effect of parathyroid hormone on the tubular reabsorption of glucose. *Acta Medica Scandinavia*, **179**, 427–432.

Hamilton, J. W., Spierto, F. W., MacGregor, R. R. & Cohn, D. V. (1971). Studies on the biosynthesis in vitro of parathyroid hormone. II. The effect of calcium and magnesium on synthesis of parathyroid hormone isolated from bovine parathyroid tissue and incubation media. *Journal of Biological Chemistry*, **246**, 3224–3233.

Hamilton, J. W., Niall, H. D., Jacobs, H. W., Keutmann, H. T., Potts, J. T., Jr., & Cohn, D. V. (1974). The N-terminal amino acid sequence of bovine proparathyroid hormone. *Proceedings of the National Academy of Science* (U.S.A.), **71**, 653–656.

Hruska, K. A., Kopelman, R., Rutherford, W. E., Klahr, S. & Slatopolsky, E. (1975). Metabolism of parathyroid hormone in the dog. The role of the kidney and the effects of chronic renal disease. *Journal of Clinical Investigation*, **56**, 39–48.

Hruska, K. A., Martin, K., Mennes, P., Greenwalt, A., Anderson, C., Klahr, S. & Slatopolsky, E. (1977). Degradation of parathyroid hormone and fragment production by the isolated perfused dog kidney. *Journal of Clinical Investigation*, **60**, 501–510.

Hughes, M. R., Brumbaugh, P. F., Haussler, M. R., Wergedal, J. E. & Baylink, D. J. (1975). Regulation of serum 1-α,25-dihydroxyvitamin D_3 by calcium and phosphate in the rat. *Science*, **190**, 578–580.

Humes, H. D., Ichikawa, I., Troy, J. L. & Brenner, B. M. (1978). Evidence for a parathyroid hormone-dependent influence of calcium on the glomerular ultrafiltration coefficient. *Journal of Clinical Investigation*, **61**, 32–40.

Kemper, B., Habener, J. F., Potts, J. T., Jr. & Rich, A. (1972). Pro-parathyroid hormone: Identification of a biosynthetic precursor to parathyroid hormone. *Proceedings of the National Academy of Science* (U.S.A.) **69**, 643–647.

Kemper, B., Habener, J. F., Rich, A. & Potts, J. T., Jr. (1975). Microtubules and the intracellular conversion of proparathyroid hormone to parathyroid hormone. *Endocrinology*, **96**, 903–912.

Kemper, B., Habener, J. F., Ernst, M. D., Potts, J. T., Jr., & Rich, A. (1976). Pre-proparathyroid hormone: Analysis of radioactive tryptic peptides and amino acid sequence. *Biochemistry*, **15**, 15–19.

Keutman, H. T., Aurbach, G. D., Dawson, B. F., Niall, H. D., Deftos, L. J. & Potts, J. T., Jr. (1971). Isolation and characterization of the bovine parathyroid isohormones. *Biochemistry*, **10**, 2779–2787.

Knox, F. G. & Lechene, C. (1975). Distal site of action of parathyroid hormone on phosphate reabsorption. *American Journal of Physiology*, **229**, 1556–1560.

Knox. F. G., Haas, J. A. & Lechene, C. P. (1976). Effect of parathyroid hormone on phosphate reabsorption in the presence of acetazolamide. *Kidney International*, **10**, 216–220.

Kuntziger, H., Amiel, C., Roinel, N. & Morel, F. (1974). Effects of parathyroidectomy and cyclic AMP on renal transport of phosphate, calcium and magnesium. *American Journal of Physiology*, **227**, 905–911.

Lorentz, W. B., Jr. (1976). Effect of parathyroid hormone on renal tubular permeability. *American Journal of Physiology*, **231**, 1401–1407.

MacCallum, W. G. & Voegtlin, C. (1909). On the relation of tetany to the parathyroid glands and to calcium metabolism. *Journal of Experimental Medicine*, **11**, 118–151.

MacGregor, R. R., Hamilton, J. W. & Cohn, D. V. (1975). The by-pass of tissue hormone stores during secretion of newly synthesized parathyroid hormone. *Endocrinology*, **97**, 178–188.

MacIntyre, I., Boss, S. & Troughton, V. A. (1963). Parathyroid hormone and magnesium homeostasis. *Nature*, **198**, 1058–1060.

Marcus, R. & Aurbach, G. D. (1969). Bioassay of parathyroid hormone in vitro with a stable preparation of adenyl cyclase from rat kidney. *Endocrinology*, **85**, 801–810.

Martin, T. J., Greenberg, P. B., & Michelangeli, V. (1973). Synthesis of human parathyroid hormone by cultured cells: Evidence for release of prohormone by some adenomata. *Clinical Science*, **44**, 1–8.

Martin, K., Hruska, K., Greenwalt, A. & Slatopolsky, E. (1976). Selective uptake of intact parathyroid hormone by the liver. Differences between hepatic and renal uptake. *Journal of Clinical Investigation*, **58**, 781–788.

Martin, K. J., Hruska, K. A., Lewis, J., Anderson, C. & Slatopolsky, E. (1977). Renal handling of parathyroid hormone. Role of peritubular uptake and glomerular filtration. *Journal of Clinical Investigation*, **60**, 808–814.

Martin, K. J., Freitag, J. J., Conrades, M. B., Hruska, K., Klahr, S. & Slatopolsky, E. (1978). Selective uptake of the synthetic amino terminal fragment of parathyroid hormone (syn b-PTH 1–34) by isolated perfused bone. *Journal of Clinical Investigation*, **62**, 256–261.

Massry, S. G., Ritz, E. & Verberckmoes, R. (1977). Role of phosphate in the genesis of secondary hyperparathyroidism of renal failure. *Nephron*, **18**, 77–81.

Muldowney, F. P., Carroll, D. V., Donohoe, J. F. & Freaney, R. (1971). Correction of renal bicarbonate wastage by parathyroidectomy. *Quarterly Journal of Medicine*, **40**, 487–498.

Neer, R. M., Holick, M. F., DeLuca, H. F. & Potts, J. T., Jr. (1975). Effects of 1-α-hydroxy vitamin D_3 and 1,25-dihydroxy vitamin D_3 on calcium and phosphorus metabolism in hypoparathyroidism. *Metabolism*, **24**, 1403–1413.

Niall, H. D., Sauer, R. T., Jacobs, J. W., Keutman, H. T., Segre, G. V., O'Riordan, J. L. H., Aurbach, G. D. & Potts, J. T., Jr. (1974). The amino-acid sequence of the amino-terminal 37 residues of human parathyroid hormone. *Proceedings of the National Academy of Science* (U.S.A.), **71**, 384–388.

Parfitt, M. A. (1976). The actions of parathyroid hormone on bone: Relation to bone remodeling and turnover, calcium homeostasis and metabolic bone diseases. *Metabolism*, **25**, 909–955.

Parsons, J. A., Neer, R. M. & Potts, J. T., Jr. (1971). Initial fall of plasma calcium after intravenous injection of parathyroid hormone. *Endocrinology*, **89**, 735–740.

Parsons, J. A., Reit, B. & Robinson, C. J. (1973). A bioassay for parathyroid hormone using chicks. *Endocrinology*, **92**, 454–462.

Potts, J. T., Jr., Keutman, H. T., Niall, H. D. & Tregear, G. W. (1971). The chemistry of parathyroid hormone and the calcitonins. *Vitamin Hormones*, **29**, 41–93.

Potts, J. T., Jr., & Deftos, L. H. (1974). Parathyroid hormone, calcitonin, vitamin D, bone and bone mineral metabolism. In *Duncan's Diseases of Metabolism*, 7/e, ed. Bondy, P. K. and Rosenburg, pp. 1339–1350, Philadelphia: W. B. Saunders.

Prein, E. L., Jr., Pyle, E. B. & Krane, S. M. (1976). Secondary hyperparathyroidism. In *Handbook of Physiology*. Vol. VII, Section 7, Endocrinology, pp. 383–410. Washington: American Physiological Society.

Pullman, T. N., Lavender, A. R., Aho, I. & Rasmussen, H. (1960). Direct renal action of purified parathyroid extract. *Endocrinology*, **67**, 570–582.

Purnell, D. C., Scholz, D. A., Smith, L. H., Sizemore, G. W., Black, B. M., Goldsmith, R. S. & Arnaud, C. D. (1974). Treatment of primary hyperparathyroidism. *American Journal of Medicine*, **56**, 800–809.

Puschett, J. B. & Zurbach, P. (1976). Acute effects of parathyroid hormone in proximal bicarbonate transport in the dog. *Kidney International*, **9**, 501–510.

Puschett, J. B. & Sylk, D. (1977). Renal tubular effects of physiologic and pharmacologic doses of parathyroid hormone. *Kidney International*, **12**, 460A.

Rasmussen, H., Sze, Y. L. & Young, R. (1964). Further studies on the isolation and characterization of parathyroid peptides. *Journal of Biological Chemistry*, **239**, 2852–2857.

Rasmussen, H. & Bordier, P. (1974). *The Physiological and Cellular Basis of Metabolic Bone Disease*. Pp. 144–164, Baltimore: Williams and Wilkins.

Reiss, E. & Canterbury, J. M. (1968) A radioimmunoassay for parathyroid hormone in man. *Proceedings of the Society for Experimental Biology*, **128**, 501–504.

Rodriguez, H. J., Villarreal, H., Jr., Klahr, S. & Slatopolsky, E. (1974). Pseudohypoparathyroidism Type II: Restoration of normal renal responsiveness to parathyroid hormone by calcium administration. *Journal of Clinical Endocrinology and Metabolism*, **39**, 693–701.

Rutherford, W. E., Bordier, P., Marie, P., Hruska, K., Harter, H., Greenwalt, A., Blondin, J., Haddad, J., Bricker, N. & Slatopolsky, E. (1977). Phosphate control and 25-hydroxycholecalciferol administration in preventing experimental renal osteodystrophy in the dog. *Journal of Clinical Investigation*, **60**, 332–341.

Short, E. M., Elsas, L. J. & Rosenberg, L. E. (1974). Effect of parathyroid hormone on renal tubular reabsorption of amino acids. *Metabolism*, **23**, 715–727.

Slatopolsky, E., Caglar, S., Pennell, J. P., Taggart, D. D., Canterbury, J. M., Reiss, E. & Bricker, N. S. (1971). On the pathogenesis of hyperparathyroidism in chronic experimental renal insufficiency in the dog. *Journal of Clinical Investigation*, **50**, 492–499.

Slatopolsky, E., Caglar, S., Gradowska, L., Canterbury, J., Reiss, E. & Bricker, N. S. (1972).

On the prevention of secondary hyperparathyroidism in experimental chronic renal disease using "proportional reduction" of dietary phosphorus intake. *Kidney International,* **2,** 147–151.

Slatopolsky, E., Rutherford, W. E., Hruska, K., Martin, K. & Klahr, S. (1978). How important is phosphate in the pathogenesis of renal osteodystrophy? *Archives of Internal Medicine,* **138,** 848–852 (special issue).

Steele, T. H. (1976). Renal resistance to parathyroid hormone during phosphorus deprivation. *Journal of Clinical Investigation,* **58,** 1461–1464.

Sutton, R. A. L., Wong, N. L. M. & Dirks, J. H. (1976). Effects of parathyroid hormone on sodium and calcium transport in the dog nephron. *Clinical Science and Molecular Medicine,* **51,** 345–351.

Talmage, R. V. & Kraintz, F. W. (1954). Progressive changes in renal phosphate and calcium excretion in rats following parathyroidectomy or parathyroid administration. *Proceedings of the Society for Experimental Biology and Medicine,* **87,** 263–267.

Wang, C. A., Potts, J. T., Jr., & Neer, R. M. (1975). Controversy of parathyroid surgery. In *Calcium Regulating Hormones; Proceedings of the Fifth Parathyroid Conference,* ed. Talmage, R. V., Owen, M. and Parsons, J. A. Pp. 82–85. Amsterdam: Excerpta Medica.

Wells, S. A., Ellis, G. J., Gunnells, J. C., Schneider, A. B. & Sherwood, L. M. (1976). Parathyroid autotransplantation in primary parathyroid hyperplasia. *New England Journal of Medicine,* **295,** 57–62.

Wen, S. F. (1974). Micropuncture studies of phosphate transport in the proximal tubule of the dog: The relationship to sodium reabsorption. *Journal of Clinical Investigation,* **53,** 143–153.

8

Renal effects of prolactin, estrogen, and progesterone

TOMAS BERL
ORI S. BETTER

Stimulated primarily by the unique changes in renal function during gestation, a considerable investigative effort has been devoted to the understanding of the renal effects of prolactin, estrogen, and progesterone. The present review will summarize the state of our knowledge of the actions of these female sex hormones on the kidney.

RENAL EFFECTS OF PROLACTIN

Frantz and Klineberg (1970) first demonstrated that the anterior pituitary hormone prolactin is present in human blood as an entity that can be distinguished clearly from growth hormone. This observation and the subsequent development of a radioimmunoassay for the human hormone (Hwang, Guyda, and Freisan, 1971) have led to the intensive investigation of the chemistry, biological actions, and metabolism of prolactin both in health and disease (Frantz, 1978). However, studies of the renal effects of prolactin have been rather sparse, particularly in vertebrates. Despite the recent elucidation of the entire amino acid sequence of human prolactin (Shome and Parlow, 1977), this substance is not readily available, and thus studies in humans are limited. Here we will attempt to summarize and review critically the studies that have been performed on the renal actions of prolactin by posing a number of questions. As will become evident, few, if any, of these questions have been answered conclusively.

1. Are there specific prolactin receptors in renal tissue? When Birkinshaw and Falconer (1972) injected prolactin labeled with radioactive iodine, they noted a considerable concentration of radioactivity in the kidney and urine. Most of the latter was shown to be accounted for by degradation products of the hormone. Likewise, other investigators using either microautoradiographic techniques (Rajaniemi, Oksanen, and VanhaPerttula, 1974) or a double-antibody technique (Donatsch and Richardson, 1975) have further localized the prolactin uptake to the proximal tubule in rodents. In contrast, Evan et al. (1977), also employing autoradiographic localization of I^{125} ovine prolactin in the rat, found the predominant radioactivity to be in the thick ascending loop of Henle, in the distal tubule, and in the cortical collecting ducts. The discrepancy between these results remains unexplained. It must be emphasized, however, that none of the abovedescribed studies provides specific evidence for a renal receptor since the renal localization may well be nonspecific and primarily related to the metabolism or excretion of the hormone. The studies of Frantz, MacIdoe, and Turkington (1974) provided an initial characterization of a specific receptor. Specific binding activity (the activity that could be displaced by prolactin but not by luteinizing hormone) was found in subcellular particles prepared from kidneys of the rat and the mouse. This binding was, however, significantly smaller than that of mammary tissue, the recognized target organ of this hormone. Subsequently, employing similar displacement methods, Marshall, Gelato, and Meites (1975) found specific prolactin binding in microsomal membranes of the rat, which could be slightly modified by dehydration but not by salt loading. Likewise, castration increased and testosterone decreased prolactin-binding activity, while progesterone was without effect (Marshall et al., 1976). On the other hand, in their extensive study on the binding of a number of hormones in various tissues, Posner et al. (1974) noted that only frog kidney displayed highly significant binding (>3 percent). However, these investigators also failed to see significant binding of prolactin to mammary tissue in most of the species studied, thus throwing some doubt on the interpretation of the negative results. We must note, however, that even the abovementioned studies suggesting the existence of specific renal prolactin receptors (Frantz et al., 1974; Marshall et al., 1975) do not provide the strictest proof for their existence. The specific renal binding sites described may be primarily related to an enzyme involved in the metabolism of the hormone and therefore are not necessarily receptors linked to its biological response. Kahn (1975) has outlined the functional characteristics of polypeptide hormone receptors, such as the existence of a finite number of binding sites on the plasma membrane, a binding that is rapid and reversible, and a relation to the biological effects of the hormone. These characteristics have yet to be defined for prolactin in renal tissue. Finally, it is interesting to speculate that because prolactin is phylogenetically a very old hormone that affects sodium and water balance in some lower forms, receptors may indeed exist in the kidney, but a functional renal role for the hormone may have been lost in the evolutionary process.

2. *Does prolactin affect renal hemodynamics?* The effects of prolactin on glomerular filtration rate and renal blood flow have been recorded in a number of experiments in which the hormone was infused into various species of animals. The results are by no means uniform. However, with the exception of one study in which the administration of large doses of ovine prolactin (40 U/kg) was associated with accelerated nephropathy in aging rats as judged by histologic criteria (Richardson and Luginbuhl, 1976), in all other cases the glomerular filtration rate and/or renal blood flow remained unchanged or even increased. Thus, in the rat neither ovine (Lockett and Nail, 1965; Miller, Van Gemert, and Moses, 1974) nor bovine (Lockett and Nail, 1965) prolactin causes changes in creatinine excretion or the clearance of inulin (Wallin and Lee, 1976). The same authors, however, noted that the infusion of the hormone caused a transient increase in glomerular filtration rate and renal blood flow in some perfused cat kidneys (Lockett, 1965). Such an effect was not observed with growth hormone despite the great structural similarities between the two hormones.

Studies on the effects of prolactin on renal hemodynamics in the dog have yielded conflicting results and have been reported primarily in preliminary form. Thus, Riley, Hagen, and Stefaniak (1976) found that the systemic administration of 6 to 13 μg/min of ovine prolactin increased the glomerular filtration rate in six anesthetized dogs from 33 to 38 ml/min (p < .025) with no change in blood flow. However, the same authors (Riley, Hagen, and Stefaniak, 1975) failed to detect changes in glomerular filtration rate or renal blood flow when an even higher dose of ovine prolactin (11–44 μg/min) was infused in the renal artery. Such results would suggest that the increase in glomerular filtration rate noted in the systemic study is mediated by an extrarenal mechanism, although neither changes in blood pressure, heart rate, or cardiac output were noted in that study (Riley et al., 1976). Furthermore, studies in awake dogs (MacCallum, Simpson, and Auld, 1975) infused with a dose of ovine prolactin that increased the blood concentration of the hormone from 5 to 26 ng/ml found a significant increase in both glomerular filtration rate (from 59 to 70 ml/min) and clearance of para-aminohippurate (from 192 to 245 ml/min). Systemic hemodynamics are not reported in this study. However, since no increase in urinary osmolality accompanied the infusion, it is unlikely that the vasopressin that frequently contaminates prolactin preparations caused elevations of systemic pressure that could have accounted for the observed changes. Because this latter study was performed under the most physiologic conditions and in a setting that minimizes errors in clearance measurements (a water diuresis), this observation deserves further substantiation.

Measurements of renal hemodynamics in response to prolactin admininstration in man are scant. The sustained administration of ovine prolactin to patients with hypopituitarism caused a decrease in blood urea nitrogen concentration that reached its nadir after the fourth day of treatment (Beck et al., 1964). In the same report, the more detailed study in one patient revealed an increase of 21 percent in the clearance of inulin and 17 percent increase in the clearance of para-aminohippurate. This tentative finding requires confirmation but suggests that the absence of prolactin may at least in part contribute to the decrease in renal hemodynamics seen in hypophysectomized animals. Other evidence in the literature for such a suggestion is at best circumstantial. The observation that neither adrenocorticotropic hormone nor triiodothyronine hormone alone, or in combination, restore glomerular filtration rate in hypophysectomized rats despite correction of systemic pressure (Bauman and Phillips, 1970) implies that the lack of some other anterior pituitary hormone is responsible for the lowering of glomerular filtration rate. Likewise, hypophysectomy appears to decrease glomerular filtration rate less in pregnant than in nonpregnant rats, perhaps pointing to placental lactogen as being responsible for the difference (Matthews, 1963). The relevance of these studies to nonpregnant humans with normal pituitary function is questionable. Thus, an increase of endogenous prolactin levels does not increase renal hemodynamics in normal volunteers (Berl et al., 1976), and patients with hyperprolactinemia have been reported to have normal glomerular filtration rates (Buckman, Peake, and Robertson, 1976). In summary, therefore, there is some suggestive, albeit preliminary, evidence that prolactin may increase renal hemodynamics in some experimental animals and in some pathophysiologic settings in humans, but probably has no such effect in healthy nonpregnant women.

3. *Does prolactin play a role in the control of sodium excretion?* The effects of prolactin on the excretion of sodium have received considerable attention since the demonstration that some hypophysectomized teleost fish lose the ability to survive in fresh water environment, an ability that can be restored by the administration of prolactin (Ensor and Ball, 1972; Pickford and Phillips, 1960). Such hypophysectomized animals become hypotonic at least in part because of an increase in the branchial efflux of sodium. It is of interest, therefore, that prolactin markedly decreases the Na-K-ATPase activity in the gills of these hypophysectomized fish, a process that would decrease branchial efflux of sodium and at the same time markedly increase the activity of the enzyme in the kidney, perhaps in an attempt to promote sodium retention (Pickford et al., 1970). Likewise, prolactin (10^{-5} to 10^{-8} M) appears to stimulate short current circuit (i.e., sodium transport) in the toad bladder in a pattern reminiscent of the action of antidiuretic hormone (Dalton and Snart, 1969).

These biochemical and in vitro studies have been complemented by a number of in vivo experiments in which prolactin preparations were administered to various species. The interpretation of these studies, however, deserves some cautionary notes. In virtually none of the studies is the purity of the administered hormone determined, and in some cases contamination with growth hormone is actually acknowledged (Horrobin et al., 1971). Such contamination is particularly bothersome because growth hormone has been reported to cause sodium retention (Biglieri, Watlington, and Forsham, 1961), although the purity of the growth hormone administered in this study is itself in doubt. The second note of caution refers to the fact that the observed effects may well represent pharmacologic rather than physiologic effects of the hormone. The blood levels of hormones attained with the infusions are almost never monitored and in most studies the doses are clearly pharmacologic.

The great majority of experiments in which the response of the mammalian nephron to prolactin administration was studied suggest that the hormone causes a decrease in sodium excretion. Such observations have been made in the isolated cat kidney (Marshall et al., 1975) as well as the awake (Lockett and Nail, 1965) and anesthetized (Lucci, Bengele, and Solomon, 1975) rat. In the latter study, it is of note that ovine prolactin (7.1 μg/hr/100 gm) had no effect on the excretion of the cation in hydropenia, but blunted the natriuresis of isotonic saline infusion. The authors postulate an effect on proximal reabsorption. Their postulate is based on the fact that prolactin inhibited the dilatation of lateral intercellular spaces that the authors observed in the proximal tubules of saline-loaded rats (Lucci et al., 1974). Such evidence for an action of prolactin on proximal sodium reabsorption is at best indirect. Further studies will thus be needed to delineate the mechanism, site of action, and physiologic significances of the antinatriuretic effect of prolactin in the rat.

Studies in ewes (Burstyn, Horrobin and Manku, 1972; Horrobin, Manku and Burstyn, 1973; Horrobin, Manku and Robertshaw, 1973) and rabbits (Burstyn et al., 1975) suggest that prolactin may have sodium-retaining properties in these species as well. However, the complexity of the experimental designs involving a number of hormonal interrelations makes the interpretation of these data somewhat difficult. As was the case with renal hemodynamics, experiments in dogs have yielded variable results. In the anesthetized dog, intrarenal prolactin administration caused no change in sodium excretion (Riley et al., 1976). In the conscious animal the infusion of the hormone yielding "physiologic" concentrations (26 ng/ml) was associated with a natriuresis, an effect probably mediated by the increase in glomerular filtration rate (MacCallum et al., 1975).

In humans, Horrobin et al. (1971) found a decrease in urinary sodium excretion following the administration of a massive dose (8 mg intramuscularly) of sheep prolactin. The physiologic significance of such an observation is rather doubtful, since an increase in endogenous prolactin levels to the supraphysiologic range by the administration of thyrotropin-releasing hormone caused no significant change in the rate of urinary sodium excretion (Berl et al., 1976; Baumann and Loriaux, 1976). Furthermore, neither patients with galactorrhea, who have markedly elevated prolactin levels, nor lactating women appear to develop significant sodium retention.

Since prolactin's circadian rhythm is characterized by peak concentrations at night (Sassin et al., 1972; Norkin et al., 1972), the possibility that this hormone, at least in part, mediates nocturnal decreases in sodium excretion has been proposed (Simpson et al., 1975). However, studies that employed a known inhibitor of prolactin secretion, 2 Br alpha ergocryptine (del Pozo et al., 1972), in ten healthy females noted no change in the excretion rhythm of sodium when the subjects were on the drug (del Pozo and Ohnhaus, 1976). Such studies provide rather strong evidence against a role of prolactin in this phenomenon. Finally, a possible role of prolactin "hypersensitivity" as a cause of premenstrual sodium retention, irritability, and mastodynia has been suggested (Horrobin, 1976). In this regard, a preliminary report (Benedek-Jaszman et al., 1975) involving a double-blind cross-over study showed improvement of premenstrual symptoms in bromocryptine-treated patients. This report requires further confirmation.

   4. Is prolactin an osmoregulating hormone in mammals, and does it affect renal water excretion? In view of the role of prolactin in the osmoregulation of teleosts (Ensor and Ball, 1972; Pickford and Phillips, 1960) as well as birds, (Ensor and Phillips, 1970), the role of the hormone as an osmoregulator in mammals has been the subject of considerable attention. Studies in which perfused cat kidney (Lockett, 1965), unanesthetized rats (Lockett and Nail, 1965), rats with congenital pituitary diabetes insipidus (Miller, Van Gemert, and Moses, 1974), and humans (Horrobin et al., 1971) have appeared to respond to exogenous prolactin administration with a decrease in renal water excretion suggest a role for the hormone in the control of fluid balance in mammals as well. The clearance studies of Wallin and Lee (1976) pointed to an effect on the collecting duct, since prolactin impaired maximal free water clearance but not maximal free water reabsorption. A mechanism similar to that of vasopressin was further postulated, since the infusion of the hormone was shown to increase urinary cyclic AMP excretion (Wallin and Lee, 1976) as well as to stimulate medullary adenylate cyclase (Evan et al., 1977).

   The significance and interpretation of these studies, which involve the administration of exogenous prolactin, have been brought into question not only because of their pharmacologic nature but also because many of the preparations appear to be contaminated with vasopressin itself (Malarkey, George, and Baehler, 1975; Bond et al., 1976). More recently Keeler and Wilson (1976) have shown with an immunoassay that National Institutes of Health prolactin is heavily contaminated with antidiuretic hormone and that the purer preparation is essentially devoid of antidiuretic properties. Likewise, Vorherr, Vorherr and Solomon (1978), employing specific antisera, have demonstrated that all the antidiuretic effects of three different prolactin preparations are eliminated by treatment with vasopressin antisera or pregnancy plasma that is rich in vasopressinase.

   Studies involving elevations of endogenous prolactin are somewhat conflicting. In a preliminary study, Buckman et al. (1974) reported that patients with hyperprolactinemia have abnormalities in the excretion of a water load. However, a more complete report by the same investigators (Buckman, Peake, and Robertson, 1976) shows that free water generation, minimal urinary osmolality, and even suppression of antidiuretic hormone levels is normal following a water load. The decrease in urine flow was entirely accounted for by an unexplained decrease in solute clearance. Likewise, neither the acute increase of endogenous prolactin levels with thyrotropin-releasing hormone (Berl et al., 1976; Baumann and Loriaux, 1976) nor the chronic elevation of prolactin levels (Baumann et al., 1977) impair the normal excretion of water.

Finally, the possibility that the control of prolactin release itself may be under osmotic control has been proposed (Buckman et al., 1973; Buckman and Peake, 1973; Relkin, 1974). Thus, an oral water load seemed to decrease pro-lactin levels to at least 50 percent of baseline in normals and in patients with "physiologic galactorrhea" but not in those with tumors (Buckman et al., 1973). Likewise, the infusion of hypertonic solutions increased serum prolactin levels both in humans (Buckman and Peake, 1973) and the rat (Relkin, 1974). More recently, our studies (Berl et al., 1976) and the very well-controlled study of Adler et al. (1975) could not confirm an effect of either hypotonic or hyper-tonic infusions on the circulating levels of prolactin. Adler et al. (1975) postu-late that failure to control for diurnal variations and for stress as well as the use of a heterologous rather than a homologous assay for prolactin in some studies (Buckman et al., 1973; Buckman and Peake, 1973) may explain the observed discrepancy. Taken together, however, all of these studies impose doubt on any physiologic role of prolactin in the control of renal water excretion and provide no solid evidence for an osmoregulation of prolactin release in humans. It appears very likely, therefore, that these properties of the hormone have been lost in the evolutionary process.

RENAL EFFECTS OF ESTROGEN

Renal estrogen receptors

The initial search for the existence of receptors for estrogen in renal tissue was stimulated by the observation that renal tumors can be induced in male or ovariectomized female hamsters by the prolonged administration of stilbes-terol (Matthews, Kirkman, and Bacon, 1947). Studies employing radioactively labeled estradiol have demonstrated uptake by renal tissue and primarily the proximal tubule but with a retention rate that is much lower than that of other "target" tissues of the hormones such as the uterus, vagina, mammary gland, and the anterior pituitary gland (King, 1967; Steggles and King, 1967). How-ever, no specific binding studies were undertaken by these authors. Since then, studies in the hamster (Li et al., 1974), adrenalectomized rats (De Vries, Ludens, and Fanestil, 1972), mice (Bullock and Bardin, 1975), and fetal guinea pigs (Pasqualini, Sumida, and Gelly, 1974) have all demonstrated the existence and even characterized a number of the physical properties of an estrogen spe-cific macromolecule present in the cytosol. It is important to note that such receptors were demonstrated in animals lacking androgen receptors (Bullock and Bardin, 1975) to which estrogen are known to bind (Fang and Liao, 1971). In addition to these cytosolic receptors, some of the above studies (De Vries et al., 1972; Bullock and Bardin, 1975) have noted binding of the hormone to nuclei as well. Such an observation is very much in line with the current view on the mechanisms whereby estrogens (as well as other steroid hormones) exert their biologic action (Jensen and DeSombre, 1972). The process involves the binding of the hormone to a cytosolic protein receptor that is then translocated by the nucleus. Here, the hormone protein complex binds to a nuclear receptor and in some way alters the biosynthetic machinery of the nucleus. While renal tissue appears to be endowed with the components that are needed to make such a process possible, all the steps in the above sequence have not been defined. Furthermore, the physiologic role of the receptor, if any, in mediating either the formation of renal tumors (Bullock and Bardin, 1975), the multiplicity of biochemical effects of estrogens in the kidney (Christy and Shaver, 1974), or the antinatriuresis that accompanies its administration (De Vries et al., 1972) remains to be determined.

Effects on renal hemodynamics

The effects of the female sex hormones on renal hemodynamics have been studied almost as early as measurements of glomerular filtration rate and renal blood flow became available. This interest was stimulated primarily in an attempt to determine whether alterations in renal hemodynamics could be mediating the changes in sodium excretion that accompany the administration of these hormones. Likewise, these measurements were stimulated by the possibility that elevations in the concentrations of estrogens and progesterones could be responsible for the marked increases in glomerular filtration rate and renal blood flow that supervene in pregnancy.

A number of early studies in which the response to pharmacologic doses of estrogenic hormones (Richardson and Houck, 1951; Dance, Lloyd, and Pickford, 1959) or ovariectomy (White, Heinbecker, and Rolf, 1947) was studied in dogs are lacking in appropriate controls and employed a small number of animals. Nonetheless, the studies revealed either no or a very slight effect on glomerular filtration rate and renal blood flow. Likewise, measurements of these parameters of renal function performed in the rat (Nocenti and Cizek, 1964), rabbit (Nocenti and Cizek, 1973), and guinea pig (Middleton and Williams, 1974) show that they remain essentially unaffected in response to a variety of estrogenic compounds given in various doses and by various routes. The studies of Johnson et al. (1972; Johnson and Davis, 1976) are the most carefully controlled dog studies in the field. These authors studied adrenalectomized female dogs maintained on fixed replacement of glucocorticoid and mineralocorticoid hormones. The administration of 1 mg/day of estradiol caused a slight increase in creatinine clearance after two days but when measured after 5 and 8 days of treatment the change was no longer significant.

Studies on the effects of estrogens on the glomerular filtration rate and renal blood flow in humans are particularly scarce. Dean et al. (1945) noted that 4–6 mg of estradiol given for 9 to 12 days to four women caused no change in either glomerular filtration rate or renal blood flow. More recently, neither postmenopausal women (Dignam, Voskian, and Assali, 1956), premenopausal women (Chesley and Tepper, 1967), nor male volunteers (Katz and Lindheimer, 1977) showed either an acute (Dignam et al., 1956; Katz and Lindheimer, 1977) or chronic (Dignam et al., 1956; Chesley and Tepper, 1967; Katz and Lindheimer, 1977) effect of the hormone on renal blood flow or glomerular filtration rate. It must be noted, however, that a recent study of normotensive women (Hollenberg et al., 1976), in which renal blood flow was measured by the xenon washout technique, showed that those who ingested oral contraceptives containing an estrogen-progesterone combination had a significantly lower blood flow than that of matched controls. A possible role of angiotensin II was proposed, but to our knowledge not yet substantiated with appropriate inhibitors.

Taken together, the above studies suggest that the effect of estrogens per se on renal hemodynamics is slight or nonexistent. Measurements of these parameters are not sensitive enough to ensure absolutely that the changes in sodium excretion that accompany the administration of the hormone are not at least in part mediated by changes in glomerular filtration rate. It is clear, however, that the large changes in glomerular filtration rate and renal blood flow that are seen in pregnancy cannot be ascribed to effects of the hormone.

Effects of estrogens of electrolyte and water excretion

Since Thorn and Engel (1938) noted that single injections of crude estrogen preparations (estradiol or estrone) were followed over the ensuing 3 days by a marked decrease in sodium chloride and water excretion, the antinatriuretic property of the hormone repeatedly has been documented in the dog (Richardson and Houck, 1951; Dance et al., 1959). The most careful balance studies in this species have demonstrated that administration of as little as 100 μg/day of estradiol results in a positive balance of sodium, but not of potassium (Johnson et al., 1970). Since the same dose of estriol, which has much less estrogenic potency than estradiol (Sealey and Sondern, 1941), was also associated with sodium retention, it appears that the sodium-retaining property of the hormone is not closely correlated with its estrogenic activity. The effect of estrogens on cation excretion in humans is similar to that in the dog. While the acute infusion of the hormone does not significantly alter sodium excretion, the administration of 8 mg/day of estradiol for 3 to 6 days to postmenopausal women is associated with sodium and water retention without associated changes in potassium balance (Dignam et al., 1956). Subsequently, Landau et al. (1957), using much smaller doses (0.5 mg of estradiol benzoate daily), also observed sodium retention. Of particular interest are the studies of Preedy and Aitken (1956a; 1956b), who noted that 10 mg/day of estradiol given for one week caused sodium chloride and water retention. This retention was only transient in normal subjects (Preedy and Aitken, 1956a) but sustained in subjects with cirrhosis (Preedy and Aitken, 1956b). Such a behavior in normals is reminiscent of the "escape" phenomenon that is observed in response to administration of mineralocorticoids. It is of note, however, that studies employing radioactive sodium to measure exchangeable sodium spaces have determined that estrogenic components bring about an increase in sodium space (± 200 mEq) that is considerably smaller than is observed in aldosteronism (± 370 mEq) (Crane and Harris, 1974a). This estrogen-associated sodium retention brings about the expected increases in extracellular fluid volume (Preedy and Aitken, 1956a; Aitken, Lindsay and Hart, 1974) with the accompanying decrease in serum proteins and hematocrit (Aitken et al., 1974). These latter authors, furthermore, have noted a significant decrease in serum sodium and osmolality in their larger group of oophorectomized women on estrogen replacement (Aitken et al., 1974). Such an observation suggests an even greater degree of water retention, perhaps involving abnormalities in the secretion or action of antidiuretic hormone. In this regard a recent preliminary observation (Vallotton et al., 1976), in which estrogens appeared to potentiate the osmotic release of vasopressin, requires further exploration. Finally, Katz and Kappas (1967) reported that an even larger dose of estradiol (20 mg/day) caused an initial (1 or 2 days) increase in sodium excretion that was then followed by a pronounced decrease in sodium excretion over the ensuing 9 to 10 days. The significance of the initial natriuresis, if any, has not been defined.

In contrast to studies in dog and humans, the effects of estrogens on sodium excretion in rats is somewhat controversial. While some investigators have noted a decrease in sodium excretion in rats treated with estradiol (De Vries et al., 1972), others have found that the hormone has little (Deming and Luetscher, 1950) or no (Dorfman, 1949; Simpson and Tait, 1952) antinatriuretic action. More carefully conducted studies in this species have shown that estrogens cause a decrease in food consumption. Such an effect on food intake may be primarily responsible for the decrease in sodium excretion (Thornborough and Passo, 1975). Thus, neither the excretion of sodium nor potassium is different in stilbesterol-treated rats when compared to their pair-fed controls (Nocenti and Cizek, 1964). In summary, therefore, it appears that estrogens possess antinatriuretic properties both in dog and humans, but may have no such effect in the rat.

The mechanisms responsible for estrogen-mediated antinatriuresis have not been fully elucidated. In view of the abovedescribed effects on renal hemodynamics it does not appear likely that decreases in glomerular filtration rate or changes in renal vascular resistance are responsible for the antinatriuresis. Furthermore, the hemodilution and decrease in serum proteins that have been reported would have the opposite effect on renal sodium handling (Schrier and de Wardener, 1971). The possibility that the effects of estrogens on sodium excretion may be mediated by mineralocorticoids is of interest. Such a mechanism is supported by the observation that ethinyl estradiol (0.5 mg/day) results in a marked increase in the urinary excretion of aldosterone, particularly in the first week of therapy (Crane and Harris, 1969), and by the ability of both estradiol and estriol to increase the secretion rate of aldosterone in humans (Katz and Kappas, 1967).

Evidence has also accrued against an aldosterone-mediated mechanism. In the first place, some investigators (Laidlaw, Ruse, and Gornall, 1962) have found that the excretion of the hormone did not rise above normal in seven of eight subjects given estrogenic hormone. However, since estradiol appears to enhance the binding of aldosterone to its renal receptor (Swaneck, Highland, and Edelman, 1969), this observation does not in itself rule out a mineralocorticoid-mediated mechanism. Stronger evidence is provided by studies in the adrenalectomized state. Thus, estrogens have been observed to cause sodium retention in an Addisonian patient (Thorn, Nelson, and Thorn, 1938) as well as in adrenalectomized dogs on a fixed replacement dose of either mineralocorticoids or glucocorticoids and, even more importantly, glucocorticoid replacement alone (Johnson et al., 1972). These studies very strongly suggest that neither increases in circulating levels of mineralocorticoids nor a potentiation of their renal action mediate the antinatriuresis associated with estrogen administration. The available evidence, therefore, points to a direct intrarenal effect of estrogens possibly involving the aforementioned receptors. Such an intrarenal mechanism is, furthermore, compatible with the observation that 17 beta-estradiol increases short circuit current in the frog skin (Tomlinson, 1971a).

A role for estrogens in the development of premenstrual edema (Thorn et al., 1938) and in the sodium retention of pregnancy (Taylor, Warner, and Welsh, 1939) has been proposed since the 1930s. In the rat, for example, the excretion of sodium and water decreases in the oestrus cycle at a time when the estrogen secretory rate is high (i.e., estrus phase) (Crocker and Hinsull, 1972). A cause-effect relationship cannot be drawn from this association because the production of mineralocorticoids also increases in the estrus phase (Hinsull and Crocker, 1970) as it does in the luteal phase of the menstrual cycle in women (Gray et al., 1968). Furthermore, since estrogen secretion is actually highest in midcycle, it is difficult to incriminate it in the pathogenesis of premenstrual edema. Likewise, the role of estrogens in the process that leads to the retention of approximately 800 mEq of sodium in pregnancy has not been defined. Clearly, it is neither the only nor the most potent of the antinatriuretic forces that control sodium excretion in this state (Lindheimer and Katz, 1973). Finally, estrogens have been implicated in the mechanism of salt retention in idiopathic cyclic edema (Ferris and Bay, 1978). However, as these authors note, no increase in estradiol levels have been documented in women with this disorder, and it occurs in both postmenopausal and oophorectomized patients. In summary, therefore, the physiologic significance of the sodium retention properties of estrogens is not clear. It is likely that they are a component of a delicate hormonal balance involving also progesterone and aldosterone, which serves to maintain external sodium homeostasis.

RENAL EFFECTS OF PROGESTERONE

Progesterone occupies a unique position among hormones inasmuch as it is an obligatory intermediary in the biosynthetic pathway leading to the production of a number of other hormones, including androgens, estrogens, aldosterone, cortisol, and desoxycorticosterone (Landau, 1973). It is likely that phylogenetically progesterone may have been a hormone early and probably prior to the evolution of other gonadal hormones. This perhaps explains the great species differences that have been observed in the renal effects of this hormone. Furthermore, the consistent failure to detect specific progesterone receptors in renal tissue (Li et al., 1974) makes it likely that many of the effects occur by an extrarenal mechanism or by the binding to the receptors of another hormone.

Effects of progesterone on renal hemodynamics

Because the synthesis of progesterone greatly increases during pregnancy (Pearlman, 1957), the possibility that it is responsible for the increases in glomerular filtration rate and renal blood flow that occurs in gestation has been considered. Large doses of the hormone, therefore, have been administered to experimental animals in an attempt to achieve levels comparable to those seen in the pregnant state.

In the rat, progesterone increases creatinine secretion (Harvey and Malvin, 1966) and, as part of its anabolic effects, causes an increase in renal mass (Hervey and Hervey, 1967). Therefore, only studies that employ clearance of inulin as an index of glomerular filtration rate and make a correction for body and kidney weight are readily interpretable. In two such studies, the prolonged administration of large amounts of the hormone did not increase either the clearance of inulin or para-aminohippurate (Lindheimer, Koeppen, and Katz, 1976; Matthews, 1963). Likewise in the dog, progesterone does not alter renal blood flow or its distribution (Barnes, 1973). In contrast to the rat and the dog, studies suggest that the hormone may have an effect on renal hemodynamics in humans. Thus, Chesley and Tepper (1967) noted that unlike estrogen administration, after 3 days of 150 mg of progesterone per day, nonpregnant women had an increase in both inulin clearance (from 108 to 122 ml/min) and para-aminohippurate clearance (from 590 to 676 ml/min). Subsequently, Oparil, Ehrlich, and Lindheimer (1975) found in men that acute as well as chronic progesterone administration in doses as high as 300 mg/day increased para-aminohippurate clearance but not inulin clearance. The magnitude of these changes is, however, small and can by no means account for the increases in renal hemodynamics observed in the pregnant state. It is possible, however, that the observed renal vasodilatation and the accompanying decrease in filtration fraction play a role in the increased sodium excretion that is associated with progesterone administration in humans.

Effects of progesterone on sodium and water excretion

The observation made in the 1920s that pregnancy protected adrenalectomized animals against volume depletion (Rogoff and Stewart, 1927) stimulated studies on the salt-retaining properties of various hormones, including progesterone. Thus, soon thereafter, progesterone was shown to be associated with increased survival in adrenalectomized ferrets and mice (Gaunt and Hays,

1938; Gaunt, Nelson, and Loomis, 1938). Likewise, Thorn and Engel (1937) noted that the administration of progesterone decreased sodium excretion in adrenalectomized dogs. However, recent studies in this species employing careful balances have failed to show any significant effect of the hormone given in doses as high as 200 mg/day on sodium balance (Johnson et al., 1970; O'Connell et al., 1969). Studies in rats have also yielded conflicting results, as an acute sodium-retaining effect was observed in one study (Fimognari, Fanestil, and Edelman, 1967) and no effect noted in a more chronic setting (Lindheimer et al., 1976). In contrast to the rather inconclusive state of our knowledge in the rat and dog, a natriuretic effect of progesterone has been repeatedly demonstrated both in acute and chronic metabolic studies in man (Oparil et al., 1975; Landau et al., 1955; Landau et al., 1957; Oelkers, Schoneshofer, and Blumel, 1974). This natriuresis results in a measurable decrease in exchangeable sodium in progesterone-treated subjects (Crane and Harris, 1974b) and is most likely responsible for the associated increases in plasma renin activity and aldosterone excretion (Oparil et al., 1975; Crane and Harris, 1974a).

The mechanism of progesterone-mediated natriuresis has not been fully elucidated. It is possible that the abovementioned vasodilatory decrease in filtration fraction that accompanies progesterone administration could be responsible for the observed increase in sodium excretion. More interest has been focused, however, on the possible interaction between progesterone and mineralocorticoids. Landau and Lugibihl (1958) thus postulated that the natriuresis was mediated by antagonism to mineralocorticoids, because no natriuresis was observed with the hormone after aldosterone was withdrawn from an Addisonian patient. However, the more recent study of Oparil et al. (1975) suggests that the acute natriuretic action of progesterone is at least in part independent of aldosterone inhibition. Such evidence is based on the observation that progesterone caused a comparable natriuresis in subjects on a sodium-depleted diet (i.e., high aldosterone state) as on a high sodium diet (i.e., low aldosterone state). Likewise, by employing clearance techniques in subjects undergoing a water diuresis, an effect of the hormone on both the proximal and distal nephron was noted. Aldosterone is not known to have an effect on proximal tubular sodium reabsorption. In view of methodologic limitations, this evidence must be viewed as indirect. Perhaps more extensive studies on the effect of the hormone in adrenalectomized or spironolactone-treated subjects will provide more final information on the in vivo interaction between progesterone and mineralocorticoids in humans.

The spironolactonelike action of progesterone would be expected to result in potassium retention. Some balance studies, however, have found no evidence for an antikaliuretic effect (Landau and Lugibihl, 1958; Landau and Lugibihl, 1961). However, Ehrlich and Lindheimer (1972) have shown that progesterone markedly attenuates the kaliuretic action of mineralocorticoids during desoxycorticosterone escape and postulate that this effect may be important in protecting women from hypokalemia during pregnancy.

Studies performed on the effects of progesterone in anuran membranes have not yielded uniform results. Thus, while progesterone appears to decrease short-circuit current and active sodium transport in the frog skin (Tomlinson, 1971a; Tomlinson, 1971b), no such effect has been seen in the isolated toad bladder (Porter and Edelman, 1964). High concentrations of progesterone $(3 \times 10^{-5}$ to 10^{-4} M), however, displace aldosterone from its binding sites in the toad bladder (Sharp, Komack, and Leaf, 1966) and antagonize the effect of aldosterone on sodium transport (Crabbe, 1964). However, Porter, Bogoroch, and Edelman (1964) found that lower doses of progesterone $(7 \times 10^{-7}$ M) do not significantly influence aldosterone-mediated sodium transport, and the abovenoted studies employing much higher concentrations of the hormone may represent a nonspecific toxic effect.

Taken together, the above studies suggest that progesterone may have a slight antinatriuretic effect in dogs and rats and a clear natriuretic property in humans. It appears likely that when circulating in very high concentrations, progesterone binds to renal mineralocorticoid receptors where it exerts an agonist action in some species and an antagonist action in others.

The significance of progesterone natriuresis has been the subject of considerable speculation, primarily in terms of its role in the increased secretion of aldosterone during the luteal phase of the menstrual cycle (Gray et al., 1968) and pregnancy (Ehrlich et al., 1976). It is of interest, in terms of the former, that when ovulation is suppressed with mestranol, aldosterone secretory rate failed to increase in five of six subjects. However, the correlation between the level of urinary pregnandiol (a marker of progesterone production) and the increase of aldosterone secretion is poor, thus, suggesting that other factors also play a role in the control of aldosterone secretion during the menstrual cycle. It has also been postulated that the hyperaldosteronism of pregnancy is a response to the "sodium-wasting" forces of pregnancy. Because the secretion of aldosterone responds to physiologic changes such as volume loading or volume depletion (Lindheimer and Katz, 1977), it seems reasonable to assume that the elevated levels of aldosterone represent a compensatory response to what is perceived by afferent pathways as a "suboptimal" extracellular fluid volume. It must be noted, however, that even when progesterone is administered to normal volunteers in a dose resembling secretion during pregnancy, the increases in aldosterone are considerably smaller than those recorded during gestation. There must, therefore, again be other factors involved in this control mechanism.

Effects of estrogens and progesterones on the renin-angiotensin system: Implications for oral contraceptive-associated hypertension

Soon after oral contraceptives came into use, their association with the development of reversible hypertension has been frequently reported. The magnitude of the problem is unclear and the incidence of this complication varies from a few percent (Kunin, McCormack, and Abernathy, 1969) to almost 20 percent (Saruta, Saade, and Kaplan, 1970). The mechanism of the hypertension has not been entirely elucidated. The contraceptives consistently produce increased plasma substrate and plasma renin activity. These changes are primarily caused by the estrogenic component of the pill (Laragh, 1974), since the effect of synthetic gestagen is extremely variable (Crane and Harris, 1974a). These alterations in the renin-angiotensin system, however, supervene in normotensive as well as hypertensive subjects on oral contraceptives. It has been suggested, however, that the decrease in plasma renin concentration (the amount of angiotensin generated in the presence of fixed amount of renin substrate), while suppressed in normotensive pilltakers, is not suppressed in those with hypertension (Saruta et al., 1970; Kaplan, 1974), suggesting failure of the normal feedback control of plasma renin concentration. Luetscher et al. (1974), however, have found no support for such a concept. This discrepancy may be accounted for by methodologic differences and needs to be resolved.

Although the activation of the renin-angiotensin system may well account for the decrease in renal blood flow described in some normotensive patients on the pill (Hollenberg et al., 1976), it is unlikely to be the sole factor in the etiology of the hypertension. As noted above, the estrogenic compounds produce sodium retention. However, because of feedback suppression of the pituitary, the antagonistic effect of progesterone does not come into play. In fact, some of the synthetic gestagens in oral contraceptives, unlike progesterone, have mineralocorticoidlike activity and thus further enhance sodium retention (Crane and Harris, 1974a). It is likely, therefore, that in the "susceptible" patient, whose characteristics are heretofore unknown, the combination of sodium retention and the volume and sodium-independent activation of the renin-angiotensin-aldosterone axis could culminate in hypertension. In view of the enormous epidemiological importance of this form of hypertension, the screening of such patients would be invaluable.

ACKNOWLEDGMENT

The authors wish to thank Dr. Robert W. Schrier for his critical review of this manuscript and Ms. Linda M. Benson for her secretarial assistance.

REFERENCES

Adler, R. A., Noel, G. L., Wartofsky, L. & Frantz, A. G. (1975). Failure of oral water loading and intravenous hypotonic saline to suppress plasma prolactin in man. *Journal of Clinical Endocrinology and Metabolism*, **41**: 383–389.

Aitken, J. M., Lindsay, R. & Hart, D. M. (1974). The redistribution of body sodium in women on long-term oestrogen therapy. *Clinical Science and Molecular Medicine*, **47**, 179–187.

Barnes, A. B. (1973). The effect of oxytocin on renal blood flow and its distribution in the dog. *Nephron*, **11**, 40–57.

Bauman, J. W. & Phillips, E. S. (1970). Failure of blood pressure restoration to repair glomerular filtration rate in hypophysectomized rats. *American Journal of Physiology*, **218**, 1605–1608.

Baumann, G. & Loriaux, D. (1976). Failure of endogenous prolactin to alter renal salt and water excretion and adrenal function in man. *Journal of Clinical Endocrinology and Metabolism*, **43**, 643–649.

Baumann, G., Marynick, S. P., Winters, S. J. & Loriaux, D. L. (1977). The effect of osmotic stimuli on prolactin secretion and renal water excretion in normal man and in chronic hyperprolactinemia. *Journal of Clinical Endocrinology and Metabolism*, **44**, 199–202.

Beck, J. C., Gonda, A., Hamic, M. A., Morgen, R. O., Rubinstein, D. & McGarry, E. E. (1964). Some metabolic changes induced by primate growth hormone and purified ovine prolactin. *Metabolism*, **13**, 1108–1134.

Benedek-Jaszman, L. J., Lequin, R. M., Thomas, C. M. G. & Sternthal, V. (1975). Letter to the editor. *European Journal of Obstetrics, Gynecology and Reproductive Biology*, **5**, 191–192.

Berl, T., Brautbar, N., Ben-David, M., Czaczkes, W. & Kleeman, C. (1976). Osmotic control of prolactin release and its effect on renal water excretion in man. *Kidney International*, **10**, 158–163.

Biglieri, E. G., Watlington, C. O. & Forsham, P. H. (1961). Sodium retention with growth hormone and its subfraction. *Journal of Clinical Endocrinology and Metabolism*, **21**, 361–370.

Birkinshaw, M. & Falconer, I. R. (1972). Localization of prolactin labelled with radioactive iodide in rabbit mammary tissue. *Journal of Endocrinology*, **55**, 323–334.

Bond, G. C., Pasley, J. N., Koike, T. I. & Llerena, L. (1976). Contamination of an ovine prolactin preparation with antidiuretic hormone. *Journal of Endocrinology*, **71**, 169–170.

Buckman, M. T., Kaminsky, N., Conway, M. & Peake, G. T. (1973). Utility of L dopa and water loading in evaluation of hyperprolactinemia. *Journal of Clinical Endocrinology and Metabolism*, **36**, 911–919.

Buckman, M. T. & Peake, G. T. (1973). Osmolar control of prolactin secretion in man. *Science*, **181**, 755–757.

Buckman, M. T., Peake, G. T. & Robertson G. (1976). Hyperprolactinemia influences renal function in man. *Metabolism*, **25**, 509–516.

Buckman, M. T., Robertson, G. & Peake, G. T. (1974). Antidiuresis of patients with hyperprolactinemia (abstract). *Proceedings of 56th Annual Endocrine Society*, #170.

Bullock, L. P. & Bardin, C. W. (1975). The presence of estrogen receptor in kidneys from normal and androgen insensitive tfm/y mice. *Endocrinology*, **97**, 1106–1111.

Burstyn, P. G., Gaynes, N., Golightly, N. & Scott, A. (1975). The effects of prolactin on renal excretion, and on voluntary intake of water and sodium in rabbits. *Journal of Physiology*, **251**, 30–31.

Burstyn, P. G., Horrobin, D. F. & Manku, M. S. (1972). Saluretic action of aldosterone in the presence of increased salt intake and restoration of normal action by prolactin or oxytocin. *Journal of Endocrinology*, **55**, 369–376.

Chesley, L. C. & Tepper, I. H. (1967). Effects of progesterone and estrogen on the sensitivity to angiotensin II. *Journal of Clinical Endocrinology and Metabolism*, **27**, 576–581.

Christy, N. P. & Shaver, J. C. (1974). Estrogens and the kidney. *Kidney International*, **6**, 366–376.

Crabbe, J. (1964). Decreased effectiveness of aldosterone on active sodium transport by the isolated toad bladder in the presence of other steroids. *Acta Endocrinology*, **47**, 419–432.

Crane, M. G. & Harris, J. J. (1974a). Effects of estrogens and gestagens on the renin-aldosterone system. In *Oral Contraceptives and High Blood Pressure*, ed. Fregly, M. J. & Fregly, M. S. Pp. 100–119. Gainesville: Dolphin.

Crane, M. G. & Harris, J. J. (1974b). Effectiveness of estrogens and gestagens on exchangeable sodium. In *Oral Contraceptives and High Blood Pressure*, ed. Fregly, M. J. & Fregly, M. S. Pp. 159–182. Gainesville: Dolphin.

Crane, M. G. & Harris, J. J. (1969). Plasma renin activity and aldosterone excretion rate in normal subjects: I. Effect of ethinyl estradiol and medroxyprogesterone acetate. *Journal of Clinical Endocrinology*, **29**, 550–557.

Crocker, A. D. & Hinsull, S. M. (1972). Renal electrolyte excretion during the oestrus cycle in the rat. *Journal of Endocrinology*, **55**, xlii–xliii.

Dalton, T & Snart, R. T. (1969). Effect of prolactin in the active transport of sodium by the isolated toad bladder. *Journal of Endocrinology*, **43**, 6–7.

Dance, P., Lloyd, S. & Pickford, M. (1959). The effects of stilboestrol on the renal activity of conscious dogs. *Journal of Physiology*, **145**, 225–240.

Dean, A. L., Abels, J. C. & Taylor, H. C. (1945). The effects of certain hormones on the renal function of man. *Journal of Urology*, **53**, 647–651.

del Pozo, E., Bru del Re, R., Varga, L. & Freisen, H. (1972). The inhibition of prolactin secretion by 2 Br alpha ergocryptin. *Journal of Clinical Endocrinology and Metabolism*, **35**, 768–771.

del Pozo, E. & Ohnhaus, E. E. (1976). Lack of effect of acute prolactin suppression on renal water, sodium and potassium excretion during sleep. *Hormone Research*, **7**, 11–15.

Deming, Q. B. & Luetscher, J. A. Jr. (1950). Bioassay of deoxycorticosterone-like material in the urine. *Proceedings of the Society for Experimental Biology and Medicine*, **73**, 171–175.

DeVries, J. R., Ludens, J. H. & Fanestil, D. D. (1972). Estradiol renal receptor molecules and estradiol-dependent antinatriuresis. *Kidney International*, **2**, 95–100.

Dignam, W. S., Voskian, J. & Assali, N. S. (1956). Effects of estrogens on renal hemodynamics and excretion of electrolytes in human subjects. *Journal of Clinical Endocrinology*, **16**, 1032–1042.

Donatsch, P. & Richardson, B (1975). Localization of prolactin in rat kidney tissue using a double-antibody technique. *Journal of Endocrinology*, **66**, 101–116.

Dorfman, R. I. (1949). Influence of adrenal cortical steroids and related compounds on sodium metabolism. *Proceedings of the Society for Experimental Biology and Medicine*, **72**, 395–398.

Ehrlich, E. N. & Lindheimer, M. D. (1972). Effect of administered mineralocorticoids or ACTH in pregnant women. Attenuation of kaliuretic influence of mineralocorticoids during pregnancy. *Journal of Clinical Investigation*, **51**, 1301–1309.

Ehrlich, E. N., Nolten, E. W., Oparil, S. & Lindheimer, M. D. (1976). Mineralocorticoids in normal pregnancy. In *Hypertension in Pregnancy*, ed. Lindheimer, M. D., Katz, A. I. & Zuspan, F. P. Pp. 189–201. New York: John Wiley & Sons.

Ensor, D. M. & Ball, J. N. (1972). Prolactin and osmoregulation in fishes. *Federal Proceedings, Federation of American Societies for Experimental Biology*, **31**, 1615–1623.

Ensor, D. M. & Phillips, J. G. (1970). The effect of salt loading on the pituitary prolactin level of domestic duck and juvenile herring or less black backed gulls. *Journal of Endocrinology*, **48**, 167–172.

Evan, A. P., Palmer, G. C., Lucci, M. & Solomon, S. (1977). Prolactininduced stimulation of rat renal adenylate cyclase and autoradiographic localization to the distal nephron. *Nephron*, **18**, 266–267.

Fang, S. & Liao, S. (1971). Androgen receptors. *Journal of Biology and Chemisty*, **246**, 16–24.

Ferris, T. F. & Bay, W. H. (1978). Idiopathic edema. In *Sodium and Water Homeostasis*, ed. Brenner, B. M. & Stein J. H. Ch. 6, pp. 131–153. New York: Churchill Livingstone.

Fimognari, G. M., Fanestil, D. D. & Edelman, I. S. (1967). Induction of RNA and protein synthesis in the action of aldosterone in the rat. *American Journal of Physiology*, **213**, 954–962.

Frantz, A. G. (1978). Prolactin. *New England Journal of Medicine*, **298**, 201–207.

Frantz, A. G. & Kleinberg, D. L. (1970). Prolactin: Evidence that it is separate from growth hormone. *Science*, **170**, 745–747.

Frantz, W. L., MacIdoe, J. H. & Turkington, R. W. (1974). Prolactin receptors: Characteristics of the particulate fraction binding activity. *Journal of Endocrinology*, **60**, 485–497.

Gaunt, R. & Hays, H. W. (1938). Life-maintaining effect of crystalline progesterone in adrenalectomized ferrets. *Science*, **88**, 576–577.

Gaunt, R., Nelson, W. O. & Loomis, E. (1938). Cortical hormone-like action of progesterone and non-effect of sex hormones on water intoxication. *Proceedings of the Society for Experimental Biology and Medicine*, **39**, 319–322.

Gray, M. J., Strausfeld, K. S., Watnabe, M., Sims, E. A. H. & Solomon, S. (1968). Aldosterone secretory rates in the normal menstrual cycle. *Journal of Clinical Endocrinology*, **28**, 1269–1275.

Harvey, A. M. & Malvin, R. L. (1966). The effect of androgenic hormones on creatinine secretion in the rat. *Journal of Physiology*, **184**, 883–888.

Hervey, E. & Hervey, G. R. (1967). The effects of progesterone on body weight and composition in the rat. *Journal of Endocrinology*, **37**, 361–364.

Hinsull, S. M. & Crocker, A. D. (1970). The effects of ovarian hormones on the activity of the adrenal cortex and on water and sodium transport. *Journal of Endocrinology*, **48**, lxxix–lxxx.

Hollenberg, N. K., Williams, G. H., Burger, B., Chenitz, W., Hoosmand, I. & Adams, D. F. (1976). Renal blood flow and its response to angiotensin II, an interaction between oral contraceptive agents, sodium intake, and the renin-angiotensin system in healthy young women. *Circulation Research*, **38**, 35–40.

Horrobin, D. F. (1976). Fluid and electrolyte metabolism. In *Prolactin 1976*. Pp. 118–124. Montreal: Eden Press.

Horrobin, D. F., Lloyd, I. J., Lipton, A., Burstyn, P. G., Durkin, N. & Muiruri, K. L. (1971). Actions of prolactin on human renal function. *Lancet*, **2**, 352–354.

Horrobin, D. F., Manku, M. S., & Burstyn, P. G. (1973). Saluretic action of aldosterone in the presence of excess cortisol: Restoration of salt-retaining action by prolactin. *Journal of Endocrinology*, **56**, 343–344.

Horrobin, D. F., Manku, M. S. & Robertshaw, D. (1973). Water-losing action of antidiuretic hormone in the presence of excess cortisol: Restoration of normal action by prolactin or by oxytocin. *Journal of Endocrinology*, **58**, 135–136.

Hwang, P., Guyda, H. & Freisen, H. (1971). A radioimmunoassay for human prolactin. *Proceedings of the National Academy of Science* (U.S.A.), **68**, 1902–1906.

Jensen, E. V. & DeSombre, E. R. (1972). Mechanism of action of the female sex hormones. *Annual Review of Biochemistry*, **41**, 203–230.

Johnson, J. A. & Davis, J. O. (1976). The effect of estrogens on renal sodium excretion in the dog. In *Hypertension in Pregnancy*, ed. Lindheimer, M. D., Katz, A. I. & Zuspan, F. P. Pp. 239–248. New York: John Wiley & Sons.

Johnson, J. A., Davis, J. O., Baumber, J. S. & Schneider, E. G. (1970). Effect of estrogens and progesterone on electrolyte balances in normal dogs. *American Journal of Physiology*, **219**, 1691–1697.

Johnson, J. A., Davis, J. O., Brown, P. R., Wheeler, P. D. & Witty, R. T. (1972). Effects of estradiol on sodium and potassium balances in adrenalectomized dogs. *American Journal of Physiology*, **223**, 194–197.

Kahn, C. R. (1975). Membrane receptors for polypeptide hormones. In *Methods in Membrane Biology 3*, ed. Korn, E. D. Pp. 81–146. New York: Plenum Press.

Kaplan, N. M. (1974). Oral contraceptives and plasma renin concentration. In *Oral Contraceptives and High Blood Pressure*, ed. Fregly, M. J. & Fregly, M. S. Gainesville: Dolphin.

Katz, F. H. & Kappas, A. (1967). The effects of estradiol and estriol on plasma levels of cortisol and thyroid hormone-binding globulins on aldosterone and cortisol secretion rates in man. *Journal of Clinical Investigation*, **46**, 1768–1777.

Katz, A. I. & Lindheimer, M. D. (1977). Actions of hormones on the kidney. *Annual Review of Physiology*, **39**, 97–134.

Keeler, R. & Wilson, N. (1976). Vasopressin contamination as a cause of some apparent renal action of prolactin. *Canadian Journal of Physiology and Pharmacology*, **54**, 887–890.

King, R. J. B. (1967). Fixation of steroids in receptors. *Archives of Anatomical Microscopic and Morphology Experiments* (Suppl. 3–4), **56**, 570–582.

Kunin, C. M., McCormack, R. C. & Abernathy, J. R. (1969). Oral contraceptives and blood pressure. *Archives of Internal Medicine*, **123**, 363–365.

Laidlaw, J. C., Ruse, J. L. & Gornall, A. G. (1962). The influence of extrogen and progesterone on aldosterone excretion. *Journal of Clinical Endocrinology and Metabolism*, **22**, 161–171.

Landau, R. L. (1973). The metabolic influence of progesterone. In *Handbook of Physiology, Endocrinology II, Part 1*. Pp. 573–589. Baltimore: Williams & Wilkins.

Landau, R. L., Bergenstal, D. M., Lugibihl, K., Dimick, D. F. & Rashid, E. (1957). The relationship of estrogen and pituitary hormones to the metabolic effects of progesterone. *Journal of Clinical Endocrinology*, **17**, 177–185.

Laudau, R. L., Bergenstal, D. M., Lugibihl, K. & Kascht, M. E. (1955). The metabolic effects of progesterone in man. *Journal of Clinical Endocrinology*, **15**, 1194–1215.

Landau, R. L. & Lugibihl, K. (1958). Inhibition of the sodium-retaining influence of aldosterone by progesterone. *Journal of Clinical Endocrinology*, **18**, 1237–1245.

Landau, R. L., Lugibihl, K. (1961). The catabolic and natriuretic effects of progesterone in man. *Recent Progress in Hormone Research*, **17**, 249–253.

Landau, R. L., Lugibihl, K., Bergenstal, D. M. & Dimick, D. F. (1957). The metabolic effects of progesterone in man: Dose response relationships. *Journal of Laboratory and Clinical Medicine*, **50**, 613–620.

Laragh, J. (1974). Oral contraceptives, female hormones, the renin axis, and blood pressure. In *Oral Contraceptives and High Blood Pressure*, ed. Fregly, M. J. & Fregly, M. S. Gainesville: Dolphin.

Li, J. J., Talley, D. J., Li, S. A. & Villee, C. A. (1974). An estrogen-binding protein in the renal cytosol of intact, castrated and estrogenized golden hamsters. *Endocrinology*, **95**, 1134–1141.

Lindheimer, M. D. & Katz, A. I. (1973). Sodium and diuretics in pregnancy. *New England Journal of Medicine*, **288**, 891–894.

Lindheimer, M. D. & Katz, A. I. (1977). *Kidney Function and Disease in Pregnancy*. Philadelphia: Lea & Febiger.

Lindheimer, M. D., Koeppen, B. & Katz, A. I. (1976). Renal function in normal and hypertensive pregnant rats. In *Hypertension in Pregnancy*, ed. Lindheimer, M. D., Katz, A. I. & Zuspan, F. P. Pp. 217–227. New York: John Wiley & Sons.

Lockett, M. F. (1965). A comparison of the direct renal actions of pituitary growth and lactogenic hormones. *Journal of Physiology*, **181**, 192–199.

Lockett, M. F. & Nail, B. (1965). A comparative study of the renal actions of growth and lactogenic hormones in rats. *Journal of Physiology*, **180**, 147–156.

Lucci, M. S., Bengele, H. H. & Solomon, S. (1975). Suppressive action of prolactin on renal response to volume expansion. *American Journal of Physiology*, **229**, 81–85.

Lucci, M. S., Evan, A., Bengele, H. H. & Solomon, S. (1974). Altered effect of saline loading on the lateral intercellular spaces of the proximal tubule during prolactin infusion. *Federal Proceedings, Federation of American Societies for Experimental Biology*, **33**, 368.

Luetscher, J. A., Beckerhoff, R., Beckerhoff, I. & Gonzalez, C. M. (1974). Changes in plasma renin substrate activity and concentration and in plasma and urinary aldosterone in normotensive and hypertensive women before and after oral contraceptives. In *Oral Contraceptives and High Blood Pressure*, ed. Fregly, M. J. & Fregly, M. S. Gainesville: Dolphin.

MacCullum, G. C., Simpson, A. & Auld, R. B. (1975). Effects of prolactin (Prl) on canine renal function (abstract). *Clinical Research*, **23**, 652A.

Malarkey, W. B., George, J. M. & Baehler, R. W. (1975). Evidence for vasopressin contamination of ovine and bovine prolactin. *IRCS Medical Science: Endocrine System: Kidneys and Urinary System; Physiology*, **3**, 291.

Marshall, S., Gelato, M. & Meites, J. (1975). Serum prolactin levels and prolactin binding activity in adrenals and kidneys of male rats after dehydration, salt loading, and unilateral nephrectomy. *Proceedings of the Society for Experimental Biology and Medicine*, **149**, 185–188.

Marshall, S., Kledzik, G. S., Gelato, M., Campbell, G. P. & Meites, J. (1976). Effect of estrogen and testosterone on specific binding in the kidneys and adrenal of rats. *Steroids*, **27**, 187–195.

Matthews, B. F. (1963). Effects of hormones, placental extracts and hypophysectomy on inulin and paraaminohippurate clearances in the anesthetized rat. *Journal of Physiology*, **165**, 1–9.

Matthews, V. S., Kirkman, H. & Bacon, R. L. (1947). Kidney damage in the golden hamster following chronic administration of diethylstilbestrol in sesame oil. *Proceedings of the Society for Experimental Biology and Medicine*, **66**, 195–196.

Middleton, E. & Williams, P. C. (1974). Electrolyte and fluid appetite and balance in male guinea-pigs: Effects of stilboestrol treatment and renal function tests. *Journal of Endocrinology*, **61**, 381–399.

Miller, M., Van Gemert, M. & Moses, A. M. (1974). Prolatin-induced antidiuresis in the rat with diabetes insipidus. *Federal Proceedings, Federation of American Societies for Experimental Biology*, **33**, 253.

Nocenti, M. R. & Cizek, L. J. (1964). Influence of estrogens on electrolyte and water exchanges in the ovariectomized rat. *American Journal of Physiology*, **206**, 476–482.

Nocenti, M. R. & Cizek, L. J. (1973). Influence of estrogen on renal function and water intake in male rabbits rendered polyuric-polydipsic by food deprivation. *Endocrinology*, **93**, 925–931.

Norkin, J., VeKemans, M., Littermite, M. & Robyn, C. (1972). Circadian periodicity of serum prolactin concentration in man. *British Medical Journal*, **111**, 561–563.

O'Connell, J. M., Boonshaft, B., Hayes, J. M. & Schreiner, G. E. (1969). Metabolic effects of progesterone in the dog. *Proceedings of the Society for Experimental Biology and Medicine*, **132**, 862–864.

Oelkers, W., Schonesshofer, M. & Blumel, A. (1974). Effects of progesterone and four synthetic progestagens on sodium balance and the renin-aldosterone system in man. *Journal of Clinical Endocrinology and Metabolism*, **39**, 882–890.

Oparil, S., Ehrlich, E. N. & Lindheimer, M. D. (1975). Effects of progesterone on renal sodium handling in man: Relation to aldosterone excretion and plasma renin activity. *Clinical Science and Molecular Medicine*, **49**, 139–147.

Pasqualini, J. R., Sumida, C. & Gelly, C. (1974). Steroid hormone receptors in fetal guinea-pig kidney. *Journal of Steroid Biochemistry*, **5**, 977–985.

Pearlman, W. H. (1957). [16-^{3}H] progesterone metabolism in advanced pregnancy and in oopherectomized hysterectomized women. *Biochemistry Journal*, **67**, 1–5.

Pickford, G. E., Griffith, R. W., Torretti, J., Hendez, E. & Epstein, F. H. (1970). Bronchial reduction and renal stimulation of [Na+ K+]-ATPase by prolactin in hypophysectomized killfish in fresh water. *Nature*, **228**, 378–379.

Pickford, G. E. & Phillips, J. G. (1960). Prolactin, a factor in promoting survival of hypophysectomized killfish in fresh water. *Science*, **130**, 454–455.

Porter, G. A., Bogoroch, R. & Edelman, I. S. (1964). On the mechanism of action of aldosterone on sodium transport: The role of RNA synthesis. *Proceedings of the National Academy of Science* (U.S.A.), **52**, 1326–1333.

Porter, G. A. & Edelman, I. S. (1964). The action of aldosterone and related corticosteroids on sodium transport across the toad bladder. *Journal of Clinical Investigation*, **43**, 611–620.

Posner, B. I., Kelly, P. A., Shiu, R. P. C. & Freisen, H. G. (1974). Studies of insulin, growth hormone and prolactin binding: Tissue distribution, species variation and characterization. *Endocrinology*, **95**, 521–531.

Preedy, J. R. K. & Aitken, E. H. (1956a). The effect of estrogen on water and electrolyte metabolism: I. The normal. *Journal of Clinical Investigation*, **35**, 423–429.

Preedy, J. R. K. & Aitken, E. H. (1956b). The effect of estrogen on water and electrolyte metabolism: II. Hepatic disease. *Journal of Clinical Investigation*, **35**, 430–442.

Rajaniemi, H., Oksanen, H. & VanhaPerttula, T. (1974). Distribution of ^{125}I-prolactin in mice and rats. Studies with whole-body and microautoradiography. *Hormone Research*, **5**, 6–20.

Relkin, R. (1974). Effects of alterations in serum osmolality on pituitary and plasma prolactin levels in the rat. *Neuroendocrinology*, **14**, 61–64.

Richardson, B. & Luginbuhl, H. (1976). The role of prolactin in the development of chronic progressive nephropathy in the rat. *Virchows Archives (Pathology Anatomy)*, **370**, 13–19.

Richardson, J. A. & Houck, C. R. (1951). Renal tubular excretory mass and the reabsorption of sodium, chloride and potassium in female dogs receiving testosterone propionate or estradiol benzoate. *American Journal of Physiology*, **165**, 93–101.

Riley, A. L., Hagen, T. C. & Stefaniak, J. (1975). Is kidney a target organ for prolactin (abstract)? *Clinical Research*, **23**, 508A.

Riley, A. L., Hagen, T. C. & Stefaniak, J. E. (1976). Effect of prolactin on glomerular filtration rate (GFR) (abstract). *Clinical Research*, **24**, 556A.

Rogoff, J. M. & Stewart, G. N. (1927). Studies on adrenal insufficiency: III. The influence of pregnancy upon the survival period in adrenalectomized dogs. *American Journal of Physiology*, **79**, 508–535.

Saruta, T., Saade, G. A. & Kaplan, N. M. (1970). A possible mechanism for hypertension-induced oral contraceptives. *Archives of Internal Medicine*, **120**, 621–626.

Sassin, J. F., Frantz, A. G., Weitzman, E. D. & Kapen, S. (1972). Human prolactin: 24 hour pattern with increased release during sleep. *Science*, **177**, 1205–1207.

Schrier, R. W. & de Wardener, H. E. (1971). Factors other than aldosterone which influence the tubular reabsorption of sodium. *New England Journal of Medicine*, **285**, 1231–1243; 1292–1303.

Sealey, J. L. & Sondern, C. W. (1941). Comparative estrogen potency of diethylstilbesterol, estrone, estradiol and estrial II. Uterine and vaginal changes in infantile rats. *Endocrinology*, **29**, 356–367.

Sharp, G. W. G., Komack, C. L. & Leaf, A. (1966). Studies on the binding of aldosterone in the toad bladder. *Journal of Clinical Investigation*, **45**, 450–459.

Shome, B. & Parlow, A. F. (1977). Human pituitary prolactin (hPRL): The entire linear amino acid sequence. *Journal of Clinical Endocrinology and Metabolism*, **45**, 1115.

Simpson, H. W., Cole, E. N., Hume, P. D., Fleming, K. A. & Tavadia, H. B. (1975). Is prolactin involved in circadian rhythm of sodium excretion? *Lancet*, **1**, 342.

Simpson, S. A. & Tait, J. F. (1952). A quantitative method for the bioassay of the effect of adrenal cortical steroids on mineral metabolism. *Endocrinology*, **50**, 150–161.

Steggles, A. W. & King, R. J. B. (1967). The uptake and localization of [6-7³H] estradiol-17 beta in tissues of male syrian hamsters. *Journal of Endocrinology*, **38**, 25–32.

Swaneck, G. E., Highland, E. & Edelman, I. S. (1969). Sterospecific nuclear and cytosol aldosterone-binding proteins of various tissues. *Nephron*, **6**, 297–316.

Taylor, H. C. Jr., Warner, R. C. & Welsh, C. A. (1939). The relationship of the estrogens and other placental hormones to sodium and potassium balance at the end of pregnancy and in the puerperium. *American Journal of Obstetrics and Gynecology*, **38**, 748–773.

Thorn, G. W. & Engel, L. L. (1937). The effect of sex hormones on the renal excretion of electrolytes. *Journal of Experimental Medicine*, **68**, 299–312.

Thorn, G. W., Nelson, K. R. & Thorn, D. W. (1938). A study of the mechanism of edema associated with menstruation. *Endocrinology*, **22**, 155–163.

Thornborough, J. R. & Passo, S. S. (1975). The effects of estrogens on sodium and potassium metabolism in rats. *Endocrinology*, **97**, 1528–1536.

Tomlinson, R. W. S. (1971a). The action of progesterone derivatives and other steroids on the sodium transport of isolated frog skin. *Acta Physiologica Scandinavica*, **83**, 407–411.

Tomlinson, R. W. S. (1971b). The action of progesterone on the sodium transport of isolated frog skin. *Acta Physiologica Scandinavica*, **83**, 463–472.

Vallotton, M. B., Dubied, M. C., Gaillard, R. & Merkelbach, U. (1976). Influence of angiotensin II (AII) and estrogen (E) on responsiveness of vasopressin (AVP) to salt loading (SL) in man (abstract). *Clinical Research*, **24**, 280A.

Vorherr, H., Vorherr, U. F. & Solomon, S. (1978). Contamination of prolactin preparations by antidiuretic hormone and oxytocin. *American Journal of Physiology*, **234**: F318–324.

Wallin, J. D. & Lee, P. A. (1976). Effect of prolactin on diluting and concentrating ability in the rat. *American Journal of Physiology*, **230**, 1524–1530.

White, H. L., Heinbecker, P. & Rolf, D. (1947). Some endocrine influences on renal function and cardiac output. *American Journal of Physiology*, **149**, 404–417.

9

Physiology of the vitamin D endocrine system and disorders of altered vitamin D metabolism

BARTON S. LEVINE
JACK W. COBURN

INTRODUCTION

Developments over the last decade indicate that the kidney is responsible for producing the most active form of vitamin D, 1,25-dihydroxyvitamin D_3. Vitamin D_3 (cholecalciferol) is relatively inactive itself, and the effects attributed to vitamin D_3 are believed to occur only after its ultimate conversion to 1,25-dihydroxyvitamin D_3 [1,25(OH)$_2$D$_3$], an event occurring exclusively in the kidney (Fraser and Kodicek, 1970). Thus, the kidney should be considered an endocrine organ that is responsible for the conversion of a steroid prohormone to its active form, a metabolic step having an important role in calcium homeostasis. A number of clinical disorders, such as renal osteodystrophy, may arise because of defective renal production of an active form of vitamin D. Other disease states, such as idiopathic hypercalciuria, may arise from excessive production of 1,25(OH)$_2$D$_3$ by the kidney. Finally, there is evidence that end-organ unresponsiveness to 1,25(OH)$_2$D$_3$ may occur and lead to bone disease. This review will consider the physiologic regulation of vitamin D metabolism, some of the actions of vitamin D, and a number of clinical disorders believed to arise because of derangement of vitamin D metabolism or action.

METABOLISM OF VITAMIN D

Humans normally acquire vitamin D from their diet or through ultraviolet irradiation of the provitamin, 7-dehydrocholesterol, present in the skin (Wheatly and Reinertson, 1958; Rauschkolb et al., 1969). The quantity of endogenous vitamin D$_3$ produced is variable, depending upon latitude, season, and climate. It may average 2.5–10.0 µg/day (100–400 IU), values that are near the minimum daily requirement. Vitamin D can also be ingested either as D$_3$ (cholecalciferol) or D$_2$ (ergocalciferol), which is produced synthetically by ultraviolet irradiation of the plant steroid, ergosterol. Vitamin D is absorbed in the proximal small bowel (Shachter et al., 1965), carried in plasma bound to a specific vitamin D-binding protein, MW 59,000 daltons (Haddad and Walgate, 1976; Imawari, Kida, and Goodman, 1976), and transported to the liver as well as other tissues (Mawer and Schaefer, 1969; Rosentreich, Rich, and Volwiler, 1971). A schema of vitamin D metabolism is shown in Figure 9.1.

Production of 25-hydroxycholecalciferol

The liver hydroxylates vitamin D$_3$ to 25-hydroxycholecalciferol [25(OH)D$_3$] (Ponchon and DeLuca, 1969), the predominant circulating form of vitamin D$_3$ (Smith and Goodman, 1971; Gray et al., 1974). The control of this conversion is not believed to be tightly regulated (Tucker, Gagnon, and Haussler, 1973), although all vitamin D$_3$ is not quantitatively converted to 25(OH)D$_3$. Mawer et al. (1971) found that a greater fraction of vitamin D$_3$ was converted to 25(OH)D$_3$ in patients with vitamin D deficiency than in vitamin D-replete individuals. However, high plasma levels of 25(OH)D* develop in life guards exposed to sunlight (Haddad and Chyu, 1971); there is a seasonal increase in plasma 25(OH)D levels late in the summer (Stamp and Round, 1974), and a marked increase in plasma levels of 25(OH)D occurs after ingestion of pharmacologic doses of vitamin D (Hughes et al., 1976). Such observations indicate that if "regulation" of hepatic 25-hydroxylation does exist, it can be overcome when the intake or production of vitamin D$_3$ is substantially increased.

In the avian species, tissues other than the liver may be capable of produc-

---

* The competitive binding assay for 25(OH)D measures both 25(OH)D$_3$ and 25(OH)D$_2$ and is not able to distinguish between the two; the abbreviation, 25(OH)D, is used to include lack of specificity for the hydroxylated forms of D$_2$ or D$_3$.

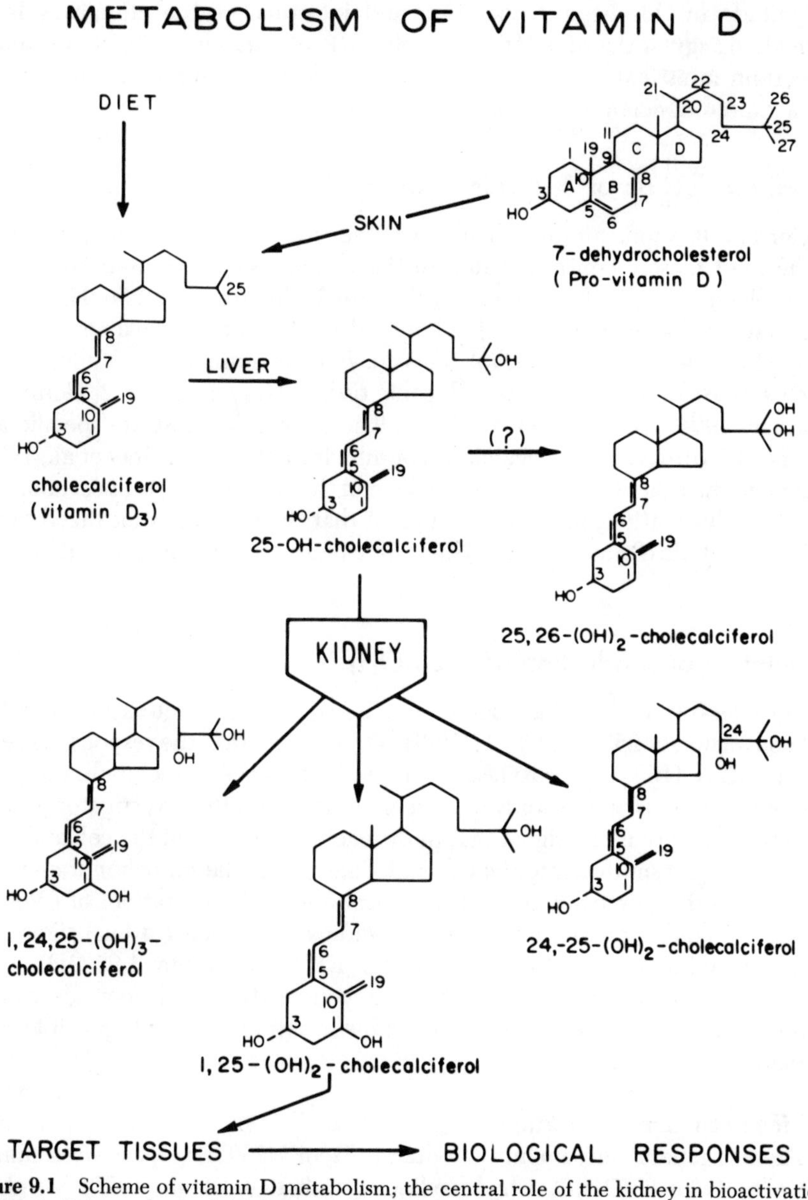

METABOLISM OF VITAMIN D

Figure 9.1 Scheme of vitamin D metabolism; the central role of the kidney in bioactivation of vitamin D is emphasized. (Coburn et al., 1974; with permission.)

ing 25(OH)D$_3$ (Tucker et al., 1973); however, the liver plays the major role in such conversion in mammals (Olson et al., 1976; Haddad and Rojanasathit, 1976). Arnaud et al. (1975) found that a sizeable fraction of radioactivity ingested as ^{3}H-25(OH)D$_3$ entered the lumen of the duodenum via bile secretion within 24 hours. Subsequently, most of the secreted radioactivity was reabsorbed, suggesting that 25(OH)D$_3$ undergoes enterohepatic circulation. The magnitude of this hepatic secretion and intestinal reabsorption was large enough to suggest that defective enterohepatic circulation of 25(OH)D$_3$, found in certain intestinal and hepatic diseases, could be an important mechanism for acquired deficiency of vitamin D.

Renal production of 1,25-dihydroxycholecalciferol

Current data indicate that the renal conversion of 25(OH)D$_3$ to 1,25(OH)$_2$D$_3$ is the most closely controlled step in the metabolism of vitamin D. The responsible enzyme, 25-hydroxycholecalciferol-1α-hydroxylase (25(OH)D$_3$-1-hydroxylase), is localized in the mitochondrial fraction of the renal cortex (Gray et al., 1972; Midgett et al., 1973). This enzyme has similarities to mixed-function oxidases found in other steroidogenic tissues (Gray et al., 1972; Henry and Norman, 1974; Ghazarian et al., 1974). The enzyme is substrate specific and will not 1-hydroxylate cholecalciferol or dihydrotachysterol (Gray et al., 1972). Although the exact location of the enzyme in the renal cortex is uncertain, preliminary observations in the chick suggest that the enzyme is localized to the proximal tubule (Brunette et al., 1978); data on its location in mammals are not available.

Regulation of production of 1,25(OH)$_2$D$_3$

Considerable interest has focused on the physiologic factors that regulate the conversion of 25(OH)D$_3$ to 1,25(OH)$_2$D$_3$. The fact that the responsible renal enzyme, 25(OH)D$_3$-1-hydroxylase, is present within the mitochondria imposes severe restrictions on the study of its regulation. Thus, the investigator is faced with the evaluation of a signal that must reach the surface of the cell and have its message transmitted into the cell and, finally, into the mitochondrion itself. Changes in the intracellular or intramitochondrial concentrations of calcium, phosphate, and hydrogen ion are each candidates for being a final signal; effectors may include parathyroid hormone (PTH), calcitonin, 1,25(OH)$_2$D$_3$, or other metabolic forms of vitamin D. Also, cyclic AMP must be considered as a potential mediator. There are data available to support or refute possible roles of many of these factors.

Effect of vitamin D status

There is general agreement that vitamin D$_3$ or 1,25(OH)$_2$D$_3$ can itself inhibit the activity of 25(OH)D$_3$-1-hydroxylase. Garabedian et al. (1972) found reduced production of ^{3}H-1,25(OH)$_2$D$_3$ from its radio-labeled precursor in vivo in thyroparathyroidectomized (TPTX) rats given small amounts of unlabeled 1,25(OH)$_2$D$_3$. Henry, Midgett, and Norman (1974) reported that enzyme activity, studied in vitro, was higher in tissues from vitamin D-deficient chicks compared to birds given 0.62 μg vitamin D$_3$/day. Also, the administration of 1,25(OH)$_2$D$_3$, 0.077 μg/day, suppressed the level of the renal enzyme. When treatment with either vitamin D$_3$ or 1,25(OH)$_2$D$_3$ was discontinued, the enzyme activity increased within 2 to 3 days. Larkins et al. (1974a) found that conversion of $25(OH)D_3$ to $1,25(OH)_2D_3$ was decreased in renal tubular suspensions following preincubation with $1,25(OH)_2D_3$; workers from the same laboratory (Larkins, MacAuley, and MacIntyre, 1974b) found that the inhibitory effect of $1,25(OH)_2D_3$ was reduced as the calcium concentration in the media was lowered, suggesting that the effect of $1,25(OH)_2D_3$ to suppress the enzyme is related to changes in transcellular calcium flux, which in turn may inhibit $25(OH)D_3$-1-hydroxylase activity. Horiuchi, Suda, and Sasaki (1974) also found that either $1,25(OH)_2D_3$ or vitamin D_3 can inhibit the enzyme activity: When chicks were given a high calcium intake to cause hypercalcemia and suppress the parathyroid glands, the enzyme activity was highest in chicks not pretreated with vitamin D_3 but was dramatically lower with the administration of even a low dose of vitamin D_3 (0.025 μg/day). Norman et al. (1973) measured the enzyme in vitamin D-deficient chicks given varying doses of vitamin D_3 that raised serum calcium to normal; they found that only the highest dose suppressed the enzyme. The reason for the discrepancy between these observations and those of Horiuchi et al. (1974) is not clear.

A possible mechanism for suppression of $25(OH)D_3$-1-hydroxylase by $1,25(OH)_2D_3$ is suggested by the work of Colston et al. (1977): The activity of $25(OH)D_3$-1-hydroxylase in D-deficient chicks decreased with $1,25(OH)_2D_3$ administration, but this negative feedback of $1,25(OH)_2D_3$ was abolished by treatment with the metabolic inhibitors, actinomycin D or by α-amatin; the latter is believed to inhibit RNA synthesis by binding to RNA polymerase II. They suggested that $1,25(OH)_2D_3$ exerted feedback inhibition on its own synthesis by a nuclear action involving changes in gene transcription. Alterations in the intracellular or mitochondrial content of calcium or phosphate are other likely possibilities.

Dietary calcium
Results of in vitro and in vivo studies on variations in dietary calcium intake suggest there is an inverse relationship between dietary calcium intake and $25(OH)D_3$-1-hydroxylase activity. In vitamin D-deficient or vitamin D-replete rats with intact parathyroid glands, feeding with a diet low in calcium was associated with an increased intestinal localization of $1,25(OH)_2D_3$ (Boyle, Gray, and DeLuca, 1971). MacIntyre et al. (1974) also showed increased $1,25(OH)_2D_3$ production with a low dietary calcium intake in both intact and parathyroid-ectomized (PTX) rats. Other data, obtained in vivo, indicated that plasma $1,25(OH)_2D$ levels rose when rats were fed a low calcium diet, but this occurred only in the presence of intact parathyroid glands (Hughes et al., 1975). Larkins et al. (1973) gave ^3H-$25(OH)D_3$ and found an increased fraction of plasma and intestinal radioactivity present as $1,25(OH)_2D_3$ in vitamin D-deficient rats fed a low compared to a normal calcium diet. Furthermore, in vitro studies using either vitamin D-replete (Omdahl et al., 1972) or vitamin D-deficient chicks (Bikle and Rasmussen, 1975; Henry et al., 1974) indicate that a reduced dietary calcium content is associated with an increase in conversion of ^3H-$25(OH)D_3$ by kidney homogenates or by mitrochondria from isolated tubules.

Such observations indicate that variations in the calcium needs of the organism can alter the activity of the $25(OH)D_3$-1-hydroxylase and have led investigators to study the effects of varying calcium concentrations in the incubation media of preparations of isolated renal tubules, homogenates of renal cortex, and isolated mitochondria (Henry and Norman, 1974, 1975; Horiuchi, 1974; Bikle and Rasmussen, 1975; Colston et al., 1973). Divergent results have arisen, possibly because of variations in the techniques employed. Moreover, pertubations in the external environment of the cell may not be reflected by the changes within the cell or the mitochondrion where the enzyme exists. Nonetheless, evidence is strong that a reduction in dietary calcium can augment the conversion of $25(OH)D_3$ to $1,25(OH)_2D_3$ by augmenting the $25(OH)D_3$-1-hydroxylase activity; however, the exact mechanism responsible has not been elucidated.

Effects of parathyroid hormone (PTH)

The conversion of $25(OH)D_3$ to $1,25(OH)_2D_3$ has been studied in various laboratory and clinical models of PTH-excess or deficit. In vivo studies by Garabedian et al. (1972) in the vitamin D-deficient rat showed a decrease in conversion of radio-labeled $25(OH)D_3$ to $1,25(OH)_2D_3$ after parathyroidectomy, and Hughes et al. (1975) found decreased plasma $1,25(OH)_2D$ levels in parathyroidectomized, vitamin D-replete rats compared to rats with intact parathyroid glands, observations suggesting that parathyroidectomy decreases the conversion of $25(OH)D_3$ to $1,25(OH)_2D_3$. Henry et al. (1974) in the vitamin D-replete chick and Booth, Tsai, and Morris (1977) in the vitamin D-deficient chick showed that the activity of the $25(OH)D_3$-1-hydroxylase decreased after parathyroidectomy. In the study of Booth et al. (1977), a decrease in serum calcium was prevented after PTX by a calcium infusion, eliminating the possibility that a fall in serum calcium level was a factor altering the enzyme activity. Galante et al. (1973) were unable to show any effect of parathyroidectomy in hypocalcemic chicks fed a low calcium diet; however, a further fall in serum calcium level after parathyroidectomy may have prevented any further decrease in $25(OH)D_3$-1α-hydroxylase after disappearance of circulating PTH.

Studies on the effects of PTH on the conversion of $25(OH)D_3$ to $1,25(OH)_2D_3$ in vivo or on the enzyme activity in vitro have yielded somewhat conflicting results: Galante et al. (1972) showed that high doses of parathyroid extract decreased the conversion of $25(OH)D_3$ to $1,25(OH)_2D_3$ in vitamin D-deficient rats, while Fraser and Kodicek (1973) found increased 25-hydroxy-D_3-1-hydroxylase in kidney homogenates from chicks treated with parathyroid hormone. The hypercalcemia present in Galante's study may have accounted for the failure to find a positive effect. Studies by Rasmussen et al. (1972) with renal tubules from vitamin D-deficient chicks revealed that the addition of parathyroid hormone increased the conversion of radio-labeled $25(OH)D_3$ to $1,25(OH)_2D_3$, although high concentrations of PTH were either without effect or they decreased the conversion.

Clinical observations provide support for a role of parathyroid hormone in stimulating the generation of $1,25(OH)_2D_3$. Haussler et al. (1975a) found increased plasma levels of $1,25(OH)_2D$ in patients with primary hyperparathyroidism, and the blood levels of $1,25(OH)_2D$ rose when normal subjects were given parathyroid extract intramuscularly for 7 days. Furthermore, blood levels of $1,25(OH)_2D$ were low in patients with hypoparathyroidism (Haussler et al., 1975b). Recently, Gray et al. (1977) reported a correlation between intestinal calcium absorption and increased levels of $1,25(OH)_2D$ in patients with primary hyperparathyroidism, an observation providing convincing evidence that increased intestinal absorption of calcium in primary hyperparathyroidism arises as a consequence of increased conversion of $25(OH)D_3$ to $1,25(OH)_2D_3$.

Effect of inorganic phosphate

Inorganic phosphate is another factor that can affect the activity of renal $25(OH)D_3$-1-hydroxylase. Interest in a role of phosphate in affecting vitamin D metabolism arose because of the similarities between the skeletal lesion of phosphate depletion and that of osteomalacia due to vitamin D deficiency (Day and McCollum, 1939; Lotz, Ney, and Bartter, 1964). A number of studies in the rat (Morrisey and Wasserman, 1971; Tanaka and DeLuca, 1973) and in man (Lotz, Zisman, and Bartter, 1968; Gray, Dominguez, and Lemann, 1975) indicate that intestinal absorption of calcium is augmented by dietary phosphate restriction, suggesting a possible effect on vitamin D metabolism. However, conflicting results have arisen with studies of phosphate restriction on vitamin D metabolism. No difference in vitamin D metabolism was found in vitramin D-replete rats given radio-labeled D_3 or $25(OH)D_3$ (Haddad, Boisseau, and Avioli, 1971). Henry et al. (1974) in the vitamin D-replete chick and Bikle and Rasmussen (1975) in the vitamin D-deficient chick found little or no increase in renal $25(OH)D_3$-1-hydroxylase after a reduction in dietary phosphate intake. However, Bikle, Murphy, and Rasmussen (1975) found a reduction in enzyme activity when dietary phosphate was increased. On the other hand, Tanaka and DeLuca (1973) and Hughes et al. (1975) found evidence for increased production of $1,25(OH)_2D_3$ when dietary phosphate intake was decreased in vitamin D-deficient rats; moreover, this effect occurred independent of the status of the parathyroid glands. Other studies of phosphate concentration, carried out in vitro, reveal an interdependency between phosphate and calcium concentrations in the incubation media (Bikle and Rasmussen, 1975).

Effect of acidosis

Chronic metabolic acidosis is associated with hypercalciuria and a negative calcium balance (Lemann, Litzow, and Lennon, 1966). The negative calcium balance is due, in part, to increased urinary losses of calcium; however, several studies have documented that there is either a decrease in intestinal absorption of calcium or the increment in absorption is insufficient to offset the negative balance produced by the urinary losses (Greenberg, McNamara, and McCrory, 1966). Impaired calcium absorption could play a role both in the production of bone disease and in the retardation of skeletal repair in disorders such as chronic renal failure or renal tubular acidosis, with long-standing metabolic acidosis. Several studies have demonstrated a reduction in the conversion of 25(OH)D$_3$ to 1,25(OH)$_2$D$_3$ in D-deficient rats (Lee, Russel, and Avioli, 1977) or chicks (Sauveur et al., 1977) with ammonium chloride-induced metabolic acidosis. One could hypothesize that metabolic acidosis, by causing a decreased production of 1,25(OH)$_2$D$_3$, may impair calcium absorption by the gut. A study in humans with ammonium chloride-induced acidosis has failed to demonstrate a decrease in the conversion of 25(OH)D$_3$ to 1,25(OH)$_2$D$_3$ (Weber et al., 1976). Normal plasma levels of 1,25(OH)$_2$D$_3$ but a reduced intestinal content of 1,25(OH)$_2$D$_3$ were reported in acidotic rats given ^{3}H-25(OH)D$_3$ (Brewer et al., 1978). Thus, the question of whether the production of 1,25(OH)$_2$D$_3$ is decreased by metabolic acidosis remains somewhat uncertain.

Action of estrogens and other sex steroids

Kenny (1976) suggested a physiologic role of gonadal hormones in the regulation of the renal production of 1,25(OH)$_2$D$_3$ in an egg-laying bird, the Japanese quail. It was subsequently found that ovariectomy and antiestrogen treatment each inhibited the renal generation of 1,25(OH)$_2$D$_3$ (Baksi and Kenny, 1976a, 1976b). In addition, parallel increments in intestinal calcium-binding protein and renal 25(OH)D$_3$-1-hydroxylase have been found in laying quail compared to premature birds (Bar et al., 1977). Moreover, the administration of estradiol or progesterone to immature Japanese quail augmented the activity of 25(OH)D$_3$-1-hydroxylase, with the estradiol being more effective (Baksi and Kenny, 1977). DeLuca et al. (1977) and Tanaka, Castillo, and De-Luca (1977) reported that the simultaneous administration of either progesterone or testosterone augmented the action of estrogen to stimulate the renal 25(OH)D$_3$-1-hydroxylase in either male Japanese quail or in castrate adult male chickens. Pike et al. (1977) found increased plasma levels of 1,25(OH)$_2$D in laying compared to nonlaying hens and higher serum levels of 1,25(OH)$_2$D in pregnant compared to nonpregnant women. Such observations provide strong evidence for a role of sex steroids in regulating the renal production of 1,25(OH)$_2$D$_3$, particularly during states with added need for calcium (e.g., pregnancy in mammals and egg-laying in birds).

Effects of pituitary hormones

Prolactin and growth hormone may affect the renal generation of 1,25(OH)$_2$D$_3$. Thus, Spanos et al. (1976) reported that prolactin stimulated renal 25(OH)D$_3$-1-hydroxylase in chicks; moreover, circulating levels of 1,25(OH)$_2$D were found to be increased in lactating humans compared to normal women and in lactating rats compared to age- and sex-matched, nonlactating controls (Spanos, 1976b). It is of interest that patients with pseudohypoparathyroidism, a disorder associated with reduced levels of 1,25(OH)$_2$D, often have reduced plasma levels of prolactin (Carlson, Brickman, and Bottazao, 1977).

There is a similarity between the amino acid sequence of prolactin and growth hormone, and preliminary data suggest that growth hormone may affect the metabolism of vitamin D. Thus, plasma levels of 1,25(OH)$_2$D were higher in young than in old rats and in young compared to older humans (Pike et al., 1977). Further evidence for a role of pituitary hormones in affecting vitamin D metabolism was reported by Spencer and Tobiassen (1977) who found that hypophysectomy reduced the conversion of 25(OH)D$_3$ to 1,25(OH)$_2$D$_3$ in rats studied in vivo, while replacement with growth hormone improved the bioconversion. These observations suggest there may be hormonal regulation of the generation of 1,25(OH)$_2$D$_3$ during growth and lactation, physiologic events associated with enhanced demands for calcium.

Effect of other hormones

Other hormonal factors may also affect the renal generation of 1,25(OH)$_2$D$_3$. Thus, there is considerable experimental evidence that a decrease or absence of insulin is associated with decreased generation of 1,25(OH)$_2$D$_3$. Rats with diabetes mellitus from treatment with streptozotocin exhibit a decrease in intestinal calcium transport, reduced intestinal calcium binding protein, and low blood levels of 1,25(OH)$_2$D; these abnormalities are corrected by insulin administration. At present, it is not known whether a counterpart of this phenomenon may exist in humans with diabetes (Schneider et al., 1977).

The mechanisms whereby cortisol and other glucocorticoids may affect vitamin D metabolism remains unclear. Most data obtained in experimental animals suggest that pharmacologic doses of glucocorticoids do not affect the metabolism or the tissue localization of active forms of vitamin D (Kimberg et al., 1971; Favus et al., 1973). Thus, an end-organ unresponsiveness has been suggested. On the other hand, studies in humans (Klein et al., 1977) suggest there may be decreased generation of 1,25(OH)$_2$D$_3$ in humans treated with large doses of glucocorticoids. Thus, therapy of glucocorticoid-treated patients with 1,25(OH)$_2$D$_3$, in doses considered to be "physiologic," restored abnormal intestinal calcium absorption to normal. Also, Chesney et al. (1978) reported reduced plasma levels of 1,25(OH)$_2$D in steroid-treated children with nephrosis and nephritis compared to levels in children with similar diseases who were not receiving steroids. Studies of Hahn (1978) suggest that administration of certain vitamin D analogs to steroid-treated patients may retard the bone loss observed in these patients.

ACTIONS OF VITAMIN D

Intestinal action

The most extensively studied and best-documented effect of vitamin D is to enhance the intestinal transport of calcium; there is good evidence that vitamin D also enhances phosphate transport. Certain segments of the intestine may have a greater response with regard to phosphorus absorption compared to calcium, while other segments may react with greater augmentation of calcium transport (Walling, 1977). Walling has reported that vitamin D-stimulated calcium absorption was greatest in the duodenum, while the ileum was next; active phosphorus absorption was highest in the jejunum. Of interest, the ratio of absorptive flux of phosphorus to the flux of calcium remained relatively constant even as their absorption was stimulated one- to twofold with $1,25(OH)_2D_3$. Data in man (Brickman et al., 1977a) indicate that net phosphorus absorption is increased in parallel to that of calcium during metabolic balance studies, indicating a significant action of vitamin D on phosphate transport in man.

Most evidence suggests that the action of vitamin D to stimulate calcium transport occurs via enhanced calcium movement across the brush border into the cell. However, some disagreement exists regarding the mechanism by which this occurs. On the one hand, considerable evidence has been raised suggesting that a specific calcium-binding protein, which is stimulated by $1,25(OH)_2D_3$, may act to augment calcium entry into the cell. The cellular production of this calcium-binding protein as well as other proteins may occur as $1,25(OH)_2D_3$ induces new protein synthesis through a nuclear action to enhance synthesis of messenger RNA. This action of vitamin D via stimulation of protein synthesis suggests a mechanism of action similar to that of other steroid hormones (Haussler and McCain, 1977).

More recent information, with the use of vesicles prepared from intestinal brush borders, suggests that the $1,25(OH)_2D_3$-stimulated influx of calcium may occur without new protein synthesis (Rasmussen et al., 1979). Such data suggest that vitamin D may have actions other than those involving the synthesis of new protein. Similarities between the action of vitamin D and polyene antibiotic, filipin, which reversibly enhances the entry of calcium into the cell of vitamin D-deficient but not vitamin D-treated chicks (Adams, Wong, and Norman, 1970) provide support for such mechanism of vitamin D action.

Actions on bone

The skeleton represents another important target tissue for vitamin D action, although the precise mechanism whereby vitamin D induces its effects on bone remains uncertain. Clinical observations indicate that vitamin D and certain of its metabolites are effective in inducing mineralization of unmineralized osteoid, with this effect often in evidence before there is a change in serum calcium and phosphorus levels. On the other hand, studies on bone cultures (Raisz et al., 1972) indicate that a major effect of $1,25(OH)_2D_3$ is to enhance bone resorption, as indicated by increased liberation of calcium from bone into the culture medium. Other observations (Raisz et al., 1972) suggest that $1,25(OH)_2D_3$ may also inhibit collagen synthesis. Thus, there is a major dilemma concerning how vitamin D heals rickets. One view maintains that rickets is healed as a consequence of an elevation in extracellular levels of calcium and phosphorus to appropriate values, which then allows the osteoid to calcify. Another view, particularly obtained from in vivo studies and clinical observations, suggests that vitamin D may have a direct effect to stimulate the maturation of collagen, which in turn lends itself to normal calcification. Current observations do not permit clarification of the mechanism for such a direct effect on bone. Moreover, certain evidence, noted below, suggests that forms of vitamin D other than $1,25(OH)_2D_3$ may be more active in stimulating bone formation.

Renal actions of vitamin D

It has been reported that $25(OH)D_3$ or $1,25(OH)_2D_3$, when given acutely and in pharmacologic quantities, can inhibit the phosphaturic actions of parathyroid hormone, calcitonin, and antidiuretic hormone (Popovtzer and Robinette, 1975; Puschett, Beck, and Jelonek, 1975; Popovtzer, Blum, and Flis, 1977). However, in long-term studies utilizing lower, more "physiologic" quantities of $1,25(OH)_2D_3$, the effect of $1,25(OH)_2D_3$ may be just the opposite. Thus, Bonjour, Preston, and Fleisch (1977) showed that $1,25(OH)_2D_3$, when given for several days in an amount that restored intestinal calcium transport to normal in thyroparathyroidectomized rats, led to an increase in urinary phosphorus excretion. The chronically parathyroidectomized animal is hyperphosphatemic, and $1,25(OH)_2D_3$ may cause serum phosphorus to fall in an animal with a high serum phosphorus level, while $1,25(OH)_2D_3$ leads to an increase in serum phosphorus level in an animal with hypophosphatemia (Garabedian et al., 1976; Steele et al., 1975). The mechanism whereby $1,25(OH)_2D_3$ can produce a decrease in phosphorus excretion under one condition and yet increase phosphate excretion in another remains uncertain. The phosphorus stores of the animal may dictate the overall action of $1,25(OH)_2D_3$ on net tubular reabsorption of phosphate.

The effect of $1,25(OH)_2D_3$ and other vitamin D sterols on the renal handling of calcium has also been the subject of considerable interest (Levine, Brautbar, and Coburn, 1978). In parathyroidectomized rats, Rizzoli, Fleisch, and Bonjour (1977) found that $1,25(OH)_2D_3$, given for several days, augmented the renal excretion of calcium. Short-term studies in dogs suggested that $25(OH)D_3$ can produce an early decrease in urinary calcium excretion (Puschett et al., 1972b). In normal humans, the administration of $1,25(OH)_2D_3$ increases urinary calcium excretion to a greater extent than may be expected from the increase in intestinal absorption of calcium (Brickman et al., 1974; Llach et al., 1977). Thus, low doses of vitamin D sterols may decrease renal tubular reabsorption of calcium in a vitamin D-replete animal. This effect may occur, in part, due to suppression of parathyroid activity; on the other hand, the acute administration of larger quantities of $1,25(OH)_2D_3$ may enhance renal tubular calcium reabsorption. From this discussion, it is apparent that the role of vitamin D sterols in affecting renal handling of calcium and phosphorus under physiological conditions is far from being understood.

Action on the parathyroid glands

Certain observations suggest that $1,25(OH)_2D_3$, or other forms of vitamin D, may affect PTH secretion via a direct action on the parathyroid glands. Chertow et al. (1975) reported that $1,25(OH)_2D_3$ caused a significant decrease in serum iPTH 4 hours after its administration to rats; also, $1,25(OH)_2D_3$ blocked the enhanced secretion of PTH that occurred in response to hypocalcemia. Henry and Norman (1975) found that radio-labeled $1,25(OH)_2D_3$ was preferentially localized in the parathyroid glands, and Braumbaugh, Hughes, and Haussler (1975) reported that $1,25(OH)_2D_3$ was specifically bound to macromolecular components in the cytoplasm and nucleus of parathyroid glands from vitamin D-deficient chicks. Such data suggest that $1,25(OH)_2D_3$ may be involved in the regulation of PTH synthesis, secretion, or both. Other data are conflicting; thus, Llach et al. (1977) found no significant change in serum iPTH in normal man over 12 hours after the oral administration of $1,25(OH)_2D_3$. Moreover, Canterbury et al. (1978) reported an acute increase in PTH secretion in response to a pulse dose of $1,25(OH)_2D_3$ in normal dogs, and Care et al. made similar observations in goats (Care et al., 1977). Moreover, Henry, Taylor, and Norman (1977) showed that either vitamin D_3 itself or a combination of $1,25(OH)_2D_3$ and $24,25(OH)_2D_3$ were necessary to reduce the size of hyperplastic parathyroid glands found in vitamin D-deficient chicks. In vitamin D-deficient puppies, Oldham et al. (1979) showed that $1,25(OH)_2D_3$ administration and a slow infusion of calcium were synergistic in decreasing plasma iPTH levels, compared to the effect of a calcium infusion alone. Such observations make it likely that vitamin D sterols exert a direct effect on the parathyroid glands; however, the nature of the process and its physiologic role remain uncertain.

Vitamin D actions on muscle and other tissues

Striking weakness of skeletal muscles, particularly of the pelvic and shoulder girdles, and a characteristic waddling, "penguin" gait are well-described features of severe vitamin D deficiency (Schott and Wills, 1976); moreover, such muscle weakness shows striking improvement following treatment with vitamin D or one of its active metabolites (Henderson et al., 1974). The mechanism whereby vitamin D produces an effect on muscle function is unknown. Heimberg, Matthews, and Ritz (1976) reported reduced calcium uptake by sarcoplasmic reticulum of skeletal muscle cells in rabbits with experimental uremia, an abnormality corrected by $1,25(OH)_2D_3$ (Matthews et al., 1977). They suggested that the lack of $1,25(OH)_2D_3$ was responsible for the abnormalities in muscle. Additional studies showed that the contraction and relaxation phases of skeletal muscle were abnormal in vitamin D-deficient rats (Rodman and Baker, 1978).

There are other poorly understood trophic effects of vitamin D; these apparent actions of vitamin D are inferred from observations made in animals or

Table 9.1   Consequences of vitamin D deficiency

Intestine
  Reduced calcium absorption
  Reduced phosphate absorption
  ? Reduced magnesium absorption
  Hypoplastic intestinal mucosa
Skeleton
  Defective collagen synthesis and maturation
  Reduced PTH responsiveness of bone
  Impaired mineralization of osteoid
  Retarded growth
Parathyroid
  Parathyroid hyperplasia
  Impaired suppression of PTH by an increase in serum calcium
Muscle
  Proximal myopathy
Plasma
  Hypocalcemia
  Elevated iPTH
  Hypophosphatemia (if kidneys are responsive to PTH)
  Elevated alkaline phosphatase

man with vitamin D deficiency (Table 9.1). Thus the administration of vitamin D enhances food intake, stimulates growth, results in an increase in mitotic activity of intestinal muscosal cells and increased thickness of the intestinal mucosa.

Actions of vitamin D sterols other than 1,25(OH)$_2$D$_3$

Most interest in the actions of vitamin D has centered around the effects of 1,25(OH)$_2$D$_3$, the most potent form of vitamin D in stimulating intestinal calcium absorption. Several studies have suggested that other vitamin D sterols (i.e., 24,25(OH)$_2$D$_3$ or a combination of 1,25(OH)$_2$D$_3$ and 24,25(OH)$_2$D$_3$) may exert effects different from 1,25(OH)$_2$D$_3$ itself. Miravet et al. (1976) found that 24,25(OH)$_2$D$_3$ given to phosphate-depleted, vitamin D-deficient rats leads to a fall in serum calcium levels. Moreover, Henry et al. (1977) reported a combination of 1,25(OH)$_2$D$_3$ and 24,25(OH)$_2$D$_3$, but not either sterol given alone, is capable of causing regression of the hyperplastic parathyroid glands found in vitamin D-deficient chicks. This occured despite the return of calcium levels to normal in the various groups. Bordier et al. (1977) found that the simultaneous oral administration of 1,25(OH)$_2$D$_3$ and 24,25(OH)$_2$D$_3$ is more effective than 1,25(OH)$_2$D$_3$ alone in stimulating bone mineralization in humans with vitamin D-deficiency osteomalacia. Also, Kanis et al. (1977c) reported that 24,-25(OH)$_2$D$_3$ stimulated intestinal calcium absorption without causing a concomitant increase in urinary calcium in normal humans, findings different from those observed during treatment with 1,25(OH)$_2$D$_3$ (Brickman et al., 1974). Finally, Henry and Norman (1978) found that a combination of 1,-25(OH)$_2$D$_3$ and 24,25(OH)$_2$D$_3$, given to chickens from the time of hatching until sexual maturity, led to normal egg production and egg hatchability, but chickens similarly treated with either $1,25(OH)_2D_3$ or $24,25(OH)_2D_3$ produced viable eggs that failed to hatch. Thus, only the combination produced results equivalent to vitamin D_3 itself. Such observations suggest that various vitamin D sterols may exert divergent biologic actions. However, the role of sterols, such as $24,25(OH)_2D_3$, in normal physiology is not clearly defined.

CLINICAL DISORDERS OF VITAMIN D METABOLISM

Our present-day knowledge of the complexities of vitamin D metabolism and the vitamin D-endocrine system suggest that many clinical conditions with altered calcium metabolism arise, in part, because of abnormal metabolism or action of vitamin D (Table 9.2). Certain conditions, such as chronic renal failure, the Fanconi syndrome, and the nephrotic syndrome, are commonly seen by the nephrologist. Others, such as pseudohypoparathyroidism, vitamin D-dependency rickets, and the osteomalacia associated with mesenchymal tumors, are seen by endocrinologists, pediatricians, or internists because of bone disease or hypocalcemia. A fundamental role of the kidney in the metabolism of vitamin D makes it mandatory that nephrologists and scientists who are interested in the kidney have a familiarity with these disorders. A discussion of certain of these disorders follows.

Disorders with decreased production of $1,25(OH)_2D_3$

Chronic renal failure

A decreased ability of the diseased kidney to generate $1,25(OH)_2D_3$ is believed to be an important factor contributing to secondary hyperparathyroidism and altered divalent ion homeostasis in uremia. The evidence that altered vitamin D metabolism contributes to abnormal calcium metabolism in renal failure is considerable: Thus, metabolic balance studies in patients with advanced renal insufficiency usually show that fecal calcium losses are equal to or greater than dietary calcium intake (Stanbury and Lumb, 1962; Stanbury and Lumb, 1966; Kopple and Coburn, 1973), and radioisotopic methods show reduced intestinal absorption of calcium in most patients with advanced renal failure (Kaye and Silverman, 1965; Ogg, 1968; Coburn et al., 1973a; Parker et al., 1974). Many years ago, Liu and Chu (1943) observed no improvement of osteomalacia or calcium balance in uremic patients treated with the usual doses of vitamin D; they conceived the idea that uremia impairs the response to vitamin D. Subsequently, it was shown that this calcium malabsorption could be overcome with the administration of vitamin D in doses as large as 100,000–300,000 IU/day (Stanbury and Lumb, 1962; Dent, Harper, and Philpot, 1961); also, the renal rickets or osteomalacia was improved. There was speculation that the intestinal absorption of calcium in uremia was unresponsive unless the serum vitamin D activity was increased to very high levels (Stanbury, Lumb, and Mawer, 1969). A link between abnormal vitamin D me-

Table 9.2 Classification of clinical disorders associated with abnormal vitamin D metabolism or action

I. **Deficient vitamin D action**
  A. Reduced availability of vitamin D_2 or D_3
    1. Inadequate sunlight
    2. Nutritional rickets/osteomalacia
      ? Chappati diet
    3. Intestinal malabsorption of vitamin D_2 or D_3
      a. Malabsorption syndromes
      b. Subtotal gastrectomy
      c. Ileal bypass surgery
  B. Reduced availability of 25 (OH) D_3
    1. Liver disease
    2. Anticonvulsant therapy
      a. Phenobarbital
      b. Phenytoin
      c. Glutethemide
    3. Reduced enterohepatic circulation
      a. Malabsorption syndromes
      b. Liver disease
    4. Nephrotic syndrome
    5. ? Acute renal failure
  C. Reduced availability of $1,25(OH)_2D_3$ (proven or probable)
    1. Vitamin D-dependency rickets
    2. Renal insufficiency
    3. Hypo- & pseudohypoparathyroidism (I)
    4. Fanconi syndrome
    5. Mesenchymal tumor-associated osteomalacia
    6. Itai-itai disease (cadmium toxicity)
    7. Diphosphonate treatment
  D. End-organ unresponsiveness
    1. Vitamin D-dependency rickets, Type II
    2. Steroid osteopenia
  E. Disorders of possible relation to vitamin D
    1. Diabetes mellitus
    2. Neonatal hypocalcemia
    3. Steroid-induced osteopenia
    4. Osteoporosis
    5. X-linked, hypophosphatemic rickets
II. **Excessive vitamin D action**
  A. Excess vitamin D_2 or D_3 (plasma 25(OH)D elevated)
    1. Exogenous ingestion
    2. ? Excess sunlight exposure
  B. Accelerated bioconversion of vitamin D
    1. Hyperparathyroidism
    2. Pregnancy
    3. Growth, acromegaly
    4. Lactation
    5. Sarcoidosis
    6. Phosphate depletion
    7. Idiopathic hypercalciuria (absorptive)
    8. Tumoral calcinosis

tabolism and the kidney was provided by the demonstration that the kidney is the only organ producing $1,25(OH)_2D_3$ from its precursor, $25(OH)D_3$ (Fraser and Kodicek, 1970; Gray, Boyle, and DeLuca, 1971; Norman et al., 1971). Reduced intestinal calcium transport in association with diminished intestinal localization of radio-labeled $1,25(OH)_2D_3$ following injection of radio-labeled precursor were found in chicks with experimental renal insufficiency (Hartenbower et al., 1974). In vivo observations utilizing radio-labeled vitamin D or $25(OH)D_3$ suggested a failure to generate $1,25(OH)_2D_3$ in patients with renal failure (Mawer, Backhouse, and Taylor, 1973; Schaefer, Von Herrath, and Stratz, 1972). Radioreceptor assays for $1,25(OH)_2D$ have uniformly revealed low or absent plasma levels of this sterol in patients with advanced renal failure (Brumbaugh et al., 1974; Eisman et al., 1976). Moreover, the administration of very small and presumably physiological amounts of $1,25(OH)_2D_3$ increased intestinal absorption of calcium to normal in patients with chronic renal disease (Brickman, Coburn, and Norman, 1972; Brickman et al., 1974; Henderson et al., 1974). Thus, there is considerable evidence that patients with advanced renal failure have little or no production of $1,25(OH)_2D_3$. From such observations it is highly likely that abnormal vitamin D metabolism plays an important role in the pathogenesis of renal osteodystrophy.

A reduced generation of $1,25(OH)_2D_3$ in patients with renal failure may lead to several pathophysiologic features commonly found in uremia; these include: (1) decreased intestinal absorption of calcium and phosphorus; (2) decreased calcemic response to the skeletal action of parathyroid hormone; (3) increased secretion of parathyroid hormone for any given level of serum calcium; (4) altered collagen synthesis; and (5) development of proximal myopathy.

In the absence of adequate production of $1,25(OH)_2D_3$, a lowered intestinal absorption of calcium and resistance of the skeleton to the calcemic action of PTH would contribute to the reduced ionized calcium in blood, thereby stimulating the secretion of PTH and leading to secondary hyperparathyroidism. Evidence cited above indicates that $1,25(OH)_2D_3$ may play a role in the feedback suppression of PTH secretion. Thus, a deficiency of $1,25(OH)_2D_3$ may lead to reduced sensitivity of the parathyroid glands to the suppressive effect of an increment in blood calcium, an abnormality that could contribute to the secondary hyperparathyroidism of uremia. By contributing to the development of hypocalcemia and impairing the feedback inhibition of PTH by blood calcium, disordered vitamin D metabolism is thus probably an important factor in the genesis of secondary hyperparathyroidism in renal failure (Stanbury, 1977).

The impressive action of $1,25(OH)_2D_3$ and $1\alpha(OH)D_3$, an analog that is converted to $1,25(OH)_2D_3$ in vivo which reverses many of the manifestations of secondary hyperparathyroidism in patients with advanced renal failure (Brickman, 1974; Henderson et al., 1974; Silverberg et al., 1975; Pierides et al., 1975, 1976, 1977; Chan et al., 1975; Kanis et al., 1977b) provides additional support for an important role of altered vitamin D metabolism in the pathogenesis of renal osteodystrophy.

When does vitamin D metabolism become abnormal in the course of progressive renal insufficiency? The answer to this question is of considerable importance in the consideration of the pathogenesis of the secondary hyperparathyroidism of uremia. The intestinal absorption of calcium has been reported to be normal in male patients with mild to moderate renal insufficiency (i.e., serum creatinine levels below 2.5 mg/dl [Coburn et al., 1973a]). Preliminary observations indicate that the plasma levels of $1,25(OH)_2D$ are normal in azotemic patients with creatinine clearances above 30 ml/min (Slatopolsky et al., 1978). On the other hand, Malluche, Werner, and Ritz (1978) reported that a small fraction of patients with mild renal insufficiency had a decrease in intestinal calcium absorption. With an increase in blood levels of parathyroid hormone in patients with mild renal insufficiency (Reiss, Canterbury, and Egdahl, 1968; Arnaud et al., 1973), one would anticipate augmented renal production of $1,25(OH)_2D_3$ with an increase in plasma levels and augmented intestinal calcium absorption, as exists in patients with primary hyperparathyroidism (Gray et al., 1977). One could postulate that a further decrease in renal function may reduce the renal generation of $1,25(OH)_2D_3$; for the reasons noted above, there would be increased PTH secretion, which would, in turn, augment the generation of $1,25(OH)D$ and result in a return of blood levels of $1,25(OH)_2D$ to normal (Figure 9.2). Indeed, one may postulate that high levels of parathyroid hormone maintain the serum levels of $1,25(OH)_2D$ at values near normal in azotemic patients until there is marked renal insufficiency. The signal for reduced renal generation of $1,25(OH)_2D_3$ in patients with mild to moderate renal insufficiency is uncertain; phosphate retention and diminished tubular reabsorption of phosphate have been noted early in the course of renal insufficiency, and it is possible that retained phosphate may reduce the renal generation of $1,25(OH)_2D_3$ for any given level of PTH secretion.

Despite strong evidence for deficient generation of $1,25(OH)_2D_3$ in most patients with advanced uremia, many of these patients lack features of vitamin D deficiency; thus, this abnormality may not be of significance in all patients with renal insufficiency. Intestinal absorption of calcium is not uniformly reduced in patients with advanced renal failure (Recker and Saville, 1971; Coburn et al., 1975), and some uremic patients actually have augmented intestinal absorption of calcium (Recker and Saville, 1971). Moreover, lesions of osteomalacia occur in only a fraction of patients with advanced renal failure (Sherrard et al., 1974; Duursma, Visser, and Nijio, 1972). Bone biopsies may lack any histologic evidence of vitamin D deficiency, even in anephric patients (Bordier et al., 1973). If such patients do not receive pharmacologic quantities of vitamin D or a similar sterol, it is not clear why signs and/or symptoms of vitamin D deficiency fail to develop more frequently. The occurrence of normal or elevated serum phosphorus levels may protect uremic patients from osteomalacia, and there is evidence that the extent of osteomalacia is inversely related to the serum phosphorus levels in patients with end-stage uremia (Kanis et al., 1977a).

Most interest has focused on the failure of the diseased kidney to generate

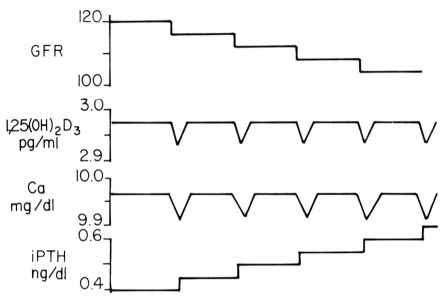

Figure 9.2 Theoretical scheme showing how alterations in the renal production of 1,25(OH)$_2$D$_3$ might lead to secondary hyperparathyroidism in early renal insufficiency. As renal mass is reduced, there may be a slight but imperceptible decrease in the renal generation of 1,25(OH)$_2$D$_3$. Serum calcium may fall leading to a rise in the secretion of PTH, which, in turn, stimulates the renal production of 1,25(OH)$_2$D$_3$, leading to normal or near normal levels of the sterol with a return of intestinal calcium absorption to normal. However, this tendency to normalization is maintained only at the expense of a sustained elevation in serum iPTH level; moreover, this process continues as long as the diseased kidney is capable of increasing its production of 1,25(OH)$_2$D$_3$ per remaining nephron. The signal leading to a decrease in the generation of 1,25(OH)$_2$D$_3$ as renal mass decreases is unknown, but phosphate retention is a reasonable candidate.

adequate quantities of 1,25(OH)$_2$D$_3$ from 25(OH)D$_3$ in azotemic patients. Any condition associated with reduced availability of 25(OH)D$_3$, the precursor to 1,25(OH)$_2$D$_3$, might exacerbate the deficiency of 1,25(OH)$_2$D$_3$. In the United Kingdom, where vitamin D intake is relatively low and sunlight exposure is reduced, Eastwood et al. (1976, 1977) reported that the plasma level of 25(OH)D is an important predictive factor for the development of osteomalacia in patients with renal insufficiency. Also, treatment with certain drugs, such as phenobarbital, phenytoin, or glutethemide, may accelerate the hepatic catabolism of 25(OH)D$_3$ and predispose to skeletal disease in uremic patients (Pierides et al., 1976b). Therefore, it seems advisable to avoid use of these drugs in renal patients, if possible.

A role of other vitamin D sterols, such as 24,25(OH)$_2$D$_3$, in the pathogenesis of renal osteodystrophy is uncertain. Although the kidney is the major organ responsible for the generation of 24,25(OH)$_2$D$_3$, this sterol may be produced in the intestine and perhaps bone as well (Garabedian et al., 1974). Reports on blood levels of 24,25(OH)$_2$D in uremic patients have been conflicting, with both reduced (Taylor and Mawer, 1977) and normal levels (Haddad and Wingate, 1977) reported. Since 24,25(OH)$_2$D$_3$ may have effects that differ from those of 1,25(OH)$_2$D$_3$ (Kanis et al., 1977, 1978; Llach et al., 1978), alterations in the generation of 24,25(OH)$_2$D$_3$ may play an as yet undefined role in the pathogenesis of altered calcium homeostasis in renal failure.

Acute renal failure

Abnormalities of calcium and phosphorus homeostasis that occur in patients with acute renal failure are of interest because the pathogenic factors are of recent onset and therefore may be evaluated more easily than is the case in chronic renal insufficiency. The possibility that the renal generation of 1,25(OH)$_2$D$_3$ is acutely reduced in patients with acute renal failure has been postulated as being a factor contributing to skeletal resistance to the calcemic action of PTH (Massry et al., 1974). Thus, the administration of 1,25(OH)$_2$D$_3$ to acutely uremic dogs partially restored the abnormal calcemic response to parathyroid extract (Massry et al., 1976). On the other hand, treating rats with acute renal failure with 1,25(OH)$_2$D$_3$ failed to restore the calcemic response to parathyroid extract (Somerville and Kaye, 1978). Thus, the mechanism for skeletal resistance in acute renal failure remains uncertain.

Pietrek, Kokot, and Kuska (1978) noted a rapid decrease in the plasma level of 25(OH)D during the course of acute renal failure. These data suggest that the turnover of 25(OH)D$_3$ may be enhanced, although the reasons for this are unclear. Such a decrease in the serum level of 25(OH)D could be a limiting factor for the generation of 1,25(OH)$_2$D$_3$ by the damaged kidney.

Hypercalcemia develops in some patients during the diuretic phase of acute renal failure. There are no firm data to implicate or to exclude an alteration of vitamin D metabolism in the pathogenesis of this hypercalcemia. Current observations suggest the cause of the hypercalcemia may be the release into the extracellular fluid of calcium previously sequestered in damaged muscle (Meroney et al., 1957; Clark and Sumerling, 1966; Siegel, Engel, and Derrer, 1977).

Fanconi syndrome

The Fanconi syndrome, characterized by proximal tubular dysfunction that results in reduced renal reabsorption of glucose, phosphate, amino acids, and bicarbonate, is commonly accompanied by metabolic bone disease, either rickets or osteomalacia (Fanconi, 1936; Schneider and Seegmiller, 1972; Morris et al., 1976). The hypophosphatemia that often exists in such patients undoubtedly contributes to the pathogenesis of such skeletal disease. However, the bone lesions often respond to treatment with pharmacologic doses of vitamin D without a measurable change in plasma phosphorus levels; such observations raise the possibility that there is reduced renal generation of 1,25(OH)$_2$D$_3$ by the kidney. Brewer et al. (1977) evaluated the bioconversion of ^{3}H-labeled-24(OH)D$_3$ in nonazotemic children with the Fanconi syndrome. These investigators could not detect ^{3}H-labeled-1,25(OH)$_2$D$_3$ in the plasma of such children despite hypophosphatemia and high serum levels of iPTH, two factors that are known to stimulate the generation of 1,25(OH)$_2$D$_3$. Unfortunately, it was not possible to carry out control studies in children lacking the Fanconi syndrome; nonetheless, such data suggest there may be reduced generation of $1,25(OH)_2D_3$ in children with the Fanconi syndrome. In a subsequent study, Brewer et al. (1977b) evaluated vitamin D metabolism in vitamin D-deficient rats given maleic acid, which induces proximal tubular dysfunction similar to that of the Fanconi syndrome. Rats treated with maleic acid failed to produce ^3H-$1,25(OH)_2D_3$ from $25(OH)D_3$. Moreover, the addition of maleic acid to suspensions of chick renal tubules inhibited the enzyme, $25(OH)D_3$-1α-hydroxylase. Such experimental studies provide support for an alteration in vitamin D metabolism in patients with the Fanconi syndrome.

Osteomalacia associated with mesenchymal tumor

Sporadic hypophosphatemic, vitamin D-resistant osteomalacia that occurs in association with a mesenchymal tumor of bone or soft tissue, a unique and potentially treatable cause of osteomalacia, may arise due to altered metabolism of vitamin D. The syndrome is characterized by skeletal lesions of osteomalacia, hypophosphatemia with normal urinary phosphate excretion, normal or slightly low serum calcium levels, elevated plasma alkaline phosphatase activity, and normal iPTH levels. Bone pain and deformity and muscle pain and weakness are often pronounced. Treatment with massive doses of vitamin D and phosphate supplementation have produced inconsistent clinical responses in most cases, although occasional patients have been reported to respond favorably. Such patients have been found eventually to have tumors of mesenchymal origin, in either bone or soft tissue; and there has been substantial improvement in the metabolic bone disease and reversal of biochemical abnormalities within weeks to months after resection of the tumor. Renal phosphate wasting is believed to play a major role in the pathogenesis of this syndrome, and certain data suggest that the tumor may generate a substance that impairs renal tubular reabsorption of phosphorus (Aschinberg et al., 1977). Thus, an extract of tumor, when injected into puppies, led to a significant fall in tubular reabsorption of phosphorus compared to extracts of normal tissue.

Drezner and Feinglos (1977) detected low plasma levels of $1,25(OH)_2D$ in one patient and found that short-term treatment of the patient with $1,25(OH)_2D_3$, 3 μg/day, led to a significant improvement in calcium and phosphorus balances with serum phosphorus rising toward normal. They postulated that a factor, which is synthesized and secreted by the tumor, reduces the synthesis of $1,25(OH)_2D_3$ by inhibiting the renal $25(OH)D_3$-1-hydroxylase; they further suggested that the deficiency of $1,25(OH)_2D_3$ causes the osteomalacia and renal phosphate wasting. If this syndrome arises simply owing to a lack of $1,25(OH)_2D_3$, it is difficult to explain the absence of hypocalcemia; moreover, most studies of the action of $1,25(OH)_2D_3$ on renal phosphate handling suggest a limited effect. Thus, it is uncertain whether hypophosphatemia can occur secondary to an isolated deficiency of $1,25(OH)_2D_3$ without concurrent secondary hyperparathyroidism. The observation that a tumor extract leads to brisk phosphaturia (Aschinberg et al., 1977) suggests that a product of the tumor may have a direct effect on tubular transport of phosphate. It would seem most attractive to postulate that a humoral substance produced by the tumor may affect renal tubular metabolism both to block phosphate reabsorption and to inhibit the tubular generation of $1,25(OH)_2D_3$.

Vitamin D-resistant rickets

Delineation of the pathways of vitamin D metabolism, therapeutic trials with forms of vitamin D, such as $25(OH)D_3$ and $1,25(OH)_2D_3$, and the ability to measure specific vitamin D sterols in plasma have clarified the pathogenesis of certain diseases associated with osteomalacia or hypocalcemia. A number of these conditions have been called, "vitamin D-resistant rickets," largely because they are recognized in children who develop rickets despite receiving normal quantities of vitamin D. A brief consideration of several of these syndromes is warranted.

Vitamin D-dependent rickets (or pseudo-vitamin D deficiency rickets) is believed to arise due to a deficiency of $1,25(OH)_2D_3$. This rare hereditary disease follows an autosomal dominant pattern; it differs from X-linked, vitamin D-resistant rickets in that afflicted children are hypocalcemic and it differs from true vitamin D deficiency in that vitamin D must be given in pharmacologic doses to correct the skeletal disease. Thus, treatment with vitamin D_2, 10,000 to 50,000 IU/day, corrects the biochemical abnormalities and leads to "catch-up" growth. Treatment with $1,25(OH)_2D_3$, 1.0 µg/day, was found to restore serum calcium to normal, while $25(OH)D_3$ (Rosen and Finberg, 1972) failed to elevate serum calcium unless it was given in pharmacological doses. Plasma levels of $1,25(OH)_2D$ (Scriver et al., 1978) were markedly depressed, even in children treated with pharmacologic doses of vitamin D. Serum $25(OH)D$ levels were generally elevated in such patients (Reade et al., 1975). These data suggest that this disorder arises as a consequence of a deficiency of the renal enzyme, $25(OH)D_3$-1-hydroxylase. Balsan et al. (1975) noted that patients with vitamin D-dependent rickets have a requirement for $1,25(OH)_2D_3$ or $1\alpha(OH)D_3$ that is approximately twice that of children with nutritional rickets, and they suggested that a factor other than deficiency of $1,25(OH)_2D_3$ is involved in the pathogenesis.

Vitamin D-dependent rickets, Type II, a variant of the syndrome described above (Brooks et al., 1978), was identified in a patient with hypocalcemia, secondary hyperparathyroidism, and skeletal changes of both secondary hyperparathyroidism and osteomalacia. This patient had normal or slightly low plasma levels of $25(OH)D$ and markedly elevated levels of $1,25(OH)_2D$. Treatment with vitamin D_3, 4,000 IU/day, increased the plasma level of $1,25(OH)_2D$ to a value 10 times that of normal; only then were the hypocalcemia and secondary hyperparathyroidism reversed. This condition appears to represent a form of end-organ resistance to the action of $1,25(OH)_2D_3$.

X-Linked hypophosphatemic rickets is a disorder that is characterized by marked hypophosphatemia, normal serum calcium levels, serum PTH levels that are usually normal, and a degree of uncertainty regarding alterations in vitamin D metabolism. As its name implies, this disorder is transmitted via the X-chromosome. A milder form of the disorder may be manifested only by hypophosphatemia with no overt skeletal disease. Treatment with $25(OH)D_3$ or $1,25(OH)_2D_3$ generally results in little correction of the hypophosphatemia, although some regression of secondary hyperparathyroidism may occur. Data on plasma levels of $1,25(OH)_2D$ are conflicting. Haussler et al. (1976a, 1977) found the plasma levels of $1,25(OH)_2D$ generally to be normal in such patients, while Scriver et al. (1978) found values to be in the low range of normal or even subnormal as compared to levels in age-matched controls. Haussler and McCain (1977) pointed out that the hypophosphatemia seen in these patients should lead to increased serum levels of $1,25(OH)_2D$; thus, normal values might be regarded as inappropriately low. From this discussion it is apparent that the pathogenesis of this disorder remains uncertain; a primary defect in renal tubular transport of phosphate seems to be most likely (Short, Binder, and Rosenberg, 1973).

Hypophosphatemic bone disease is the name given by Scriver et al. (1977) to another clinical subgroup of children with severe hypophosphatemia but only modest bone disease, not typically rachitic in nature. Serum levels of $1,25(OH)_2D$ were "normal" but inappropriately low for the degree of hypophosphatemia in these patients. Scriver et al. (1978) suggested that normal serum levels of $1,25(OH)_2D$ may prevent severe skeletal demineralization in such patients, and they suggest that the development of "true" rickets may require both hypophosphatemia and an absence of $1,25(OH)_2D_3$.

Disease states with enhanced loss of vitamin D sterols

Nephrotic syndrome

Certain features of vitamin D deficiency (e.g., hypocalcemia, hypocalciuria, and impaired intestinal absorption of calcium) commonly occur in patients with the nephrotic syndrome. Moreover, these abnormalities may be seen in patients with the nephrotic syndrome who have normal glomerular filtration rates. The hypocalcemia has been generally ascribed to a reduction in protein-bound fraction of plasma calcium which occurs as a consequence of hypoalbuminemia. Recently, Lim et al. (1976) and Goldstein et al. (1977) reported reduced plasma ionized calcium levels in patients with the nephrotic syndrome, indicating that hypoalbuminemia does not account for the hypocalcemia.

Recent evidence suggests that altered vitamin D homeostasis may be responsible for many of the alterations in calcium metabolism present in such patients. Thus, serum levels of $25(OH)D$ were found to be low in nephrotic patients, even those with normal renal function (Schmidt-Gayk et al., 1977; Barragry et al., 1977; Goldstein et al., 1977). A positive correlation was reported between serum levels of $25(OH)D$ and those of albumin, while an inverse correlation existed between serum $25(OH)D$ levels and urinary protein excretion (Goldstein et al., 1977). As previously noted, $25(OH)D_3$ circulates in the plasma attached to a specific vitamin D-binding protein (DBP). In the nephrotic syndrome, increased permeability of the glomerular wall for proteins of a molecular size similar to albumin make it likely that large quantities of the vitamin D-binding protein pass through the glomerulus and are lost in the urine. Indeed, a decrease in serum levels of vitamin D-binding protein has been reported in hypoproteinemic disorders including the nephrotic syndrome (Haddad and Walgate, 1976; Schmidt-Gayk et al., 1977; Barragry et al., 1977). Moreover, substantial excretion of vitamin D-binding protein has been reported in the urine of nephrotic patients, while this protein could not be detected in urine from normal subjects (Schmidt-Gayk et al., 1977; Barragry et al., 1977). Studies utilizing radio-labeled vitamin D have demonstrated enhanced urinary excretion of injected radioactivity in patients with the nephrotic syndrome, and the estimated loss of 25(OH)D in the urine of these patients approximates the minimal daily requirements of vitamin D (Schmidt-Gayk et al., 1977; Barragry et al., 1977).

Such data provide strong support for the view that significant urinary losses of 25(OH)D occur in the nephrotic syndrome, although the role of this abnormality in altering calcium homeostasis is uncertain. Abnormal intestinal absorption of calcium was found in nephrotic patients with marked proteinuria, while nephrotic patients in remission showed no abnormality (Lim et al., 1976; Emerson and Beckman, 1945); such observations suggest a relation between protein loss and altered calcium absorption. However, other investigators, who measured intestinal calcium absorption by a double radioisotope method, reported that a reduction in absorption was limited to nephrotic patients with significantly decreased glomerular filtration rate (Mountokalakis et al., 1977). In one study with bone biopsies in seven patients having the nephrotic syndrome, there was no evidence of osteomalacia or osteitis fibrosa (Collier, Mitch, and Walser, 1978); in contrast, other investigators reported biopsy evidence of early osteomalacia in several nephrotic patients (Malluche, Goldstein, and Massry, 1979). The use of more precise quantitative histomorphometric methods may have accounted for the positive findings in the latter study.

The existence of low blood levels of 25(OH)D in nephrotic patients who subsequently develop renal insufficiency could place such patients at greater risk for developing severe renal osteodystrophy. At present, data are not available for comparing the degree of skeletal disease in uremic patients having a past history of nephrotic syndrome with that of renal failure in other patients having no history of nephrosis.

Conditions associated with increased generation of vitamin D

An excess of vitamin D may result from an increased ingestion of vitamin D, as in vitamin D overdosage, or from alterations in vitamin D metabolism leading to the generation of excess quantities of active forms of vitamin D (i.e., 1,25-dihydroxyvitamin D_3). With vitamin D overdosage, the hypercalcemia is associated with increased quantities of circulating levels of 25(OH)D while the plasma levels of 1,25(OH)$_2$D remain normal (Hughes et al., 1976). In addition, there may be certain acquired or hereditary conditions with augmented generation of $1,25(OH)_2D_3$.

Idiopathic hypercalciuria

Many patients with calcium-containing kidney stones are classified as having "idiopathic hypercalciuria." Such patients demonstrate increased urinary calcium excretion, particularly when their dietary calcium intake is high; the levels of serum phosphorus may be normal, slightly low or overtly decreased; and serum calcium levels are normal (Edwards and Hodgkinson, 1965; Parfitt et al., 1964). By definition, such patients lack the usual evidence for primary hyperparathyroidism or other endocrine abnormalities causing hypercalciuria; hence, the term "idiopathic hypercalciuria" has been applied. Studies of radiocalcium absorption indicate that most of these patients show increased intestinal absorption of calcium (Albright et al., 1953; Henneman et al., 1958). The augmented intestinal absorption of calcium has been classified as either primary (primary absorptive hypercalciuria), with increased intestinal calcium absorption leading to excess urinary calcium excretion, or secondary, when calcium absorption is augmented as a consequence of excess renal calcium loss (renal leak hypercalciuria). A third category of hypercalciuria, appearing as absorptive hypercalciuria, may arise from excess renal generation of $1,25(OH)_2D_3$; in some instances this may be secondary to a mild degree of renal phosphate wasting and hypophosphatemia. Elaborate procedures have been developed for the separation and classification of patients with hypercalciuria (Bordier et al., 1977a); in general, the separation is on the basis of levels of serum iPTH. In renal leak hypercalciuria, iPTH levels should be high (Coe, 1977), while patients with primary hyperabsorptive hypercalciuria would be expected to have low levels of serum iPTH, whether this is due to an abnormality in the intestine, per se, or due to increased generation of $1,25(OH)_2D_3$.

Shen et al. (1975) noted that certain patients with idiopathic hypercalciuria had high plasma levels of $1,25(OH)_2D$; they suggested that the high level of $1,25(OH)_2D_3$ augments intestinal absorption of calcium, which in turn suppresses PTH secretion leading to decreased renal tubular reabsorption of calcium and consequent hypercalciuria. Indeed, studies in normal humans given $1,25(OH)_2D_3$ have demonstrated an increase in intestinal absorption of calcium and striking augmentation in urinary calcium, features similar to those of idiopathic hypercalciuria (Brickman et al., 1972). Subsequently, Gray et al. (1977) and Kaplan et al. (1977) each studied patients with hypercalciuria; in both studies, approximately one-third of patients with hyperabsorption of calcium demonstrated increased plasma levels of $1,25(OH)_2D$.

A major question concerns the mechanism for augmented production of $1,25(OH)_2D_3$. Shen et al. (1975) proposed that a renal leak of phosphate and consequent hypophosphatemia were responsible for increased renal generation of $1,25(OH)_2D_3$. Gray et al. (1977) also found somewhat low serum phosphorus levels in some patients. On the other hand, Kaplan et al. (1977) found normal levels of serum phosphorus; they felt that a renal phosphate leak was not responsible for the altered levels of $1,25(OH)_2D$. At present, it is not certain whether the patients reported represent separate pathogenic factors causing idiopathic hypercalciuria or whether a spectrum of "risk factors" may exist with some patients having a greater intestinal sensitivity to $1,25(OH)_2D_3$ while others have inappropriately increased renal generation of the sterol and still others have a combination of both factors operative.

Patients with hypercalciuria owing to renal calcium leak would also be expected to have increased plasma levels of $1,25(OH)_2D$, as a consequence of the secondary hyperparathyroidism. Of interest, Bordier et al. (1977a) have added a subgroup of patients with renal calcium leak in whom the secondary hyperparathyroidism may have become so protracted as to behave in a "nonsuppresible" manner after they were given $25(OH)D_3$.

It has been suggested that treatment of hypercalciuria should vary according to the pathogenic factor present (Pak, 1976). However, a large number of patients with renal stones have been successfully treated with thiazide diuretics, which primarily act to reduce urinary calcium excretion; the success of treatment did not have any apparent relationship to the mechanism responsible for hypercalciuria (Coe, 1977). The development of more refined techniques and further studies of stone patients may help clarify the pathogenesis of recurrent nephrolithiasis because of "idiopathic hypercalciuria."

Sarcoidosis

Sarcoidosis represents another condition characterized by an apparent increased sensitivity to vitamin D. Hypercalciuria and hypercalcemia, usually associated with increased intestinal calcium absorption, occur not uncommonly in patients with sarcoidosis (Anderson et al., 1954). The hypercalcemia of sarcoidosis is aggravated when patients are given relatively low doses of vitamin D_3 (Bell, Gill, and Bartter, 1964; Bell and Bartter, 1967), and the incidence of hypercalcemia is increased during seasons of the year with greater hours of sunlight each day (Taylor, Lynch, and Wyson, 1963). Moreover, when a patient with hypercalcemia of sarcoidosis had no exposure to ultraviolet light over a prolonged period, the hypercalcemia resolved (Anderson et al., 1954). Such observations led to the theory that sarcoidosis is associated with increased sensitivity to vitamin D. Subsequently, normal plasma levels of $25(OH)D$ have been reported, and patients appear to have a normal sensitivity to exogenously administered $1,25(OH)_2D_3$ (Bell, Sinha, and DeLuca, 1976). An elevated plasma level of $1,25(OH)_2D$ was reported in one hypercalcemic patient with sarcoidosis, suggesting that the hypercalcemia may arise owing to enhanced production of $1,25(OH)_2D_3$ from its precursor. Further observations on vitamin D metabolism in this disorder are needed to clarify this matter.

SUMMARY

Vitamin D_3 undergoes hydroxylation in both the liver and kidney before attaining its most active form, $1,25(OH)_2D_3$. Initial conversion from D_3 to

25(OH)D$_3$ is not tightly controlled, while the production of 1,25(OH)$_2$D$_3$ appears to be under strong regulatory influences including PTH, calcium, and phosphorus. The body appears to be able to respond to an increased calcium demand such as occurs in pregnancy, etc., by increasing the production of 1,25(OH)$_2$D$_3$. A high dietary calcium, on the other hand, can inhibit production of 1,25(OH)$_2$D$_3$.

1,25-dihydroxycholecalciferol appears to act at several sites including bone, intestine, kidney, and the parathyroid glands; as yet, the physiologic significance of its actions on certain of these target organs has yet to be determined. A number of pathological conditions that arise, in part, from alterations occurring at various steps in the bioconversion of vitamin D have been described. Some of these disorders, such as chronic renal failure and vitamin D-dependent rickets, result from deficient production of 1,25(OH)$_2$D$_3$ by the kidney. Other pathological conditions may occur as a consequence of increased loss of D$_3$ sterols, such as occurs in the nephrotic syndrome. Still others arise as a consequence of end-organ resistance to action of the D$_3$ metabolites. As our knowledge of the metabolism and action of vitamin D grows, the list of disease states with altered vitamin D metabolism will expand, and our ability to treat such conditions will have a more rational basis.

ACKNOWLEDGMENT

This study was supported, in part, by Veterans Administration Research Funds and USPHS grant AM-14750.

The authors gratefully acknowledge the valuable assistance of Patti Kentor and Harriet Goldware-Sorkin.

REFERENCES

Adams, T. H., Wong, R. G. & Norman, A. W. (1970). Studies on the mechanism of action of calciferol. II. Effects of the polyene antibiotic, filipin, on vitamin D-mediated calcium transport. *Journal of Biological Chemistry*, **245**, 4432.

Albright, F., Henneman, P., Bennedict, P. H. & Forbes, A. D. (1953). Idiopathic hypercalciuria. *Journal of Clinical Endocrinology* **13**, 860.

Anderson, J., Dent, C. E., Harper, C. & Philpot, G. R. (1954). Effect of cortisone on calcium metabolism in sarcoidosis with hypercalcaemia, possibly antagonistic actions of cortisone and vitamin D. *Lancet*, **2**, 720.

Arnaud, C. D. (1973). Hyperparathyroidism and renal failure. *Kidney International*, **4**, 89.

Arnaud, S. B., Goldsmith, R. S., Lambert, P. W. & Go, V. L. W. (1975). 25-hydroxyvitamin D$_3$. Evidence for an enterohepatic circulation in man. *Proceedings of the Society for Experimental Biology and Medicine*, **149**, 570.

Aschinberg, L. C., Solomon, L. M., Zeis, P. M., Justice, P. & Rosenthal, I. M. (1977). Vitamin D-resistant rickets associated with epidermal nevus syndrome: Demonstration of a phosphaturic substance in the dermal lesions. *Journal of Pediatrics*, **91**, 56.

Baksi, S. N. & Kenny, A. D. (1976a). Effect of antiestrogen (ICI 46,474) on renal metabolism of 25-hydroxyvitamin D$_3$ in vitro in female Japanese quail. *Pharmacologist*, **18**, 234.

Baksi, S. N. & Kenny, A. D. (1976b). Ovarian influence on 25-hydroxy-vitamin D$_3$ metabolism in Japanese quail. *Federation Proceedings, Federation of American Societies for Experimental Biology*, **35**, 665.

Baksi, S. N. & Kenny A. D. (1977). Vitamin D$_3$ metabolism in immature Japanese quail: Effects of ovarian hormones. In *Vitamin D: Biochemical, Chemical and Clinical Aspects Re-*

lated to Calcium Metabolism, ed. Norman, A. W., Schaefer, K., Coburn, J. W., DeLuca, H. F., Fraser, D., Grigoleit, H. G. & Herrath, D. V. P. 89. Berlin: W. de Gruyter.

Balsan, S., Garabedian, M., Sorgniard, R., Holick, M. F. & DeLuca, H. F. (1975). 1,25-dihydroxyvitamin D_3 and 1,alpha-hydroxyvitamin D_3 in children: Biologic and therapeutic effects in nutritional rickets and different types of vitamin D resistance. *Pediatric Research*, **9**, 586.

Bar, A., Cohen, A., Monteuccoli, G., Edelstein, S. & Horowitz, S. (1977). Relationship of intestinal calcium and phosphorus absorption during reproductive activity of birds. In *Vitamin D: Biochemical, Chemical and Clinical Aspects Related to Calcium Metabolism*, ed. Norman, A. W., Schaefer, K., Coburn, J. W., DeLuca, H. F., Fraser, D., Grigoleit, H. G. & Herrath, D. V. P. 93. Berlin: W. de Gruyter.

Barragry, J. M., France, M. W., Carter, N. D., Auton, J. A., Beer, M., Boucher, B. J. & Cohen, R. D. (1977). Vitamin D metabolism in nephrotic syndrome. *Lancet*, **2**, 629.

Bell, N. H. & Bartter, F. C. (1967). Studies of 47-Ca metabolism in sarcoidosis: Evidence for increased sensitivity of bone to Vitamin D. *Acta Endocrinology*, **54**, 173.

Bell, N. H., Gill, J. R. & Bartter, F. C. (1964). On the abnormal calcium absorption in sarcoidosis. Evidence for increased sensitivity to Vitamin D. *American Journal of Medicine*, **36**, 500.

Bell, N. H., Sinha, T. K. & DeLuca, H. F. (1976). Mechanism for abnormal calcium metabolism in sarcoidosis. *Clinical Research*, **24**, 484A.

Bikle, D. D. & Rasmussen, H. (1975). The ionic control of 1,25-dihydroxy-vitamin D_3 production in isolated chick renal tubules. *Journal of Clinical Investigation*, **55**, 292.

Bikle, D. D., Murphy, E. W. & Rasmussen, H. (1975). The ionic control of 1,25-dihydroxyvitamin D_3 synthesis in isolated chick renal mitochondria. *Journal of Clinical Investigation*, **55**, 299.

Bonjour, J. P., Preston, C. & Fleisch, H. (1977). Effects of 1,25-dihydroxyvitamin D_3 on the renal handling of Pi in thyroparathyroidectomized rats. *Journal of Clinical Investigation*, **60**, 1419.

Booth, B. E., Tsai, H. C. & Morris, R. C. (1977). Parathyroidectomy reduces 25-hydroxyvitamin D_3-1α-hydroxylase activity in the hypocalcemic vitamin D-deficient chick. *Journal of Clinical Investigation*, **60**, 1314.

Bordier, P., Ryckewart, A., Gueris, J. & Rasmussen, H. (1977a). On the pathogenesis of so-called idiopathic hypercalciuria. *American Journal of Medicine*, **63**, 398.

Bordier, P., Ryckwaert, A., Marie, P., Miravet, L., Norman, A. W. & Rasmussen, H. (1977b). Vitamin D metabolites and bone mineralization in man. In *Vitamin D: Biochemical, Chemical and Clinical Aspects Related to Calcium Metabolism*, ed. Norman, A. W., Schaefer, K., Coburn, J. W., DeLuca, H. F., Fraser, D., Grigoleit, H. G. & Herrath, D. V. P. 897. Berlin: W. de Gruyter.

Bordier, P. J., Tun-Chot, S., Eastwood, J. B., Fournier, A. & De Wardener, H. E. (1973). Lack of histological evidence of vitamin D abnormality in the bones of anephric patients. *Clinical Science*, **44**, 33.

Boyle, I. T., Gray, R. W. & DeLuca, H. F. (1971). Regulation by calcium of *in vivo* synthesis of 1,25-dihydroxycholecalciferol and 21,25-dihydroxycholecalciferol. *Proceedings of the National Academy of Sciences* (U.S.A.), **68**, 2131.

Brewer, E. D., Tsai, H. C. & Morris, R. C. (1977a). Fanconi syndrome and its relationship to vitamin D. In *Vitamin D: Biochemical, Chemical and Clinical Aspects Related to Calcium Metabolism*, ed. Norman, A. W., Schaefer, K., Coburn, J. W., DeLuca, H. F., Fraser, D., Grigoleit, H. G. & Herrath, D. V. P. 937. Berlin: W. de Gruyter.

Brewer, E. D., Tsai, H. S., Szeto, K. S. & Morris, R. C. (1977b). Maleic acid-induced impaired conversion of $25(OH)D_3$ $1,25(OH)_2D_3$, implication for Fanconi's syndrome. *Kidney International*, **12**, 244.

Brewer, E. D., Tsai, H. C., Hendrick, L. W. & Morris, R. C., Jr. (1978). Effect of NH_4Cl-induced acidosis on the metabolism of $25(OH)D_3$ in the rat. *Clinical Research*, **26**, 458A.

Brickman, A. S., Coburn, J. W. & Norman, A. W. (1972). Action of 1,25-dihydroxycholecalciferol, a potent kidney-produced metabolite of vitamin D_3, in uremic man. *New England Journal of Medicine*, **287**, 891.

Brickman, A. S., Coburn, J. W., Massry, S. G. & Norman, A. W. (1974). 1,25-dihydroxy-vitamin D_3 in normal man and patients with renal failure. *Annals of Internal Medicine*, **80**, 161.

Brickman, A. S., Hartenbower, D. L., Norman, A. W. & Coburn, J. W. (1977a). Actions of

1α-hydroxyvitamin D_3 and 1,25-dihydroxyvitamin D_3 on mineral metabolism in man. *American Journal of Clinical Nutrition*, **30**, 1064.

Brickman, A. S., Norman, A. W. & Coburn, J. W. (1977b). Vitamin D and pseudohypoparathyroidism. In *Vitamin D: Biochemical, Chemical and Clinical Aspects Related to Calcium Metabolism*, ed. Norman, A. W., Schaefer, K., Coburn, J. W., DeLuca, H. F., Fraser, D., Grigoleit, H. G. & Herrath, D. V. P. 867. Berlin: W. de Gruyter.

Brooks, M. H., Bell, N. H., Love, L., Stern, P. H., Orfei, E., Queener, S. F., Hamstra, A. J. & DeLuca, H. F. (1978). Vitamin D-dependent rickets Type II resistance of target organs to 1,25-dihydroxyvitamin D. *New England Journal of Medicine*, **298**, 996.

Brumbaugh, P. F., Haussler, D. H., Bressler, R. & Haussler, M. R. (1974). Radioreceptor assay for 1α,25-dihydroxyvitamin D_3. *Science*, **183**, 1089.

Brumbaugh, P. F., Hughes, M. R. & Haussler, M. R. (1975). Cytoplasmic and nuclear binding components for 1-alpha, 25-dihydroxyvitamin D_3 in chick parathyroid glands. *Proceedings of the National Academy of Science* (U.S.A.), **72**, 4871.

Brunette, M. G., Chan, M., Ferriere, C. & Roberts, D. K. (1978). The site of synthesis of 1,25(OH)$_2$-vitamin D_3 in the kidney. *Kidney International*, **14**, 636.

Canterbury, J. M., Lerman, S., Claflin, A. J., Henry, H., Norman, A. W. & Reiss, E. (1978). Inhibition of parathyroid hormone secretion by 25-hydroxycholecalciferol and 24,25-dihydroxycholecalciferol in the dog. *Journal of Clinical Investigation*, **61**, 1375.

Care, A. D., Bates, R. F. L., Pickard, D. W., Peacock, M., Tomlinson, S., O'Riordan, J. L. H., Mawer, E. B., Taylor, C. M., DeLuca, H. F. & Norman, A. W. (1976). The effects of vitamin D metabolites and their analogues on the secretion of parathyroid hormone. *Calcified Tissue Research*, **21**, 142.

Care, A. D., Pickard, D. W., Peacock, M., Mawer, B., Taylor, C. M., Redel, J. & Norman, A. W. (1977). Reduction of parathyroid hormone secretion by 24,25-dihydroxycholecalciferol. In *Vitamin D: Biochemical, Chemical and Clinical Aspects Related to Calcium Metabolism*, ed. Norman, A. W., Schaefer, K., Coburn, J. W., DeLuca, H. F., Fraser, D., Grigoleit, H. G. & Herrath, D. V. P. 105. Berlin: W. de Gruyter.

Carlson, H. E., Brickman, A. S. & Bottazzao, G. F. (1977). Prolactin deficiency in pseudohypoparathyroidism. *New England Journal of Medicine*, **296**, 140.

Chan, J. C. M., Oldham, S. B., Holick, M. F. & DeLuca, H. F. (1975). 1α-hydroxyvitamin D_3 in chronic renal failure. A potent analogue of the kidney hormone, 1,25-hydroxycholecalciferol. *Journal of the American Medical Association*, **234**, 47.

Chertow, B. S., Baylink, D. J., Wergedal, J. W., Su, M. H. H. & Norman, A. W. (1975). Decrease in serum immunoreactive parathyroid hormone in rats and in parathyroid hormone secretion in vitro by 1,25-dihydroxycholecalciferol. *Journal of Clinical Investigation*, **56**, 668.

Chesney, R. W., Hamstra, A. J., Mazess, R. B., DeLuca, H. F. & O'Reagan, S. (1978). Reduction of serum 1,25-dihydroxy-vitamin D_3 in children receiving glucocorticoids. *Lancet*, **2**, 1123.

Clark, J. G. & Sumerling, M. D. (1966). Muscle necrosis and calcification in acute renal failure due to barbiturate intoxication. *British Medical Journal*, **2**, 214.

Coburn, J. W., Hartenbower, D. L. & Massry, S. G. (1973a). Intestinal absorption of calcium and the effect of renal insufficiency. *Kidney International*, **4**, 96.

Coburn, J. W., Koppel, M. H., Brickman, A. S. & Massry, S. G. (1973b). Study of intestinal absorption of calcium in patients with renal failure. *Kidney International*, **3**, 264.

Coburn, J. W., Hartenbower, D. L. & Norman, A. W. (1974). Metabolism and action of the hormone, Vitamin D and its relation to calcium homeostasis. *Western Journal of Medicine*, **121**, 22.

Coe, F. L. (1977). Treated and untreated recurrent calcium nephrolithiasis in patients with idiopathic hypercalciuria, hyperuricosiuria, or no metabolic disorder. *Annals of Internal Medicine*, **87**, 404.

Collier, V. U., Mitch, W. & Walser, M. (1978). The effect of spontaneous or induced lowering of plasma Ca X P product on progression of chronic renal failure. *Clinical Research*, **26**, 564A.

Colston, K. W., Evans, I. M. A., Spelsberg, T. C. & MacIntyre, I. (1977). Feedback regulation of vitamin D metabolism by 1,25-dihydroxycholecalciferol. *Biochemical Journal*, **164**, 83.

Colston, K. W., Evans, I. M. A., Galante, L., MacIntyre, I. & Moss, D. W. (1973). Regulation of vitamin D metabolism: Factors influencing the rate of formation of 1,25-dihydroxycholecalciferol by kidney homogenates. *Biochemical Journal*, **134**, 817.

Day, H. G. & McCollum, E. V. (1939). Mineral metabolism, growth, and symptomatology of rats on a diet extremely deficient in phosphorus. *Journal of Biological Chemistry*, **130**, 269.

DeLuca, H. F., Tanaka, Y., Costillo, L. & Kumar, R. (1977). 1,25-dihydroxyvitamin D_3: Its further metabolism and the regulation of its biogenesis. In *Vitamin D: Biochemical, Chemical and Clinical Aspects Related to Calcium Metabolism*, ed. Norman, A. W., Schaefer, K., Coburn, J. W., DeLuca, H. F., Fraser, D., Grigoleit, H. G. & Herrath, D. V. P. 113. Berlin: W. de Gruyter.

Dent, C. E., Harper, C. N. & Philpot, G. R. (1961). Treatment of renal-glomerular osteodystrophy. *Quarterly Journal of Medicine*, **30**, 1.

Drezner, M. K. & Feinglos, M. N. (1977). Osteomalacia due to 1α,25-dihydroxycholecalciferol deficiency. *Journal of Clinical Investigation*, **60**, 1046.

Duursma, S. A., Visser, W. J. & Nijio, L. (1972). A quantitative histological study of bone in 30 patients with renal insufficiency. *Calcified Tissue Research*, **9**, 216.

Eastwood, J. B., Harris, E., Stamp, T. C. B. & DeWardener, H. E. (1976). Vitamin D-deficiency in the osteomalacia of chronic renal failure. *Lancet*, **2**, 1209.

Eastwood, J. B., Stamp, T. C., DeWardener, H. E., Bordier, P. J. & Arnaud, C. D. (1977). The effect of 25-hydroxy-vitamin D_3 in osteomalacia of chronic renal failure. *Clinical Science and Molecular Medicine*, **52**, 499.

Edwards, N. A. & Hodgkinson, A. (1965). Metabolic studies in patients with idiopathic hypercalciuria. *Clinical Science*, **29**, 143.

Eisman, J. A., Hamstra, A. J., Kream, B. E. & DeLuca, H. F. (1976). 1,25-dihydroxyvitamin D in biological fluids: A simplified and sensitive assay. *Science*, **193**, 1021.

Emerson, K. & Beckman, W. W. (1945). Calcium metabolism in nephrosis. I. A description of an abnormality in calcium metabolism in children with nephrosis. *Journal of Clinical Investigation*, **24**, 564.

Fanconi, G. (1936). Der fruhinfantile Nephrotischglycosurischie. *Jahrbuch fuer Kinderheilkunde*, **147**, 299.

Favus, M. J., Kimberg, D. V., Millar, B. N. & Gersham, E. (1973). Effects of cortisone administration on the metabolism and localization of 25-hydroxycholecalciferol in the rat. *Journal of Clinical Investigation*, **52**, 1328.

Fraser, D. R. & Kodicek, E. (1973). Regulation of 25-hydroxycholecalciferol-1-hydroxylase activity in kidney by parathyroid hormone. *Nature: New Biology* (London), **241**, 163.

Fraser, D. R. & Kodicek, E. (1970). Unique biosynthesis by kidney of a biologically active vitamin D metabolite. *Nature* (London), **228**, 764.

Galante, L., Colston, K. W., Evans, I. M. A., Byfield, P. G. H., Matthews, E. W. & MacIntyre, I. (1973). The regulation of vitamin D metabolism. *Nature* (London), **244**, 438.

Galante, L., Colston, K., MacAuley, S. & MacIntyre, I. (1972). Effect of parathyroid extract on vitamin D metabolism. *Lancet*, **1**, 985.

Garabedian, M., Holick, M. F., DeLuca, H. F. & Boyle, I. T. (1972). Control of 25-hydroxycholecalciferol metabolism by parathyroid glands. *Proceedings of the National Academy of Science* (U.S.A.), **69**, 1673.

Garabedian, M., Pavlovitch, H., Fellot, L. & Balsan, S. (1974). Metabolism of 25-hydroxyvitamin D_3 in anephric rats: A new active metabolite. *Proceedings of the National Academy of Science* (U.S.A.), **71**, 554.

Garabedian, M., Pezant, E., Miravet, L., Fellot, C. & Balsan, S. (1976). 1,25-dihydroxycholecalciferol effect on serum phosphorus homeostasis in rats. *Endocrinology*, **98**, 794.

Ghazarian, J. G., Jefcoate, C. R., Knutson, J. C., Orme-Johnson, W. H. & DeLuca, H. F. (1974). Mitochondrial cytochrome P-450, a component of chick kidney 25-hydroxycholecalciferol-lα-hydroxylase. *Journal of Biological Chemistry*, **249**, 3026.

Goldstein, D. A., Oda, Y., Kurokawa, K. & Massry, S. G. (1977). Blood levels of 25-hydroxyvitamin D in hephrotic syndrome: Studies in 26 patients. *Annals of Internal Medicine*, **87**, 664.

Gray, R. W., Wilz, D. R., Caldos, A. E. & Lemann, J., Jr. (1977). The importance of phosphate in regulating plasma 1,25$(OH)_2$-vitamin D levels in humans: Studies in healthy subjects, in calcium-stone formers and in patients with primary hyperparathyroidism. *Journal of Clinical Endocrinology and Metabolism*, **45**, 299.

Gray, R. W., Omdahl, J. L., Ghazarian, J. G. & DeLuca, H. F. (1972). 25-hydroxycholecalciferol-1-hydroxylase. *Journal of Biological Chemistry*, **247**, 7528.

Gray, R., Boyle, I. & DeLuca, H. F. (1971). Vitamin D metabolism: The role of kidney tissue. *Science*, **172**, 1232.

Gray, R. W., Weber, H. P., Dominguez, J. H. & Lemann, J. (1974). The metabolism of vitamin D$_3$ and 25-hydroxyvitamin D$_3$ in normal and anephric humans. *Journal of Clinical Endocrinology and Metabolism,* **39,** 1045.

Gray, R. W., Dominguez, J. H. & Lemann, J. (1975). 25-hydroxyvitamin D metabolism during dietary phosphate deprivation in humans. In *Vitamin D and Problems Related to Uremic Bone Disease,* ed. Norman, A. W., Schaefer, K., Grigoleit, H. G., Herrath, D. V. & Ritz, E. P. 331. Berlin: W de Gruyter.

Greenberg, A. J., McNamara, H. & McCrory, W. W. (1966). Metabolic balance studies in primary renal tubular acidosis: Effects of acidosis on external calcium and phosphorus balances. *Journal of Pediatrics,* **69,** 610.

Haddad, J. G., Boisseau, V. & Avioli, L. V. (1971). Phosphorus deprivation: The metabolism of vitamin D$_3$ and 25-hydroxycholecalciferol in rat. *Journal of Nutrition,* **102,** 269.

Haddad, J. G. & Chyu, K. J. (1971). Competitive protein-binding radioassay for 25-hydroxycholecalciferol. *Journal of Clinical Endocrinology,* **33,** 992.

Haddad, J. G., Jr. & Rojansathit, S. (1976). Acute administration of 25-hydroxycholecalciferol in man. *Journal of Clinical Endocrinology and Metabolism,* **42,** 284.

Haddad, J. G., Jr. & Walgate, J. (1976). Radioimmunoassay of the binding protein for vitamin D and its metabolites in human serum: Concentrations in normal subjects and patients with disorders of mineral homeostasis. *Journal of Clinical Investigation,* **58,** 1217.

Haddad, J. G., Jr. & Walgate, J. (1977). Radioimmunoassay of human serum DBP and competitive binding protein radioassay of 24,25(OH)$_2$D. In *Vitamin D: Biochemical, Chemical and Clinical Aspects Related to Calcium Metabolism,* ed. Norman, A. W., Schaefer, K., Coburn, J. W., DeLuca, H. F., Fraser, D., Grigoleit, H. G. & Herrath, D. V. P. 463. Berlin: W. de Gruyter.

Hahn, T. J. (1978). Corticosteroid-induced osteopenia. *Archives of Internal Medicine,* **138,** 882.

Hartenbower, D. L., Coburn, J. W., Reddy, C. R. & Norman, A. W. (1974). Calciferol metabolism and intestinal calcium transport in the chick with reduced renal function. *Journal of Laboratory and Clinical Medicine,* **83,** 38.

Haussler, M. R., Bursac, K. M., Bone, H. & Pak, C. Y. C. (1975a). Increased circulating 1α,25-dihydroxyvitamin D$_3$ in patients with primary hyperparathyroidism. *Clinical Research,* **23,** 322A.

Haussler, M. R., Lightner, E. S., Brumbaugh, P. F., Hughes, M. R. & Bursac, K. (1975b). 1α,25-dihydroxyvitamin D$_3$ in idiopathic hypoparathyroidism: Assay of circulating concentrations and therapeutic effect of the sterol. *Clinical Research,* **23,** 155A.

Haussler, M. R., Baylink, D. J., Hughes, M. R., Brumbaugh, P. F., Wergedal, J. E., Shen, F. H., Nielson, R. L., Counts, S. J., Bursac, K. M. & McCain, T. A. (1976a). The assay of 1-alpha-25-dihydroxy-vitamin D$_3$; physiologic and pathologic modulation of circulating hormone levels. *Clinical Endocrinology,* **5,** 151s.

Haussler, M., Hughes, M., Baylink, D. J., Littledike, E. T., Cork, D. & Pitt, M. (1976b). Influence of phosphate depletion on the biosynthesis and circulating level of 1α,25-dihydroxyvitamin D. In *Phosphate Metabolism,* ed. Massry, S. G. & Ritz, E. P. 233. New York: Plenum Press.

Haussler, M. R. & McCain, T. A. (1977). Basic and clinical concepts related to vitamin D metabolism and action. *New England Journal of Medicine,* **297,** 974 and 1041.

Heimberg, K. W., Matthews, C. & Ritz, E. (1976). Calcium transport of sarcoplasmic reticulum during experimental uremia. *Calcified Tissue Research,* **21,** S53.

Henderson, R. G., Russell, R. G. G., Ledingham, J. G. G., Smith, R., Oliver, D. O., Walton, R. J., Small, D. G., Preston, C., Warner, G. T. & Norman, A. W. (1974). Effects of 1,25-dihydroxycholecalciferol on calcium absorption, muscle weakness, and bone disease in chronic renal failure. *Lancet,* **1,** 379.

Henneman, P. H., Benedict, P. H., Forbes, A. P. & Dudley, H. R. (1958). Idiopathic hypercalciuria. *New England Journal of Medicine,* **259,** 802.

Henry, H. L., Midgett, R. J. & Norman, A. W. (1974a). Regulation of 25-hydroxy-vitamin D$_3$-1-hydroxylase in vivo. *Journal of Biological Chemistry,* **249,** 7584.

Henry, H. L. & Norman, A. W. (1974b). Studies on calciferol metabolism. IX. Renal 25-hydroxyvitamin D$_3$-1-hydroxylase. Involvement of cytochrome P-450 and other properties. *Journal of Biological Chemistry,* **249,** 7529.

Henry, H. L. & Norman, A. W. (1975). Studies on the mechanism of action of calciferol. VII. Localization of 1,25-dihydroxy-vitamin D$_3$ in chick parathyroid glands. *Biochemical and Biophysical Research Communications,* **62,** 781.

Henry, H. L. & Norman, A. W. (1976). Studies on calciferol metabolism. XIII. Regulation of 25-hydroxy-vitamin D_3-1-hydroxylase in isolated renal mitrochondria. *Archives of Biochemistry and Biophysics*, **172**, 582.

Henry, H. L. & Norman, A. W. (1978). Vitamin D: Two dihydroxylated metabolites are required for normal chicken egg hatchability. *Science*, **201**, 835.

Henry, H. L., Taylor, A. N. & Norman, A. W. (1977). Response of chick parathyroid glands to the vitamin D metabolites, 1,25-dihydroxycholecalciferol and 24,25-dihydroxycholecalciferol. *Journal of Nutrition*, **107**, 1918.

Horiuchi, N., Suda, T. & Sasaki, S. (1974). Direct involvement of vitamin D in the regulation of 25-hydroxycholecalciferol metabolism. *FEBS Letters*, **43**, 353.

Hughes, M. R., Haussler, M. R., Wergedal, J. & Baylink, D. J. (1975). Regulation of plasma 1α,25-dihydroxyvitamin D_3 by calcium and phosphate. *Clinical Research*, **23**, 323A.

Hughes, M. R., Baylink, D. J., Jones, P. G. & Haussler, M. R. (1976). Radioligand receptor assay for 25-hydroxyvitamin D_2D_3. *Journal of Clinical Investigation*, **58**, 61.

Imawari, M., Kida, K. & Goodman, D. S. (1976). The transport of vitamin D and its 25-dihydroxy metabolite in human plasma: Isolation and partial characterization of vitamin D and 25-hydroxyvitamin D-binding protein. *Journal of Clinical Investigation*, **58**, 514.

Kanis, J. A., Adams, N. D., Earnshaw, M., Heynen, G., Ledingham, J. G. G., Oliver, D. O., Russell, R. G. G. & Woods, C. G. (1977a). Vitamin D, osteomalacia, and chronic renal failure. In *Vitamin D: Biochemical, Chemical and Clinical Aspects Related to Calcium Metabolism*, ed. Norman, A. W., Schaefer, K., Coburn, J. W., DeLuca, H. F., Fraser, D., Grigoleit, H. G. & Herrath, D. V. P. 671.

Kanis, J. A., Earnshaw, M., Henderson, R. G., Heynen, G., Ledingham, J. G. G., Naik, R. B., Oliver, D. O., Russell, R. G. G., Smith, R., Wilkinson, R. H. & Woods, C. G. (1977b). Correlation of clinical, biochemical and skeletal responses to 1α-hydroxyvitamin D_3 in renal bone disease. *Clinical Endocrinology*, **7**, 45S.

Kanis, J. A., Heynen, G., Russell, R. G. G., Smith, R., Walton, R. J. & Warner, G. T. (1977c). Biological effects of 24,25-dihydroxycholecalciferol in man. In *Vitamin D: Biochemical, Chemical and Clinical Aspects Related to Calcium Metabolism*, ed. Norman, A. W., Schaefer, K., Coburn, J. W., DeLuca, H. F., Fraser, D., Grigoleit, H. G. & Herrath, D. V. P. 793. Berlin: W. de Gruyter.

Kanis, J. A., Russell, R. G. G., Naik, R. B., Earnshaw, M., Smith, R., Heynen, G. & Woods, C. G. (1977d). Factors influencing the response to 1α-hydroxyvitamin D_3 in patients with renal bone disease. *Clinical Endocrinology*, **7**, 51S.

Kanis, J. A., Cundy, T., Bartlett, M., Smith, R., Heynen, G., Warner, G. T. & Russell, R. G. (1978). Is 24,25-dihydroxycholecalciferol a calcium regulating hormone in man? *British Medical Journal*, **1**, 1382.

Kaplan, R. A., Haussler, M. R., Keftos, L. J., Bone, H. & Pak, C. Y. C. (1977). The role of 1α,25-dihydroxyvitamin D in the mediation of intestinal hyperabsorption of calcium in primary hyperparathyroidism and absorptive hypercalciuria. *Journal of Clinical Investigation*, **59**, 756.

Kaye, M. & Silverman, M. (1965). Calcium metabolism in chronic renal failure. *Journal of Laboratory and Clinical Medicine*, **66**, 535.

Kenny, A. D. (1976). Vitamin D metabolism: Physiologic regulation in egg-laying Japanese quail. *American Journal of Physiology*, **230**, 1609.

Kimberg, D. V., Baers, R. D., Gershon, E. & Gravdusius, R. T. (1971). Effect of cortisone treatment on the active transport of calcium by the small intestine. *Journal of Clinical Investigation*, **50**, 1309.

Klein, R. G., Arnaud, S. G., Gallagher, J. C., DeLuca, H. F. & Riggs, B. L. (1977). Intestinal calcium absorption in exogenous hypercorticism. *Journal of Clinical Investigation*, **60**, 253.

Kopple, J. D. & Coburn, J. W. (1973). Metabolic studies of low protein diets in uremia: II. Calcium, phosphorus and magnesium. *Medicine*, **52**, 597.

Larkins, R. G., Colston, K. W., Galante, L. S., MacAuley, S. J., Evans, I. M. A. & MacIntyre, I. (1973). Regulation of vitamin D metabolism without parathyroid hormone. *Lancet*, **2**, 289.

Larkins, R. G., MacAuley, S. J., Rapoport, A., Martin, T. J., Tulloch, B. R., Byfield, P. G. H., Matthews, E. W. & MacIntyre, I. (1974a). Effects of nucleotides, hormones, ions, and 1,-25-dihydroxycholecalciferol on 1,25-dihydroxycholecalciferol production in isolated chick renal tubules. *Clinical Science and Molecular Medicine*, **46**, 569.

Larkins, R. G., MacAuley, S. J. & MacIntyre, I. (1974b). Feedback control of vitamin D metabolism by a nuclear action of 1,25-dihydroxycholecalciferol on the kidney. *Nature* (London), **252**, 412.

Lee, S. W., Russel, J. & Avioli, L. V. (1977). 25-hydroxycholecalciferol to 1,25-dihydroxycholecalciferol: Conversion impaired by systemic metabolic acidosis. *Science*, **195**, 994.

Lemann, J., Jr., Litzow, J. R. & Lennon, E. J. (1966). The effects of chronic acid loads in normal man: Further evidence for the participating of bone mineral in the defense against chronic metabolic acidosis. *Journal of Clinical Investigation*, **45**, 1608.

Levine, B. S., Brautbar, N. & Coburn, J. W. (1978). Does vitamin D affect the renal handling of calcium and phosphorus? *Mineral Electrolyte Metabolism*, **1**, 295.

Lim, P., Jacob, E., Chio, L. F. & Pwee, H. S. (1976). Serum-ionized calcium in nephrotic syndrome. *Quarterly Journal of Medicine*, **45**, 421.

Liu, S. H. & Chu, H. I. (1943). Studies of calcium and phosphorus metabolism with special reference to pathogenesis and effects of dihydrotachysterol (A.T.10) and iron. *Medicine* (Baltimore), **22**, 103.

Llach, F., Brickman, A. S., Gerszi, K., Norman, A. W. & Coburn, J. W. (1978). Actions of 24,25-dihydroxy-vitamin D_3 in uremic patients. *Clinical Research*, **26**, 543A.

Llach, F., Coburn, J. W., Brickman, A. S., Kurokawa, K., Norman, A. W. & Reiss, E. (1977). Acute actions of 1,25-dihydroxy-vitamin D_3 in normal man: Effect on calcium and parathyroid status. *Journal of Clinical Endocrinology and Metabolism*, **44**, 1054.

Lotz, M., Ney, R. & Bartter, F. C. (1964). Osteomalacia and debility resulting from phosphorus depletion. *Transactions of the Association of American Physicians*, **77**, 281.

Lotz, M., Zisman, E. & Barttner, F. C. (1968). Evidence for a phosphorus depletion syndrome in man. *New England Journal of Medicine*, **278**, 409.

MacIntyre, I., Galante, L. S., Evans, I. M. A., Colston, K. W., Moss, D. W., Matthews, E. W., Byfield, P. G. H., MacAuley, S. J., Larkins, R. G., Hillyard, C. J. & Greenberg, P. B. (1974). The regulation of vitamin D metabolism. In *Endocrinology 1973*, ed. Taylor, S. P. 26. London: Heinemann Medical Books.

Malluche, H. H., Goldstein, D. A. & Massry, S. G. (1979). Osteomalacia and hyperparathyroid bone disease in patients with nephrotic syndrome. *Journal of Clinical Investigation*, **63**, 494.

Malluche, H. H., Werner, E. & Ritz, E. (1978). Intestinal absorption of calcium and whole body calcium retention in incipient and advanced renal failure. *Mineral and Electrolyte Metabolism*, **1**, 263.

Massry, S. G., Arieff, A. I., Coburn, J. W., Palmieri, G. & Kleiman, C. R. (1974). Divalent ion metabolism in patients with acute renal failure: Studies on the mechanism of hypocalcemia. *Kidney International*, **5**, 437.

Massry, S. G., Stein, R., Garty, J., Arieff, A. I., Coburn, J. W., Norman, A. W. & Friedler, R. M. (1976). Skeletal resistance to the calcemic action of parathyroid hormone in uremia: Role of $1,25(OH)_2D_3$. *Kidney International*, **9**, 467.

Matthews, C., Heimberg, K. W., Ritz, E., Agostini, B., Fritzsche, J., & Hasselback, W. (1977). Effect of 1,25-dihydroxycholecalciferol on impaired calcium transport by the sarcoplasmic reticulum in experimental uremia. *Kidney International*, **11**, 227.

Mawer, E. B. & Schaefer, K. (1969). The distribution of vitamin D_3 metabolites in human serum and tissues. *Biochemistry Journal*, **114**, 74.

Mawer, E. B., Backhouse, J. & Taylor, C. M. (1973). Failure of formation of 1,25-dihydroxycholecalciferol in chronic renal insufficiency. *Lancet*, **1**, 626.

Mawer, E. B., Lumb, G. A., Schaeffer, K. & Stanbury, S. W. (1971). The metabolism of isotopically labeled vitamin D_3 in man: The influence of the state of vitamin D nutrition. *Clinical Science*, **40**, 39.

Meroney, W. H., Arney, G. K., Segan, W. E. & Balch, H. H. (1957). The acute calcification of traumatized muscle with particular reference to acute post-traumatic renal insufficiency. *Journal of Clinical Investigation*, **36**, 825.

Midgett, R. J., Spielvogel, A. M., Coburn, J. W. & Norman, A. W. (1973). Studies of calciferol metabolism. VII. The renal production of the biologically active form of vitamin D, 1,25-dihydroxycholecalciferol; species, tissue and subcellular distribution. *Journal of Clinical Endocrinology*, **36**, 1153.

Miravet, L., Redel, J., Carre, M., Queille, M. L. & Bordier, P. (1976). The biological activity of synthetic 25,26-dihydroxycholecalciferol and 24,25-dihydroxycholecalciferol in vitamin D-deficient rats. *Calcified Tissue Research*, **21**, 145.

Morris, R. C., Jr., McInnes, R. R., Epstein, C. J., Sebastian, A. & Scriver, C. R. (1976). Genetic and metabolic injury of the kidney. In *The Kidney*, ed. Brenner, B. M. & Rector, F. C. P. 1193. Philadelphia: W. B. Saunders.

Morrissey, R. L. & Wasserman, R. H. (1971). Calcium absorption and calcium-binding protein in chicks on differing calcium and phosphorus diets. *American Journal of Physiology*, **220**, 1509.

Mountokalakis, T. H., Virvidakis, C., Singhellakis, P., Alevizaki, C. & Ikkos, D. (1977). Intestinal calcium absorption in the nephrotic syndrome. *Annals of Internal Medicine*, **86**, 746.

Norman, A. W., Midgett, R. J., Myrtle, J. F., & Nowicki, H. G. (1971). Studies on calciferol metabolism. I. Production of vitamin D metabolite 4B from 25-OH-cholecalciferol by kidney homogenates. *Biochemical and Biophysical Research Communications*, **42**, 1082.

Norman, A. W., Tsai, H. C., Spielfovel, A. M., Henry, H. L. & Midgett, R. J. (1973). Studies on the biological production and mode of action of 1,25-dihydroxycholecalciferol, the hormonally active form of vitamin D. In *Endocrinology 1973*, ed. Taylor, S. P. 52. London: Heinemann Medical Books.

Nseir, N. I., Szramowski, H. & Puschett, J. B. (1978). Mechanism of the renal tubular effects of 25-hydroxy and 1,25-dihydroxyvitamin-D_3 in the absence of parathyroid hormone. *Mineral and Electrolyte Metabolism*, **1**, 48.

Ogg, C. S. (1968). The intestinal absorption of ^{47}Ca by patients in chronic renal failure. *Clinical Science*, **34**, 467.

Olson, E. B., Jr., Knutson, J. C., Bhattacharyya, M. H. & DeLuca, H. F. (1976). The effect of hepatectomy on the synthesis of 25-hydroxyvitamin D_3. *Journal of Clinical Investigation*, **57**, 1213.

Omdahl, J. L., Gray, R. W., Boyle, I. T., Knutson, J. & DeLuca, H. F. (1972). Regulation of metabolism of 25-hydroxycholecalciferol by kidney tissue in vitro by dietary calcium. *Nature: New Biology* (London), **237**, 63.

Oldham, S. B., Smith, R., Hartenbower, D. L., Henry, H. L., Norman, A. W. & Coburn, J. W. (1979). The acute effects of 1,25-dihydroxycholecalciferol on serum immunoreactive parathyroid hormone (iPTH) in the dog. *Endocrinology*, **104**, 248.

Pak, C. Y. C. (1976). Disorders of stone formation. In *The Kidney*, ed. Brenner, B. M. & Rector, F. C., Jr., P. 1326. Philadelphia: W. B. Saunders.

Parfitt, A. M., Higgins, B. A., Massin, J. R., Collins, J. & Hilb, A. (1964). Metabolic studies in patients with hypercalciuria. *Clinical Science*, **27**, 463.

Parker, T. F., Vergne-Marini, P., Hull, A. R., Pak, C. Y. C. & Fordtran, J. S. (1974). Jejunal absorption and secretion of calcium in patients with chronic renal disease on hemodialysis. *Journal of Clinical Investigation*, **54**, 358.

Peil, C. E., Roof, B. S. & Avioli, L. V. (1973). Metabolism of tritiated 25-hydroxycholecalciferol in chronically uremic children before and after successful renal transplantation. *Journal of Clinical Endocrinology*, **37**, 944.

Pierides, A. M., Ellis, H. A., Simpson, W., Dewar, J. H., Ward, M. K. & Kerr, D. N. S. (1976a). Variable response to long-term 1α-hydroxy-cholecalciferol in haemodialysis osteodystrophy. *Lancet*, **1**, 1092.

Pierides, A. M., Ellis, H. A., Ward, M., Simpson, W., Peart, K. M., Alverez-Ude, F., Uldall, P. R. & Kerr, D. N. S. (1976b). Barbiturate and anticonvulsant treatment in relation to osteomalacia with haemodialysis and renal transplantation. *British Medical Journal*, **1**, 190.

Pierides, A. M., Ellis, H. A., Simpson, W., Cook, D. & Kerr, D. N. S. (1977a). The effect of 1α-hydroxyvitamin D_3 in predialysis renal bone disease. *Clinical Endocrinology*, **7**, 109S.

Pierides, A. M., Ellis, H. A., Ward, M. K., Simpson, W. & Kerr, D. N. S. (1977b). 1α-hydroxycholecalciferol in renal osteodystrophy. *Calcified Tissue Research*, **22**, S105.

Pierides, A. M., Ward, M. K., Ude-Alvarez, F., Ellis, H. A., Peart, K. M., Simpson, W., Kerr, D. N. S. & Norman, A. W. (1975). Long-term therapy with 1,25$(OH)_2D_3$ in dialysis bone disease. In *Proceedings, European Dialysis and Transplant Association*, ed. Moorhead, J. F. Vol. 12, p. 237. New York: Putnam Medical and Scientific Publishers.

Pietrek, J., Kokot, F. & Kuska, J. (1978). Serum 25-hydroxyvitamin D and parathyroid hormone in patients with acute renal failure. *Kidney International*, **13**, 178.

Pike, J. W., Toverud, S., Baass, A., McCain, T. & Haussler, M. R. (1977). Circulating 1α,25-$(OH)_2D$ during physiological states of calcium stress. In *Vitamin D: Biochemical, Chemical and Clinical Aspects Related to Calcium Metabolims*, ed. Norman, A. W., Schaefer, K., Coburn, J. W., DeLuca, H. F., Fraser, D., Grigoleit, H. G. & Herrath, D. V. P. 187. Berlin: W. de Gruyter.

Ponchon, G. & DeLuca, H. F. (1969). The role of the liver in the metabolism of vitamin D. *Journal of Clinical Investigation*, **48**, 1273.

Popovtzer, M. M. & Robinette, J. B. (1975). The effect of 25-OH-vitamin D₃ on renal handling of phosphorus: Evidence for inhibition of cyclic adenosine monophosphate formation. *American Journal of Physiology*, **229**, 907.

Popovtzer, M. M., Blum, M. S. & Flis, R. S. (1977). Evidence for interference of 25(OH)vitamin D₃ with phosphaturic action of calcitonin. *American Journal of Physiology*, **232**, E515.

Puschett, J. B., Fernandez, P. C., Boyle, I. T., Gray, R. W., Omdahl, J. L. & DeLuca, H. F. (1972a). The acute renal tubular effects of 1,25-dihydroxycholecalciferol. *Proceedings of the Society for Experimental Biology and Medicine*, **141**, 379.

Puschett, J. B., Moranz, J. & Kurnick, W. S. (1972b). Evidence for a direct action of cholecalciferol and 25-hydroxycholecalciferol on the renal transport of phosphate, sodium and calcium. *Journal of Clinical Investigation*, **51**, 373.

Puschett, J. B., Beck, W. S. & Jelonek, A. (1975). Parathyroid hormone and 15-hydroxy-vitamin D₃: Synergistic and antagonistic effects on renal phosphate transport. *Science*, **190**, 473.

Raisz, L. G., Trummel, C. L., Holick, M. F. & DeLuca, H. F. (1972). 1,25-dihydroxycholecalciferol: A potent stimulator of bone resorption in tissue culture. *Science*, **175**, 768.

Rasmussen, H. (1968). The parathyroids. In *Textbook of Endocrinology*, ed. Williams, R. H., p. 847. Philadelphia: W. B. Saunders.

Rasmussen, H., Fontaine, O., Goodman, D. & Matsumoto (1979). The fundamental action of 1,25(OH)₂D₃ on intestinal calcium transport does not involve gene activation. *Abstracts, Fourth Workshop on Vitamin D* (Berlin), p. 181.

Rasmussen, H., Wong, M., Bikle, D. & Goodman, D. B. P. (1972). Hormonal control of the renal conversion of 25-hydroxycholecalciferol to 1,25-dihydroxycholecalciferol. *Journal of Clinical Investigation*, **51**, 2502.

Rauschkolb, E. W., Davis, H. W., Fenimore, D. C., Black, H. S. & Fabre, L. F. (1969). Identification of vitamin D₃ in human skin. *Journal of Investigations in Dermatology*, **53**, 289.

Reade, L. M., Scriver, C. R., Glorieux, F. H., Nogrady, B., Delvin, E., Poirier, R., Holick, M. F. & DeLuca, H. F. (1975). Response to crystalline 1α-hydroxyvitamin D₃ in vitamin D dependency. *Pediatric Research*, **9**, 593.

Recker, R. R. & Saville, P. D. (1971). Calcium absorption in renal failure: Its relationship to blood urea nitrogen, dietary calcium intake, time on dialysis, and other variables. *Journal of Laboratory and Clinical Medicine*, **78**, 380.

Reiss, E., Canterbury, J. M. & Egdahl, R. H. (1968). Experience with a radioimmunoassay of parathyroid hormone in human sera. *Transactions of the Association of American Physicians*, **81**, 104.

Rizzoli, R., Fleisch, H. & Bonjour, J. P. (1977). Effect of thyroparathyroidectomy on calcium metabolism in the rat: Role of 1,25-dihydroxyvitamin D₃. *American Journal of Physiology*, **223E**, 160.

Rodman, J. S. & Baker, T. (1978). Changes in the kinetics of muscle contraction in vitamin D-depleted rats. *Kidney International*, **13**, 189.

Rojanasathit, S. & Haddad, J. G. (1976). Hepatic accumulation of vitamin D₃ and 25-hydroxyvitamin D₃. *Biochimica and Biophysica Acta*, **421**, 12.

Rosen, J. F. & Finberg, L. (1972). Vitamin D-dependent rickets: Action of parathyroid hormone and 25-hydroxycholecalciferol. *Pediatrics Research*, **6**, 552.

Rosenstreich, S. J., Rich, C. & Volwiler, W. (1971). Deposition in and the release of vitamin D₃ from body fat: Evidence for a storage site in the rat. *Journal of Clinical Investigation*, **50**, 679.

Sauveur, B. M., Garabedian, M., Fellot, L., Mongin, P. & Balsan, S. (1977). The effect of induced metabolic acidosis on vitamin D₃ metabolism in rachitic chicks. *Calcified Tissue Research*, **23**, 121.

Schachter, D., Finkelstein, J. D. & Kowarski, S. (1965). Metabolism of vitamin D. I. Preparation of radioactive vitamin D and its intestinal absorption in the rat. *Journal of Clinical Investigation*, **43**, 787.

Schaefer, K., Von Herrath, D. & Stratz, R. (1972). Metabolism of 1,2 H³-4-C¹⁴-cholecalciferol in normal, uremic and anephric subjects. *Israeli Journal of Medical Science*, **8**, 80.

Schmidt-Gayk, H., Schmitt, W., Grawunder, C., Ritz, E., Tschöpe, W., Pietsch, V., Andrassy, K. & Bouillon, R. (1977). 25-hydroxy-vitamin D in nephrotic syndrome. *Lancet*, **2**, 105.

Schneider, J. A. & Seegmiller, J. E. (1972). Cystinosis and the Fanconi syndrome. In *The Metabolic Basis of Inherited Disease*, ed. Stanbury, J. B., Wyngaarden, J. B. & Fredrickson, D. S., P. 1581. San Francisco: McGraw-Hill.

Schneider, L. E., Schedl, H. P., McCain, T. & Haussler, M. R. (1977). Experimental diabetes reduces circulating 1,25-dihydroxyvitamin D in the rat. *Science*, **196**, 1452.

Schott, G. D. & Wills, M. R. (1976). Muscle weakness in osteomalacia. *Lancet*, **1**, 626.

Scriver, C. R., Reade, T. M., DeLuca, H. F. & Hamstra, A. J. (1978). Serum 1,25-dihydroxyvitamin D levels in normal subjects and in patients with hereditary rickets or bone disease. *New England Journal of Medicine*, **299**, 976.

Scriver, C. R., MacDonald, W., Reade, T., Glorieux, R. H. & Nogrady, B. (1977). Hypophosphatemic nonrachitic bone disease: An entity distinct from X-linked hypophosphatemia in the renal defect, bone involvement and inheritance. *American Journal of Medical Genetics*, **1**, 101.

Shen, F., Baylink, D., Nielson, R., Hughes, M. & Haussler, M. (1975). Increased serum 1,25-dihydroxycholecalciferol (1,25-diHD₃) in patients with idiopathic hypercalciuria (II). *Clinical Research*, **23**, 423A.

Sherrard, D. J., Baylink, D. J., Sergedal, J. E. & Maloney, N. (1974). Quantitative histological studies on the pathogenesis of uremic bone disease. *Journal of Clinical Endocrinology*, **39**, 119.

Short, E. M., Binder, H. J. & Rosenberg, L. E. (1973). Familial hypophosphatemic rickets: Defective transport of inorganic phosphate by intestinal mucosa. *Science*, **179**, 700.

Siegel, B. A., Engel, W. K. & Derrer, E. C. (1977). Localization of technicium-99m diphosphonate in acute injured muscle. Relationship to muscle calcium deposition. *Neurology*, **27**, 230.

Silverberg, D. S., Higgins, K. B., Dossetor, M. R. & DeLuca, H. F. (1975). Use of 1α-hydroxy and 1,25-dihydroxy vitamin D₃ in renal osteodystrophy. In *Abstracts of Free Communications, VI International Congress of Nephrology, Florence* (June 8–12, 1975), p. 789.

Slatopolsky, E., Gray, R., Adams, N. D., Lewis, J., Hruska, K., Martin, K., Klahr, S., DeLuca, H. & Lemann, J. (1978). Low serum levels of 1,25(OH)₂D₃ are not responsible for the development of secondary hyperparathyroidism in early renal failure. *Kidney International*, **14**, 733.

Smith, J. E. & Goodman, D. S. (1971). The turnover and transport of vitamin D and a polar metabolite with the properties of 25-hydroxycholecalciferol in human plasma. *Journal of Clinical Investigation*, **50**, 2159.

Somerville, P. J. & Kaye, M. (1978). Resistance to parathyroid hormone in renal failure: Role of vitamin D metabolites. *Kidney International*, **14**, 245.

Spanos, E., Colston, K. W., Evans, I. M. S., Galante, L. S., MacAuley, S. J. & MacIntyre, I. (1976a). Effect of prolactin on vitamin D metabolism. *Molecular and Cellular Endocrinology*, **5**, 163.

Spanos, E., Pike, J. W., Haussler, M. R., Colston, K. W., Evans, I. M. A., Goldner, A. M., McCain, T. A. & MacIntyre, I. (1976b). Circulating 1α,25-dihydroxyvitamin D in the chick: Enhancement by injection of prolactin and during egg laying. *Life Sciences*, **19**, 1751.

Spanos, E., Colston, K. W. & MacIntyre, I. (1977). Effect of glucocorticoids on vitamin D metabolism. *FEB Letters*, **75**, 73.

Spencer, E. M., & Tobiassen, O. (1977). The effects of hypophysectomy on 25-hydroxyvitamin D₃ metabolism in the rat. In *Vitamin D: Biochemical, Chemical and Clinical Aspects Related to Calcium Metabolism*, ed. Norman, A. W., Schaefer, K., Coburn, J. W., DeLuca, H. F., Fraser, D., Grigoleit, H. G. & Herrath, D. V. P. 197. Berlin: W de Gruyter.

Stamp, T. C. B. & Round, J. M. (1974). Seasonal changes in human plasma levels of 25-hydroxyvitamin D. *Nature* (London), **247**, 563.

Stanbury, S. W. (1968). Bone disease in uremia. *American Journal of Medicine*, **44**, 714.

Stanbury, S. W. (1977). The role of vitamin D in renal bone disease. *Clinical Endocrinology*, **7**, 25S.

Stanbury, S. W. & Lumb, G. A. (1962). Metabolic studies of renal osteodystrophy: I. Calcium, phosphorus and nitrogen metabolism in rickets, osteomalacia and hyperparathyroidism complicating chronic uremia and in the osteomalacia of the adult Fanconi syndrome. *Medicine*, **41**, 1.

Stanbury, S. W. & Lumb, G. A. (1966). Parathyroid function in chronic renal failure: A statistical survey of the plasma biochemistry in azotaemic renal osteodystrophy. *Quarterly Journal of Medicine*, **35**, 1.

Stanbury, S. W., Lumb, G. A. & Mawer, E. B. (1969). Osteodystrophy developing sponta-neously in the course of chronic renal failure. *Archives of Internal Medicine*, **124**, 274.

Steele, T. H., Engle, J. E., Tanaka, Y., Lorenc, R. S., Dudgeon, K. L. & DeLuca, H. F. (1975). On the phosphatemic action of 1,25-dihydroxyvitamin D_3. *American Journal of Physiology*, **229**, 489.

Tanaka, Y. & DeLuca, H. F. (1973). The control of 25-hydroxy-vitamin D metabolism by in-organic phosphorus. *Archives of Biochemistry and Biophysics*, **154**, 566.

Tanaka, Y., Castillo, L. & DeLuca, H. F. (1976). Control of renal vitamin D hydroxylase in birds by sex hormones. *Proceedings, National Academy of Science* (U.S.A.), **73**, 2701.

Tanaka, Y., Castillo, L. & DeLuca, H. F. (1977). Sex hormonal control of the renal vitamin D hydroxylases. In *Vitamin D: Biochemical, Chemical, and Clinical Aspects Related to Calcium Metabolism*, ed. Norman, A. W., Schaefer, K., Coburn, J. W., DeLuca, H. F., Fraser, D., Grigoleit, H. G. & Herrath, D. V. P. 215. Berlin: W. de Gruyter.

Taylor, C. M. (1977). The measurement of 24,25-dihydroxycholecalciferol in human serum. In *Vitamin D: Biochemical, Chemical and Clinical Aspects Related to Calcium Metabolism*, ed. Norman, A. W., Schaefer, K., Coburn, J. W., DeLuca, H. F., Fraser, D., Grigoleit, H. G. & Herrath, D. V. P. 541. Berlin: W. de Gruyter.

Taylor, R. L., Lynch, H. J. & Wysor, W. G. (1963). Seasonal influence of sunlight on the hy-percalcemia of sarcoidosis. *American Journal of Medicine*, **34**, 221.

Tucker, G., Gagnon, R. E. & Haussler, M. R. (1973). Vitamin D_3-25-hydroxylase: Tissue oc-currence and apparent lack of regulation. *Archives of Biochemistry and Biophysics*, **155**, 47.

Walling, M. S. (1977). Intestinal calcium and phosphate transport: Differential responses to vitamin D_3 metabolites. *American Journal of Physiology*, **233**, E488.

Weber, H. P., Gray, R. W., Dominguez, J. H. & Lemann, J., Jr. (1976). The lack of effect of chronic metabolic acidosis on 25-OH-vitamin D metabolism and serum parathyroid hor-mone in humans. *Journal of Endocrinology and Metabolism*, **43**, 1047.

Wheatley, V. R. & Reinertson, R. P. (1958). The presence of vitamin D precursors in the human epidermis. *Journal of Investigation in Dermatology*, **31**, 51.

10

Cyclic nucleotides in renal pathophysiology

THOMAS P. DOUSA

INTRODUCTION

In recent years, biomedical investigations dealing with the regulatory role of cyclic nucleotides (cNMP)* have undergone both intensive and extensive development. As an organ that is subject to the regulatory action of numerous hormones and other humoral agents,† the kidney has attracted the attention of many investigators, and the scientific literature dealing with the role of cNMP

---

* The term "cyclic nucleotides" will be used (as it is currently an accepted practice) to refer to cyclic 3′5′-nucleoside monophosphates (abbreviated here cNMP) and does not include the other forms of nucleotides with cyclic structure which are known in various areas of biochemistry.

† Hormone and/or humoral agents encompass all natural organic compounds, formed outside or within the kidney, which act on renal cells from the extracellular fluid compartment and which are known to, or are assumed to, regulate cell function. For the sake of simplicity in the present discussion, the term "hormone" will include all these agents (ranging from "classical hormones" such as parathyroid hormone through kinins and prostaglandins up to biogenic amines such as histamine).

in regulation of kidney function is accumulating at a rapid and accelerating rate. The purpose of this review is to summarize what appears to be, in the authors' opinion, the basic relevant information available to date and to explore the possible implications of our present basic knowledge on renal cNMP for renal physiology and pathophysiology of renal diseases.

The specific reports dealing with the present topic are so numerous that the bibliography must by necessity be selective; thus references will frequently be made to summaries in recent symposia, reviews, and monographs. First, we would like to review briefly the general principles of metabolism and dynamics* of cNMP in the kidney and the methodologies currently used; then, we will discuss the involvement of cNMP in various specific disorders of kidney function.

BASIC FEATURES OF RENAL CYCLIC NUCLEOTIDE DYNAMICS

Overview of cNMP metabolism in kidney

Two major cNMP found in the kidney are adenosine 3′,5′-cyclic monophosphate (cAMP)† and guanosine 3′,5′-cyclic monophosphate (cGMP) (Dousa and Barnes, 1977b). Evidence for the presence of other cyclic nucleotides is scanty; enzymatic formation from CTP (Cech and Ignarro, 1977) and degradation (Kuo et al., 1978) of cytosine 3′,5′-cyclic monophosphate by kidney homogenates was recently reported, and at least the capacity of kidney extracts to hydrolyze cyclic 3′,5′-inosine monophosphate was also observed (Dousa and Rychlik, 1970). The unique feature of the kidney is that cNMP, both extrarenal and those formed in the renal cells, are excreted in huge quantities in urine, which allows one to use measurement of urinary cNMP in a variety of experimental and clinical studies (Murad, 1973; Broadus, 1977).

Enzymes of synthesis and degradation of cNMP in kidney

The two major metabolic determinants of cellular cNMP dynamics are the enzymatic synthesis of cNMP from the corresponding nucleotide triphosphates by cyclases, namely the adenylate cyclase (AdC) for cAMP (Dousa and Barnes, 1977a; Dousa, 1976) and the guanylate cyclase (GnC) for cGMP (Dousa and Barnes, 1977a), and the enzymatic hydrolysis to corresponding

---

* The term "dynamics of cyclic nucleotides" is used, for the sake of further discussion, to encompass information on basal values as well as changes in tissue levels, metabolic transformation, transmembrane movement, excretion, and actions of cNMP.

† Abbreviations: Adenylate cyclase, AdC; guanylate cyclase, GnC; cNMP-PDIE, cyclic nucleotide phosphodiesterase; cAMP-phosphodiesterase, cAMP-PDIE; cGMP phosphodiesterase, cGMP-PDIE; calcium, Ca^{2+}; magnesium, Mg^{2+}; cyclic 3′,5′-AMP, cAMP; cyclic 3′,5′-GMP, cGMP; protein kinase, PK; protein phosphatase, PPase; cAMP-dependent protein kinase, cAMP-PK; cGMP-dependent protein kinase, cGMP-PK; VP, vasopressin; PTH, parathyroid hormone, CT, calcitonin; PG, prostaglandin; GFR, glomerular filtration rate; ALH, ascending limb of Henle's loop; vit-D, vitamin D.

5′-nucleotides by cyclic nucleotide phosphodiesterases (cNMP-PDIE). Some general properties of the above-mentioned enzymes in the mammalian kidneys are similar to those found in extrarenal tissues.

The renal AdC is an intrinsic membrane-bound enzyme, located in cell surface membranes (plasma membranes) (Dousa, 1976); the presence of AdC in cytoplasm or in endocellular membranes has never been conclusively demonstated for kidney cells. AdC, as an enzyme, requires Mg^{2+} as a cofactor; there are some other natural compounds such as guanyl nucleotides (GTP, GDP, etc.), or Ca^{2+}, the presence of which were shown to influence AdC activity in vitro, namely, its activation by hormones; however, the obligatory nature of these factors in vivo has not been established. The most outstanding feature of AdC is the fact that it is almost always associated in plasma membrane with receptor for hormones via a yet unknown coupling mechanism (Dousa and Barnes, 1977a; Dousa, 1976). AdC activity could be stimulated (or inhibited) by hormones in intact cells, or in cell-free systems, ranging from crude homogenates to highly purified fractions of plasma membranes (Dousa, 1976).

In contrast to AdC, guanylate cyclase (GnC) is found both in the fraction of soluble proteins as well as in membrane fractions of the kidney tissue homogenate. Reports on the proportion of the membrane-bound versus soluble GnC vary widely; it appears to be different in various species (Kim et al., 1977a), zones of kidney (Craven and DeRubertis, 1976) and stages of ontogenetic development (Schlondorff and Weber, 1976). It is still unresolved whether membrane-associated renal GnC, which differs from the soluble form in some properties (Mittal and Murad, 1977), is an intrinsic (but loosely associated) membrane enzyme or whether it is only a soluble enzyme absorbed on the membranes in the course of the preparative procedures. GnC requires the presence of Mg^{2+} or other divalent cations (Mn^{2+} is the most potent in vitro) as a cofactor for its activity; the obligatory nature of some other cofactors that are known to influence GnC activity in vitro for in vivo situation has not yet been proven (Goldberg and Haddox, 1977). In sharp contrast to AdC, GnC can be stimulated by hormones only in intact cells, not in cell-free systems, suggesting that the stimulation by hormones is indirect. The majority of experimental evidence seems to favor a hypothesis that the hormones stimulate cGMP biosynthesis in the intact cell by indirect mechanism, associated with, or dependent on transmembranous fluxes of Ca^{2+} (or Na^+) which are elicited by hormones (Goldberg and Haddox, 1977).

cAMP and cGMP phosphodiesterases (cAMP-PDIE, cGMP-PDIE) are abundant in kidney tissue; multiple forms of these enzymes have been described in this organ (Dousa and Barnes, 1977a; Dousa, 1976; Strada and Thompson, 1978; Wells and Hardman, 1977). Most of the cAMP-PDIE and cGMP-PDIE activities are found in the fraction of soluble proteins. While some activity of cNMP-PDIE is invariably found in membrane fractions of renal homogenates, it remains to be resolved whether membrane-associated cNMP-PDIE is an intrinsic membrane enzyme. Some cNMP-PDIE have been shown to hydrolyze specifically cAMP, some cGMP, others are capable of the hydrolysis of both cNMP (Strada and Thompson, 1978; Wells and Hardman,

1977). The diversity in cNMP-PDIE applies not only to their substrate specificity (Strada and Thompson, 1978) but also to their response to the modulatory effects produced by such intracellular components as Ca^{2+}, acting via a heat-stable protein activator (Wells and Hardman, 1977), or a heat-labile protein activator (Strewler, Manganiello, and Vanghan, 1978), ATP, pyrophosphate (Dousa and Rychlik, 1970), or other factors (Dousa, 1976; Strada and Thompson, 1978; Wells and Hardman, 1977; Strewler and Orloff, 1977). Mg^{2+} is invariably required as a cofactor for the activity of all cNMP-PDIE.

Mode of action of cNMP within renal cells

The biochemical mechanisms by which cAMP and cGMP, formed within the renal cells, exert their ultimate functional effects are virtually unknown. It is the generally accepted working hypothesis that, in vertebrates many (Kuo and Greengard, 1969), if not all, actions of cNMP may be mediated by reversible phosphorylation of specific cellular proteins involved in regulation of the various specific cellular functions (Nimmo and Cohen, 1977; Rubin and Rosen, 1975; Lincoln and Corbin, 1978), including transport processes in kidney (Strewler and Orloff, 1977). While the cNMP-sensitive protein kinases—that is, cAMP-sensitive PK (cAMP-PK) and cGMP-sensitive PK (cGMP-PK), which are protein-phosphorylating enzymes—are virtually ubiquitous (Nimmo and Cohen, 1977; Rubin and Rosen, 1975), their exact role in regulation of cellular functions has been documented so far only in the mechanisms regulating some enzymes of intermediary metabolism (Nimmo and Cohen, 1977; Rubin and Rosen, 1975). It is only assumed, but not proven with certainty, that such mechanisms will be analogous for other functional effects. Kidneys are rich in cAMP-PK, and the majority of cAMP-PK are found in the fraction of soluble proteins (Dousa and Valtin, 1976; Knox et al. 1978; Dousa, Barnes, and Kim, 1977). However, cAMP-PK were also found in various membrane fractions from kidney tissue, and it thus appears that at least some renal cAMP-PK may be an intrinsic component of membranes (Dousa and Valtin, 1976; Knox et al., 1978; Dousa et al., 1977a). Protein phosphatases (PPase), enzymes, which catalyze the dephosphorylation of proteins, were also detected in the kidney (Dousa and Valtin, 1976; Knox et al., 1978; Dousa et al., 1977a), but the influence of cyclic nucleotides on these enzymes has not yet been documented.

As with cAMP-PK, cGMP-PK appears to be ubiquitous (Shoji and Kuo, 1978), and although it has not yet been investigated in detail in the kidney, its presence may be anticipated. Of interest is the presence of cGMP-PK in renal artery and renal vein, especially in the inner muscle layer of renal artery (Kuo et al., 1977). cGMP-PK is expected to have less specific and versatile function than cAMP-PK (Lincoln and Corbin, 1978). Potentially very important in regulation of protein phosphorylations are heat-stable proteins that serve as modulators of PK, activators of cGMP-PK, and inhibitors of cAMP-PK (Nimmo and Cohen, 1977; Rubin and Rosen, 1975; Shoji and Kuo, 1978).

That cAMP-PK is indeed involved in cAMP actions in intact renal cells is supported by the findings that the in situ activity of cAMP-PK was found to be increased in response to hormones (Dousa and Valtin, 1976; Edwards, Jackson and Dousa, 1979; Knox et al., 1978; Dousa and Barnes, 1977b). The major question that remains unsolved is the existence and nature of the natural protein substrates for PK. It is assumed that these natural protein substrates are associated with structures involved in the functional response, such as membranes, cytoplasmic or membrane-associated enzymes, but they have not yet been positively identified in the kidney (Nimmo and Cohen, 1977; Rubin and Rosen, 1975; Strewler and Orloff, 1977; Dousa and Valtin, 1976; Knox et al., 1978; Dousa et al., 1977a). The multiple possibilities of how cAMP-PK can be involved in mediation of renal action has been recently discussed for the specific case of VP (Dousa et al., 1977) or PTH (Knox et al., 1978); similar general considerations seem to apply to other cAMP-regulated renal systems. While most of the cAMP and cGMP binding proteins found in the kidney are PKs or regulatory subunits of PK, it is quite possible that some protein(s), binding cyclic nucleotides specifically, are not associated with PK systems (Ueland and Doskeland, 1977; Lincoln and Corbin, 1978; Lincoln et al. 1976) and that these distinct cNMP-binding proteins may exert their cellular effects through yet unknown mechanisms.

Extracellular cNMP and kidney

In addition to cNMP generated in the kidney, an appreciable quantity of cNMP are delivered to the kidney via the blood supply. cNMP from arterial blood are in part filtered by glomeruli (Murad, 1973; Broadus, 1977) and actively taken up by tubules, most likely by the organic acid transport system (Coulson, 1976; Dousa, 1976); this latter portion of cNMP appears to be catabolized mostly within tubular cells (Coulson, 1976). A portion of arterial blood cNMP passes to venous renal outflow, and a portion of cNMP generated in renal cells, so-called nephrogenous cNMP (N-cNMP), effluxes into the tubular fluid and venous blood (Murad, 1973; Broadus, 1977; Dousa, 1976).

Since the primary site of cNMP generation and action is intracellular, it is generally not expected that cNMP, which appears in very low concentrations in extracellular fluids, have functional significance, but the kidney may be an exception. cNMP in tubular fluid achieve a high concentration by water reabsorption in distal segments of tubules and, as originally proposed by Butlen and Jard (1972), tubular cNMP may conceivably have a regulatory effect (Knox et al., 1978). This intriguing possibility remains to be proven.

Otherwise, since cNMP are freely filtered by glomeruli (Murad, 1973; Broadus, 1977) and since the factors determining tubular handling of cNMP are at least in part known, it is possible to use the measurement of urinary N-cNMP to assess, in the intact organism, the renal handling of nephrogenous and extrarenal cNMP in a number of clinical and experimental situations (Murad, 1973; Broadus, 1977), as discussed in the following sections. Known, or at least theoretically anticipated, components of cNMP dynamics (metabolism and fluxes) in renal cell in general are schematically outlined in Figure 10.1.

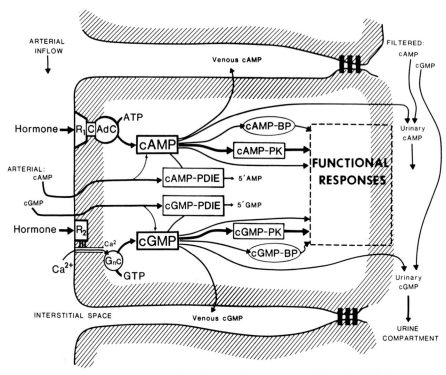

Figure 10.1 General schematic outline of major directions of cAMP and cGMP dynamics in renal cells. Position of individual factors in the figure does not denote necessarily a specific location in cell; arrows show only directionality of possible changes, without implicating their quantitative significance. However, thicker lines denote pathways currently believed to be of major importance.

Abbreviations:

R_1 = receptors for hormones acting via cAMP
R_2 = receptors for hormones acting via cGMP
cAMP = cyclic AMP
cGMP = cyclic GMP
cAMP-PK = cAMP-sensitive protein kinase
cGMP-PK = cGMP-sensitive protein kinase
cAMP-PDIE = cAMP phosphodiesterase
cGMP-PDIE = cGMP phosphodiesterase
cAMP-BP = cAMP binding proteins other than cAMP-PK
cGMP-BP = cGMP binding proteins other than cGMP-PK
AdC = adenylate cyclase
C = coupling mechanism of AdC
GnC = guanylate cyclase
Ca^{2+} = calcium
GTP = guanosine 5′-triphosphate
ATP = adenosine 5′-triphosphate
5′AMP = adenosine 5′-monophosphate (noncyclic)
5′GMP = guanosine 5′-monophosphate (noncyclic)
Functional = encompass all cellular changes regulated via cNMP systems under normal or
Responses   pathologic situations, related to cell membrane or to other endocellular structures.

Methodologies for studies on cNMP in kidney

Basic methodological approaches to study the dynamics of cAMP in kidney has been recently reviewed (Murad, 1973; Broadus, 1977; Dousa, 1976) and the principles of studies on cGMP do not differ basically from those employed for other tissues (Goldberg and Haddox, 1977). We will mention only several methods developed recently for studies of cNMP in renal tissue. Employing improved sensitivity of the AdC assay, Morel and associates developed a technique for the measurement of AdC activity in isolated, individual microdissected segments of nephrons (Morel, Chabardes, Imbert, 1975; Morel, Chabardes, and Imbert-Teboul, 1978b). With use of this technique, they found a number of major specific locations of hormone-sensitive AdC in glomeruli (Imbert, Chabardes, and Morel, 1974) and in the tubular system (Morel, Chabardes, and Imbert, 1975; Morel, Imbert, and Chabardes, 1976), some previously unsuspected. Similar approaches could be extended to GnC and other components of cNMP metabolism in the kidney (Edwards, Jackson and Dousa, 1979; Jackson, Edwards and Dousa, 1978).

Increased sensitivity of the radioimmunoassay (Steiner, Parker, and Kipnis, 1972) by preacylation of samples (Harper and Brooker, 1975; Frandsen and Krishna, 1976) allows one to measure cNMP content in small tissue samples such as isolated glomeruli or tubules (Torres et al., 1978) and, could be applied to various isolated nephron components, including measurements of cAMP level in isolated segments of tubules (Edwards, R. M., Jackson, B. A. and Dousa, T. P.; unpublished results). Heterogeneity of the kidney as an organ warrants analysis of cNMP dynamics in specific functional and structural units of the nephron. While studies done on the whole kidney (or preparations of major anatomic zones such as cortex, medulla, and papilla) are of value to detect the presence and directionality of changes in cNMP systems elicited by hormones, or occurring in different pathological states, such information can only be cautiously interpreted in relation to a specific nephron function or functions.

In many studies, unfractionated total renal tissue (or renal zones) are used as starting material to isolate subcellular components of renal cells such as specific plasma membranes (e.g., luminal brush border of proximal tubules), specific soluble proteins (such as protein kinases or tubulin). It should be realized, that if the whole kidney (or tissue from gross kidney zones) is employed as starting material, the final preparation could easily contain admixtures coming from different cell populations. For example, cAMP-PDIE in preparations from whole kidney is stimulated by the addition of cGMP (Van Inwegen et al., 1977). However, if the renal cortical tissue is separated into tubuli and glomeruli, only cAMP-PDIE in glomeruli, and not that from tubules, is subject to the stimulatory effect of cGMP (Torres et al., 1978a). Vasopressin (VP)-sensitive AdC found in the renal medulla and papilla was for a long time assumed to be derived only from collecting ducts. Imbert et al. (1975) and Imbert-Teboul et al. (1978) have recently shown that VP-sensitive AdC is in many species also present in the ascending limbs of Henle's loop (ALH)—also contained in renal medullary tissue. Likewise, VP causes activation of cAMP-PK in both segments (Edwards, Jackson, and Dousa, 1979). While the exact role of a VP-sensitive cAMP system in Henle's loop is not yet defined, studies dealing with VP effects on whole renal medulla or papilla can no longer be related simply to collecting tubules and ducts.

Immunohistochemical techniques, developed by Steiner, Ong, and Wedner (1976), could be applied on the kidney (Dousa et al., 1977) to approach the question of intracellular localization of cNMP. Similar immunocytochemical analysis could be extended to localize within the single cell protein kinase (or its subunits) and tubulin (Earp and Steiner, 1978). Immunocytochemical methods in conjunction with electronmicroscopy are expected to add further finesse to this technique (Steiner, et al., 1976). Another promising approach to study the homogeneous cell populations of mammalian kidney appears to be investigations of hormone-responsive kidney cells grown in tissue culture (Ishizuka et al., 1978; Goldring et al., 1978).

The use of exogenous cNMP and/or cNMP analogues to mimic the effects of endogenous cNMP poses a special problem in kidney—again mostly because of heterogeneity (Dousa, 1976). When infused into the systemic circulation, cNMP and/or analogs can trigger a cascade of extrarenal responses that obscure changes observed in the kidney. Even if infused into one renal artery, cNMP may act indiscriminately and simultaneously on renal vasculature, glomeruli, and various tubular segments equipped with different specific hormone-regulated and cNMP-mediated functions. Thus, while some tentative conclusions may be drawn from experiments using infusions of cNMP or analogs—mostly in relation to responses of the proximal nephron (glomerulus, early proximal tubule)—the effects of infused cNMP for more distal segments is very difficult, or perhaps impossible, to interpret. On the other hand, in isolated renal structures (isolated perfused tubules), exogenous cNMP or analogs could duplicate hormonal effects quite well (Strewler and Orloff, 1977; Hall, Barnes, and Dousa, 1977; Hall, 1979).

The use of synthetic cNMP analogs poses the question, whether these derivatives have exactly the same effect as natural cNMP, as assumed. Diacylated analogs of cNMP, such as N^6-O^2-dibutyrated cAMP or cGMP (dibutyryl cAMP, dibutyryl cGMP) should first be converted to active metabolites (N^6-monobutyryl derivatives) or natural cNMP (Dousa, 1976; Boumendil-Podevin and Podevin, 1977; Hall et al., 1977) prior to exerting the desired effect. Analogs of cNMP could have a number of other effects, such as the inhibition of cNMP-PDIE, metabolic effects due to the split-off of fatty acid residues, and so on. Other types of analogs, such as those substituted at C-8 carbon of the adenine or guanine moiety of cAMP or cGMP respectively, seem to have a distinct advantage over butyrated ones (Hall et al., 1977). Not all 8-substituted cNMP analogs need to be equally effective; the most potent derivative so far known is 8-[p-chlorophenylthio]-cyclic AMP (Hall et al., 1977; Stadel and Goodman, 1978). However, caution should be exercised in assuming that 8-substituted analogs duplicate all the effects of natural cNMP, as in the case of VP (Hall et al., 1977). For example, 8-[p-chlorophenylthio]-cyclic GMP or dibutyryl cGMP do not duplicate the stimulatory effect of natural cGMP on cAMP-PDIE in kidney cortex (Torres et al., 1978a).

In assessment of cNMP dynamics in vivo (with the exception of studies on renal biopsy samples, which could rarely be justified in human studies), a major volume of information is obtained by measurements of extracellular parameters, urinary excretion, and plasma levels of cNMP. Since cNMP appear in the urine in high quantity and can easily be measured without extensive purification (Murad, 1973), many shortcut conclusions on cNMP dynamics in the kidney have been made in the past from simple measurements of total cNMP excretion per unit of time. As discussed in a recent review (Broadus, 1977) the exact measurements of renal cAMP dynamics should be parametric and involve simultaneous determinations of cAMP clearance and glomerular filtration rate (GFR); the cAMP excretion should be expressed in relation to GFR because filtered cAMP is, at least in humans, a major extrarenal component of total urinary cAMP (Broadus, 1977). The most precise parameter to measure involves calculation of urinary nephrogenous cAMP excretion,[*] but it appears that, as a minimum, urinary cAMP excretion should be expressed as a function of GFR (Broadus, 1977). Such measurements (without determining plasma cAMP) are especially helpful for clinical studies (Broadus, et al. 1977) or in experiments on small laboratory animals when multiple sampling for plasma cAMP may require prohibitively high amounts of blood. Some other factors should be also taken into consideration for renal cNMP dynamics. It appears that cAMP can be reabsorbed by tubules (Dousa, 1976; Butlen and Jard, 1972; Czekalski, et al. 1974) and that the rate of tubular reabsorption may depend on the pH of tubular fluid (Czekalski et al., 1974), since cAMP behaves, in terms of tubular transport, as a weak organic acid. The rate of urine flow does not appear to be a factor (Broadus, 1977) in cAMP excretion; extracellular volume expansion has been reported to increase N-cAMP (Friedler, et al., 1977). The criteria for judicious and meaningful uses of urinary cNMP excretion measurements in human studies are summarized in detail in a recent excellent review (Broadus, 1977).

In animal studies, the factor of species difference should be kept in mind. For example, human, dog, rat, and rabbit kidney cortex all contain a renal cAMP system sensitive to PTH in vitro (detectable by in vitro activation of AdC and tissue accumulation of cAMP). On the other hand, while human (Murad, 1973; Broadus, 1977) or rat kidney (Knox et al., 1978; Aurbach et al., 1972) responds readily to PTH administration with rise in N-cAMP, in rabbit

---

[*] Nephrogenous cNMP are by definition cNMP generated in kidney cells. Since a part of cNMP is released not only to tubular urine, but also to renal venous blood (Blonde, Wehmann, and Steiner, 1974; Friedler et al., 1977), total nephrogenous cNMP includes venous nephrogenous cNMP and urinary nephrogenous cNMP. However, for practical purposes, by "nephrogenous cNMP" is meant the urinary component. Nephrogenous cNMP is abbreviated here N-cNMP, and unless specified otherwise, it denotes urinary nephrogenous cNMP.

(Berndt et al., 1978) or dog (Davis et al., 1969; Blonde et al., 1974; Knox and Dousa, unpublished observations) no changes in N-cAMP occur or are barely detectable even after high doses of PTH.

An approach not yet widely employed is measurement of N-cAMP in venous outflow blood (Friedler et al., 1977; Nakajima, Niatoh, and Kuruma, 1977); this may be suitable for testing the renal effects of those agents which increase renal tissue cAMP but which do not cause cAMP to efflux into the tubule lumen and consequently to appear in urine. For example, while VP does not increase consistently urinary N-cAMP (Dousa and Barnes, 1977a; Murad, 1973; Broadus, 1977; Dousa, 1976), VP could lead to a marked increase in N-cAMP in renal vein outflow (Nakajima et al., 1977); this may offer a way to assess the renal response to VP whenever renal vein catheterization is feasible.

Much less is known about renal dynamics of extracellular cGMP (Murad, 1973; Broadus, 1977), but it appears that as in the case of cAMP similar, if not greater, caution (Broadus, 1977) should be exercised in the planning and interpretation of in vivo experiments.

Diversity of cNMP dynamics in kidney

Many observations on renal cNMP dynamics have been made on whole kidney in vivo or on in vitro preparations from whole kidney. Because the kidney is extremely diversified both morphologically and functionally, it is not surprising that cAMP and cGMP content and metabolism also differ in various structural and functional units and subunits of the nephron.

The most striking diversity in cNMP dynamics relates to the responsiveness to hormones, as summarized in the following section of this review. However, even the basal properties of the elements of cNMP dynamics are different in different parts of the kidney and are also different from one mammalian species to another.

The basal activities of AdC, GnC, and cAMP-PDIE or cGMP-PDIE are different in the three major anatomical zones: cortex, medulla, and papilla (Craven and DeRubertis, 1976; Wald, Gutman, and Czaczkes, 1977; Jackson, Northrup, and Dousa, 1978). Major differences exist even between different segments of the nephron. For example, within renal cortex, GnC (Helwig et al., 1975) and cGMP content (Torres et al., 1978b) as well as cGMP-PDIE (Torres et al., 1978b) were found to be much higher in glomeruli than in cortical tubules. Likewise, the basal activity of AdC differs substantially between different segments of the tubular system in cortex and medulla (Morel, Chabardes, and Imbert, 1975; Morel, Imbert, and Chabardes, 1976; Imbert et al., 1975). Immunohistochemical techniques (Steiner et al., 1976) suggest differential distribution of cAMP and cGMP within nephron units in cortex such as in glomeruli and tubules, and initial results also suggest specific localization of cNMP within single renal cell types (Dousa et al., 1977b).

Major species differences exist at least in some aspects of cNMP metabolism in kidneys of various mammals frequently used as experimental models; these relate both to basic enzyme properties, to tissue cNMP levels as well as to hormonal stimulation. Such differences are detected even when studied with the use of exactly the same techniques. For example, although the highest specific activity of renal cortical GnC in rat is in the cytoplasmic fraction (Craven and DeRubertis, 1976; Kim et al., 1977a; Criss, Murad, and Kimura, 1976), in human renal cortex most of the GnC activity is membrane-bound (Kim et al., 1977a). In rat, dog, and rabbit kidney, VP markedly stimulates AdC in outer medulla; on the other hand, while in the renal papilla of rat and dog the stimulation of AdC by VP is striking, in rabbit papilla it is almost non-existent (Jackson et al., 1978). In papillary sections of the kidney, PTH has no effect on AdC in rabbit, but it stimulates AdC in rat and actually inhibits AdC in dog (Jackson et al., 1979a). Prominent species differences in AdC were found in studies on individual nephron segments (Morel, Chabardes, and Imbert-Teboul, 1978a). The abovementioned species and hormone responsiveness diversity is encountered also in dynamics of N-cNMP, as mentioned in the preceding section. Caution should thus be exercised in the extrapolation of findings from one experimental model to another and to human kidney.

Effect of hormones on cNMP in kidney

Numerous hormones, which play a role in renal physiology and pathology, affect in one way or another cNMP dynamics, and it is therefore assumed that cNMP are involved in the cellular action of these agents. In considering whether the action of a given hormonal stimulus is mediated by cNMP, it is helpful to consider the time-honored criteria (perhaps broadened and modified) set forth originally by Sutherland and associates (Robison, Butcher, and Sutherland, 1971). Briefly, based on these criteria, which are discussed in detail elsewhere (Dousa, 1976; Robison et al., 1971), the hormonal stimulus in question (1) should increase (or decrease) the rate of cNMP generation or cNMP tissue levels. In case of AdC, it (2) should activate (or inhibit) this enzyme in a cell-free system. Such change in cNMP (3) should precede or be concomitant in time with the hormone-elicited functional event. The hormonal effects involving cNMP mediation (4) should be duplicated by exogenous cNMP (or their active chemical analogues), and the hormonal response (5) should be potentiated by cNMP-PDIE inhibitors.

In reviewing all hormones and agents that have so far been reported to influence renal cNMP, it should be realized that the depth of evidence for their involvement in hormone action differs vastly, ranging from instances where all the abovementioned criteria have been fulfilled and documented independently, up to the isolated preliminary reports exploring only one of the abovementioned criteria. To recount briefly the present information about the hormones acting on kidney via cNMP, a summary is provided in Table 10.1. Specific reviews dealing with individual hormones or group of hormones can also be found in several recent periodicals and books (Dousa and Barnes, 1977a; Murad, 1973; Broadus, 1977; Dousa, 1976; Strewler and Orloff, 1977;

Table 10.1 Hormones acting on cyclic nucleotides in the kidney

	Action				Localization		
	change in tissue level of		adenylate cyclase	inhibited by specific antagonists	in major renal zones		
Hormone	cAMP	cGMP			Cortex	Medulla	Papilla
Parathyroid hormone (and analogs)	↑↑↑	↑(?)	↑↑↑	+	+++	+	+?
Calcitonin	↑↑		↑↑		+	++	⊖
Glucagon	↑	⊖	↑			++	
Vasopressin (and analogs)	↑↑↑	⊖	↑↑↑		+	++	+++
Angiotensin-II	↓	⊖			+		
Bradykinin	⊖	↑			+	+	+
Insulin	↓				+		
Somatostatin	↓				+		
β-adrenergic agonists	↑		↑	+	+	+	+
α-adrenergic agonists	↓				+(?)	+(?)	
Dopamine	↑		↑		+(?)		
Histamine	↑↑↑	↑		+	+		+
Cholinergic agents	⊖	↑↑↑		+	+	+	+
Serotonin	↑↑↑	⊖		+	+	⊖	⊖
Prostaglandins	↑		↑		+	+	+
Thyroid hormones	↑		↑		+	+	
Glucocorticoids	↓		↑			+	+
Aldosterone			↑(?)			+	+
Vitamin-D	↑		↑		+		

Legend: Summary of known effects of hormones on cyclic nucleotides in the kidney. ↑ denotes increase or activation; ↓ denotes decrease or inhibition; O denotes no effect found. Without symbols denotes no data available. Relative magnitude of hormonal response is approximated by + to ++++.

Dousa and Valtin, 1976; Knox et al., 1978; Morel et al., 1975; Aurbach et al., 1972; Aurbach and Heath, 1974; Dousa et al. 1980). The table will likely be outdated by the time it is published since progress in this field is so rapid.

DYNAMICS OF cNMP IN DISEASE

Endocrinopathies and kidney

Virtually all disorders of the endocrine regulation of kidney function fall into the category of either hyporesponsiveness or hyperresponsiveness to a given hormone; the former category is much more frequent. It is now recognized that the responsiveness of target tissue is frequently determined by the

Major localization in nephron

Glomeruli	Tubules	Comments	
+	++++ (Pt,ℓH,Dt)	Major species differences	↑ urinary and venous NcAMP
	+++ (Pt,ℓH,Dt)	Major species differences	↑ urinary NcAMP
	++	Species differences	
±?	++++(ℓH,Dt,Cd)	Species differences	May increase venous NcAMP
++	++		
+		May inhibit action of PTH	
		May inhibit action of PTH	
+	++ (Dt)		
		Inhibits action of VP?	
0			May increase venous NcAMP
++++	+	Acts on H_2 receptors	
++	+	Dependent on Ca^{2+}, acts on muscarinic receptor	May increase urinary NcAMP
++++	+		
+	++	Also reported to antagonize cAMP increases by other hormones; mainly prostaglandins E are effective	
+		Effect is likely indirect; direct inhibition of cAMP-PDIE	
		Effect probably indirect, reported to lower cAMP levels elevated by hormones	
		Reported to inhibit cAMP-PDIE; potentiate ↑ cAMP by VP	
		Effect perhaps indirect	

Abbreviations of tubular segments: (Pt) proximal tubule; (ℓH) loop of Henle; (Dt) distal convoluted tubule; (Cd) collecting ducts (and also collecting tubules).

previous exposure to hormones (Bradshaw and Frazier, 1977; Kahn, 1976). In general, sustained low levels of hormones lead to an increased tissue sensitivity to the same hormone (Bradshaw and Frazier, 1977; Kahn, 1976), while previous exposure to consistently high plasma levels of hormones causes diminution of responsiveness. The molecular basis of this desensitization or sensitization is not yet established, but it appears to be specific for a given hormone (Kahn, 1976) and has been described for a number of hormones including those acting on the kidney (Sraer, Ardaillou, and Couette, 1974; Rajerison et al., 1977; Tomlinson et al., 1976). It should also be realized that besides the abovementioned sensitization or desensitization by previous exposure to the hormone (Sraer, Ardaillou, and Couette, 1974; Rajerison et al., 1977; Tomlinson et al., 1976), functional consequences of hormone action, such as changes in calcium levels (e.g., hypercalcemia owing to PTH action on bone and gut) or changes in acid-base balance (e.g., acidosis) induced by a hormone, may consequently influence the sensitivity of renal tissue to the same hormone.

Parathyroid hormone (PTH)

Major renal actions of PTH (Raisz et al., 1977; Aurbach and Heath, 1974) include hypocalciuria, phosphaturia, 1-α hydroxylation of 25-OH vitamin D$_3$ to final 1,25-dihydroxyvitamin D^3 (Raisz et al., 1977; Horiuchi et al., 1977), inhibition of isotonic fluid reabsorption in the proximal tubule (Knox, et al., 1978), and also changes in glomerular dynamics (Ichikawa et al., 1978). Although some evidence exists that all of the abovementioned actions may be mediated by cAMP, only in the case of proximal isotonic fluid reabsorption and of the phosphaturic effect, the evidence for a mediatory role of cAMP is close to substantive (Knox et al., 1978; Aurbach and Heath, 1974).

One favorable feature of human kidney is that it responds to small doses in PTH by marked changes in the urinary excretion of N-cAMP (Broadus, 1977); this feature was successfully employed for detecting the renal response to PTH in a number of clinical situations (Broadus, Deftos and Bartter, 1978), namely, in the differential diagnosis of hypercalcemic syndromes (Broadus, 1977; Shaw, 1977; Broadus et al., 1977).

Anomalous functional responses of the kidney to PTH have been monitored so far mostly as an increase in the fractional excretion of phosphate, a phosphaturic response to PTH. One of the first-recognized, and to date most extensively studied, disease involving renal responsiveness to PTH is pseudohypoparathyroidism (PHP), a pleiotropic genetic syndrome of variable expression, in which the kidney does not respond to PTH by phosphaturia (Chase, Melson, and Aurbach, 1969) and in which also the generation of 1,25-dihydroxyvitamin D$_3$ is sometimes (Metz et al., 1977; Sinha, DeLuca, and Bell, 1977), but perhaps not always (Drezner and Haussler, 1978), defective. When Chase and Aurbach first discovered that the PHP kidney responds to high doses of exogenous PTH by no or miniscule increases in urinary cAMP (Chase et al., 1969), a pathogenetic anomaly in the regulatory role of cAMP was immediately suspected. However, to date, the specific point of defect in the renal PTH-dependent cAMP system has not yet been identified, although the most straightforward explanation would be a defective PTH-dependent formation of cAMP in kidney tubules. Since levels of circulating PTH are high in PHP, receptor desensitization by PTH should be considered (Kahn, 1976; Tomlinson et al. 1976), but this mechanism seems unlikely since, in primary hyperparathyroidism with high circulating PTH, the response to exogenous PTH (in terms of N-cAMP increase) is not defective (Chase et al., 1969). While vitamin D deficiency (Forte, Nickols, and Anast, 1976) and/or accompanying hypocalcemia (Carnes, Anast, and Forte, 1978; Kakuta et al., 1978) could decrease responsiveness of renal cortical AdC to PTH, normalization of Ca and vitamin D supplements in PHP do not restore the urinary response in terms of N-cAMP (Chase et al., 1969; Murad, 1973). Finally, in two cases where AdC from kidneys of PHP patients was directly assayed in vitro, in one case, no anomalous response to PTH was detected (Marcus, Wilber, and Aurbach, 1971), and in the other, only a partial decrease of AdC responsiveness to PTH was observed at lower ATP substrate level (Drezner and Burch, 1978), suggesting decreased affinity of AdC for ATP (Drezner and Burch, 1978). While it thus seems unlikely that PHP is due to a complete absence of PTH receptors or PTH-sensitive AdC, many observations still point to a possible insufficiency in renal PTH-dependent cAMP formation. Absence of normal increases in N-cAMP after PTH could also, in principle, be due to defects in the cAMP efflux into tubule lumen. However, such a defect of luminal tubular plasma membranes without defective cAMP formation could hardly explain the findings that PHP patients also do not increase plasma cAMP in response to PTH (Murad, 1973). Reports that functional impairments (lack of phosphaturia) can be improved by the administration of drugs with a capacity to inhibit cAMP-PDIE also raises the possibility that the deficient cAMP accumulation in cells may be due not only to decreased cAMP formation but also to accelerated cAMP degradation (Murad, 1973). Observations that infusions of the cAMP analogs (DB-cAMP) induce phosphaturic responses in PHP patients seem to favor the view that steps in the cellular action of PTH subsequent to cAMP formation may not be impaired (Bell et al., 1972). Thus, on balance, it appears that in PHP the defective formation of cAMP in response to PTH is responsible for, or associated with, the functional unresponsiveness of kidney. The point of cAMP dynamics at which the defect lies remains to be elucidated.

The problem is further compounded by the discovery of a PHP variant in which N-cAMP increases in response to PTH normally but in which the renal functional response (in terms of phosphaturia) is absent. In this type of PHP (operationally called pseudohypoparathyroidism type-II [PHP-II] as distinguished from the abovementioned classic form called PHP type-I), a defect in steps distal to PTH-dependent renal cAMP generation seems likely (Drezner et al., 1973; Rodriguez et al., 1974).

Regardless of the molecular mechanisms involved, the absence of N-cAMP elevation after PTH in PHP (PHP type-I) as originally described (Chase et al., 1969) has proven to be a most sensitive diagnostic test to discriminate clinically this entity from X-linked hypophosphatemia (Glorieux and Scriver, 1972), pseudo-pseudohypoparathyroidism, PHP type-II, Gardner syndrome (Aurbach et al., 1970), and other syndromes all characterized by a defect in the renal phosphaturic response to PTH (Aurbach et al., 1970).

So far, no satisfactory animal model of PHP has been found. It is interesting to note that a functional constellation of PTH unresponsiveness resembling PHP type-I is encountered in the rabbit. Its kidney does not respond to exogenous PTH by increased phosphaturia or N-cAMP (Berndt et al., 1978), but rabbit cortex contains AdC sensitive to PTH in vitro (Berndt et al., 1978; Jackson et al., 1978). And the administration of acetazolamide uncovered a phosphaturic response to PTH without increasing N-cAMP (Berndt et al., 1978), as was reported in humans (Baran et al., 1978). The major functional features of

PHP type-II—lack of phosphaturic response to PTH but normal increase in N-cAMP—have been observed under certain experimental circumstances in hamster (Knox et al., 1977) or in organisms deprived of dietary phosphorus (Steele, 1976; Beck, 1976) or dietary magnesium (Hahn, Chase, and Avioli, 1972; Chase and Slatopolsky, 1974).

In a number of experimental situations, partially decreased functional responsiveness to PTH, associated with diminished cAMP generation, was reported both in hypercalcemia (Beck et al., 1974) and in calcium depletion (Carnes, et al., 1978; Kakuta, et al., 1978), in hypermagnesemia (Slatopolsky et al., 1976) in metabolic acidosis (Beck, Mim, and Kim, 1975), and in potassium depletion (Beck and Davis, 1975b).

Finally, it has been reported recently that high doses of PTH decrease GFR at least in a certain subpopulation (superficial cortical) of nephrons (Humes et al., 1978; Ichikawa et al., 1978). PTH stimulates glomerular AdC (Imbert, Chabardes, and Morel, 1974; Schlondorff, Yoo, and Alpert, 1978; Sraer et al., 1974b; Edwards et al., 1978) and increases cAMP and, to a lesser degree cGMP (Dousa et al., 1977b; Torres et al., 1978b), in glomeruli. It should thus be considered that the glomerular effects of PTH may be mediated by cNMP.

It should be recalled that these experimental models may not be caused by a simple, isolated abnormality of one factor (hormone) and that concomitant, sometimes secondary, pathophysiologic changes may potentially contribute to the overall picture of defective responsiveness to PTH. For example, disorders of potassium metabolism can cause anomalous renal acidification; adaptation to a low phosphorous diet is attended by large urinary losses of Mg^{2+} and Ca^{2+}. It is difficult to relate, at the present time, these observations on animal models directly to the interpretation of pathogenesis of the clinical disorders.

Calcitonin (CT)

The physiologic role of CT in the kidney is presently uncertain; some renal effects of pharmacological high doses of CT, such as phosphaturia, are similar to PTH and are associated with increased cAMP formation in renal cortex and increased N-cAMP (Aurbach and Heath, 1974; Knox et al., 1978). On the other hand, CT does not have a hypocalciuric effect, or an effect on renal vitamin D 1-α-hydroxylation as does PTH (Knox et al., 1978). In certain experimental conditions (e.g., in hamster; Knox et al., 1977) and also in the renal adaptation to low phosphorous intake (Kurokawa et al., 1977), the kidney responds to CT with increased cAMP formation and accumulation but without a phosphaturic effect, analogous to the dissociation of N-cAMP increase and phosphaturia in response to PTH. Of potential interest is a recent report that, in mice with a syndrome resembling X-linked hypophosphatemic rickets, AdC in certain segments of the distal nephron is hyperresponsive to CT (Brunette et al., 1977).

Vitamin D (Vit-D)

Although many studies indicate that vit-D diminishes phosphate execretion, in some observations the infusion of vit-D is, on the contrary, phosphaturic

(Bonjour, Preston, and Fleisch, 1977). The exact physiologic effect of vit-D on renal mineral metabolism remains to be defined, and no direct effect of vitamin D on renal cNMP has been reported. In vitamin D-depleted animals, the renal responses to PTH were diminished in terms of increases both in N-cAMP and in fractional excretion of phosphate. Likewise, the stimulation of renal cortical AdC by PTH was found to be decreased. All these changes proved to be reversible by treatment with vit-D (Forte et al., 1976). On the other hand, in vitamin D depletion with osteomalacia, the urinary excretion of cAMP was reported to be increased rather than decreased (Sovik and Apold, 1976; Vainsel, Manderlier, and Otten, 1976). In other series of experiments, in Ca^{2+}-depleted and Vit-D-depleted animals, the hyporesponsiveness of renal cortical cAMP system cannot be corrected by the administration of vit-D without calcium repletion (Carnes et al., 1978; Kakuta et al., 1978). Thus, while vitamin D may be a factor in cNMP-mediated regulations of renal mineral metabolism, its exact role remains to be established.

Vasopressin (VP)

The role of cAMP in the pathogenesis of renal concentrating defects has been considered some years ago (Dousa, 1974b); several recent findings should be taken into account in current discussions about the pathophysiology of the cellular action of VP.

First, it has been found in many species, although to a different degree (Morel et al., 1978a), that a VP-sensitive cAMP system leading to the activation of PK (Edwards, Jackson, and Dousa, 1979) exists not only in collecting tubules and ducts but also in the ascending limb of Henle's loop (ALH) (Morel, Imbert, and Chabardes, 1976; Imbert-Teboul et al., 1978). VP-sensitive cAMP system in ALH may well be associated, in one way or another, with renal concentrating mechanisms. Direct evidence that VP influences, *via* cAMP the function of both ALH and collecting tubule was provided recently by studies showing that VP and cAMP analogue increases the lumen—positive membrane potential difference across ALH (Hall, 1979). This finding strongly suggests that VP acts on the collecting tubule to increase water permeability and, independently, it also acts on ALH to stimulate solute transport from the lumen to peritubular fluid; in both tubular segments VP stimulates cAMP formation and also increases PK activity (Edwards, Jackson and Dousa, 1979). It has also been reported that VP stimulates the release of arachidonic acid and consequently the formation of prostaglandins (PG) or PG-like compounds in cells of renal medulla (Zusman and Keiser, 1977) as well as in toad bladder (Zusman, Keiser, and Handler, 1977b). These VP effects on PG metabolism seem to be independent of cAMP generation (Zusman et al., 1977b). Thus, it should be kept in mind that in renal medullary tissue VP acts not only to activate AdC-cAMP systems in collecting ducts and in ALH but also to stimulate the formation of PG compounds from arachidonic acid. In amphibian bladder, the inhibitory effect of prostaglandins type E on the hydroosmotic action of VP can be readily demonstrated (Handler and Orloff, 1973); in mammalian kidney has been directly detected only in initial observations on perfused collecting tubules (Grantham and Orloff, 1968). Otherwise, evidence for such PG action in kidney is based almost solely on indirect data showing that the administration of PG synthesis inhibitors potentiate the VP action (Anderson et al., 1976; Dousa and Northrup, 1978). It is of interest that PG synthesis inhibitor ibuprofen potentiates AdC stimulation by VP in collecting tubule but inhibits AdC stimulation in ALH (Jackson, Edwards and Dousa, 1979c). These drugs, which have multiple effects, were recently reported to be antidiuretic, even in animals lacking endogenous VP (e.g., in rats with cerebral diabetes insipidus* [CDI]; Stoff et al., 1978).

In light of these new findings, some previous observations might warrant reconsideration, and in the design and interpretation of future studies, the above-mentioned factors should be taken into account.

Anomalous responsiveness to VP—nephrogenic diabetes insipidus (NDI)

From clinical observations of NDI in humans, it has not yet been possible to deduce whether the impairment of VP-sensitive cAMP systems may be involved and at which point, since the antidiuretic response to VP is not accompanied by consistent increases in urinary N-cAMP (Broadus, 1977). The small increases that have been reported may be due to PTH released in response to VP infusion (Humes, Simmons, and Brenner, 1978). Infusion of cAMP or analogs, either intravenously or in the renal artery, has not yet resulted in clear-cut antidiuretic responses commensurate to that of VP (Dousa and Valtin, 1976; Dousa, 1974b). Thus far, information on the pathogenesis of NDI is based on observations in experimental animals.

The animal model that seems to resemble most closely the human hereditary NDI is the hereditary urinary concentrating defect in mice (Valtin, Sokol, and Sunde, 1975). In this NDI strain of mice a lower response of AdC from renal medulla and papilla to VP, which is proportional to the degree of functional impairment, has been found (Dousa and Valtin, 1974); it seems that this hyporesponsiveness of AdC did not prevent VP-stimulated cAMP accumulation and protein kinase activation in intact renal medullary slices (Kim et al., 1977b). However, recent studies on isolated tubules revealed that AdC in medullary ascending limb of Henle's loop is stimulated by VP to a much lesser degree in NDI mice than in controls (Edwards, Jackson, and Dousa, 1979a). In addition, VP failed to increase cAMP levels in microdissected medullary collecting tubules of NDI mice in the absence of cAMP-PDIE inhibitor (Edwards, Jackson, Valtin, and Dousa, unpublished results).

The lithium (Li)-induced polyuric syndrome is in part due to a renal resistance to VP (Singer and Forrest, 1976). The most prominent finding related to

---

* The term "cerebral diabetes insipidus" (CDI) denotes a syndrome caused by lack of the circulating ADH, regardless of whether the primary impairment is in a synthesis and/or a release in relevant cerebral structures (hypothalamus, hypophysis). The term "nephrogenic diabetes insipidus" (NDI) denotes the state of renal unresponsiveness to either endogenous or exogenous VP.

Li-induced NDI seems to be an inhibitory effect of Li on VP-sensitive renal medullary AdC. Other observed effects of Li, such as stimulation of cAMP-PDIE (Beck and Davis, 1975a), inhibition of PK (Dousa, 1974a), or microtubule polymerization (Dousa, Hui, and Barnes, 1978), which were found in various experiments, all seem quantitatively minor, although they could contribute to the overall impairment of VP-sensitive cAMP system. Overproduction of PG in this syndrome has also been invoked recently as a possible pathogenic factor (Rutecki et al., 1977).

It appears that NDI induced by demethylchlortetracycline (Declomycin) could be due both to an inhibition of VP-sensitive cAMP formation and to cAMP action in subsequent steps (Singer and Forrest, 1976). An observation from the toad bladder system suggests that the anti-VP effects of some tetracyclines may be related to their ability to bind to cellular proteins (Feldman and Singer, 1974). The usefulness of Declomycin in the treatment of water intoxication caused by inappropriately high VP levels has been observed on several occasions (de Troyer and Demanet, 1975; Singer and Forrest, 1976).

Studies on NDI occurring in K^+ deficiency yielded somehow conflicting results (Dousa, 1974b). Deficient cAMP accumulation in response to VP, low AdC activity (Beck and Webster, 1976), and/or high cAMP-PDIE (Beck, Reed, and Davis, 1973) have all been implicated in the pathogenesis of NDI, sometimes no cAMP abnormality in cAMP system in K^+ depletion (Pawlson et al., 1970) was found. A recent observation suggests indirectly that enhanced renal PG synthesis may play a role: In K^+ depletion the renal synthesis of PG was reported to be increased and treatment with PG synthesis inhibitors improved the urinary concentrating capacity as well as inhibited PG synthesis (Galvez et al., 1976). It should be recalled that in K^+-depleted urinary bladders, the hydroosmotic response to both VP and exogenous cAMP was abolished, suggesting the possibility of a defect in steps subsequent to cAMP generation (Finn, Handler, and Orloff, 1966).

The pathogenesis of NDI in hypercalcemia (Dousa, 1974b) has not been much further elucidated. Conceivably calcium can inhibit VP-dependent cAMP formation and accumulation, activate cAMP-PDIE, interfere with microtubule integrity, etc. (Dousa, 1974b). The pathogenesis may be multifactorial, and conclusions from current studies should thus be guarded.

The role of VP-PG antagonism in the pathogenesis of renal concentrating abnormalities, if applicable to mammalian kidney, may offer a possible explanation of the well-known effect of chloropropamide (and similarly acting sulphonylureas) to potentiate the effects of small antidiuretic doses of VP. Studies on amphibian bladder support the possibility (Zusman et al., 1977a) that chloropropamide acts by diminishing PG synthesis and, thus, potentiating the antidiuretic effects of small VP doses.

NDI also develops after chronic fluoride administration (Wallin and Kaplan, 1977); a preliminary report suggests that anomalously low cAMP levels in renal medulla can be due to a deficient amount of ATP substrate (Wallin et al., 1978).

Concentrating defect in cerebral diabetes insipidus (CDI)

Clinical and laboratory observations show that in long-standing CDI the kidney is hyporesponsive to exogenous VP. In homozygotes of the Brattleboro strain of rats, an animal model probably closest to human hereditary CDI (Valtin et al., 1975), the activity of VP-sensitive AdC in renal medulla was found to be diminished (Rajerison et al., 1977; Dousa, Hui, and Barnes, 1975); this AdC activity could be increased and the concentrating defect corrected after a course of treatment with exogenous VP. According to a recent preliminary report, the lower VP-sensitive AdC activity is found only in the ascending limb of Henle's loop, while in the collecting ducts, the VP-sensitive AdC is not different from control animals (Imbert-Teboul, et al. 1978b). This finding, if validated, would not only further elucidate cellular defects in CDI but also suggest a role for VP-sensitive AdC in the loop of Henle in the overall regulation of urine concentration.

Disorders of thyroid and adrenals

Abnormalities of the renal handling of water and electrolytes in thyroid disorders are complex, and probably several simultaneous changes in different segments of nephrons may cause the anomalous excretion of water, especially in hypothyroidism (Bradley et al., 1974). In hypothyroid rats the activity of VP-stimulated AdC was found to be decreased and cAMP-PDIE increased (Harkcom et al., 1978). Low renal medullary cAMP levels in hypothyroid rats (Zenser et al., 1978) and a lower degree of cAMP-PK activation by VP was observed (Harkcom et al., 1978); even in the presence of high levels of circulating VP, hypothyroid rats had a subnormal concentrating ability (Seif et al., 1977). Thyroxin added in vitro did not influence renal medullary AdC. Enzyme changes as well as depressed activation of cAMP-PK could be restored by short-term treatment with thyroxin (Harkcom et al., 1978). In hypothyroid rats, the response of cortical AdC to PTH is diminished, and this decreased PTH response is not restored by short treatment with thyroxin as in the case of renal medulla (Harkcom et al., 1978). These observations suggest that thyroid hormones may have trophic, likely indirect, effects on renal AdC, different in cortex than in medulla. This factor should be taken into account in the interpretation of studies on the regulation of kidney function by VP or PTH, namely, in studies on chronically thyroparathyroidectomized animals that may develop hypothyroidism, or in hypothyroid patients (Ashby, MacPherson, and Strong, 1977). Recent micropuncture findings in hypothyroid rats indicate a specific decreased ability to reabsorb Na and to generate free water in the ALH (Michael et al., 1976). In view of the presence of VP-sensitive AdC in this nephron segment (Imbert-Teboul et al., 1978), a possible association between these two phenomena should be considered.

Deficiency of adrenal steroids in rats has been found to result in decreased stimulation of renal medullary AdC with VP (without changes in basal, NaF-stimulated activity or in PTH-sensitive AdC), probably owing to lower binding and less efficient coupling of VP receptor with AdC (Rajerison it al., 1974). In another study, aldosterone administration to adrenalectomized animals was not found to have an affect on renal adenylate cyclase (Lang and Edelman, 1972). In yet another report, higher levels of cAMP, (basal or those increased in the presence of VP) in renal medullary tubules have been found in glucocorticoid deficiency; this has been interpreted to mean that increased levels of cAMP could contribute to impaired urinary dilution (Kurokawa et al., 1978). On the other hand, in toad bladder, treatment with aldosterone inhibited cAMP-PDIE and potentiated cAMP accumulation in response to VP as well as the hydroosmotic response to VP (Stoff, Handler, and Orloff, 1972); perhaps via inhibition of PG synthesis (Zusman, Keiser, and Handler, 1978). Adrenalectomy did not change cAMP-PDIE activity but the administration of glucocorticoid dexamethasone led to a decrease in cAMP-PDIE activity in ALH and also in medullary collecting tubules (Jackson, Edwards, Heublein, and Dousa, 1979b). It remains to be seen whether or not adrenal steroids play a definite role in cellular VP action in mammalian kidney, and at which site.

cNMP in renal growth and its disorders

The role of cNMP in cell growth and differentiation is one of the most controversial topics dealing with the cellular function of cNMP (Goldberg et al., 1976; Friedman, 1976). Although numerous exceptions have been reported, the prevailing notion is that increased levels of cGMP promote, or are associated with, accelerated cell growth and decreased differentiation; increased cAMP levels are associated with slower cell growth rate and promote cell differentiation. Changes of cellular cGMP and cAMP are frequently simultaneous and reciprocal, and cAMP/cGMP ratios may perhaps serve as a more important regulatory signal for growth than changes in either cAMP or cGMP levels alone (Goldberg et al., 1976).

In relation to normal postnatal renal growth, Schlondorff and Weber (1976) found in rat at an early developmental period that the renal tissue levels of cGMP were higher and decreased with maturation while cAMP levels appeared to be lower and increased with time. Thus, the cAMP/cGMP ratio increases with age. Several reports tend to agree that in early postnatal period the response of renal AdC to VP and PTH is not fully developed and that the responsiveness to these hormones gradually increases in the early adult age, at least in some species of experimental animals (Rajerison, Butlen, and Jard, 1976; Gengler and Forte, 1972; Schlondorff et al., 1978).

cNMP were studied in compensatory renal growth in response to unilateral nephrectomy, a situation reminiscent of hypertrophy of remnant kidney in living kidney transplant donors. Early after unilateral nephrectomy, a rise in cGMP and decrease in cAMP levels has been recorded (Schlondorff and Weber, 1976; Dicker and Greenbaum, 1977); these changes were of short duration. While cGMP-PDIE was not changed, soluble guanylate cyclase paralleled changes in tissue cGMP levels from the whole kidney (Schlondorff and Weber, 1976).

As far as neoplastic renal tissue growth is concerned, somehow paradoxical results have been achieved in experimental animals with transplanted tumors. GnC activity was found to be lower in tumors than in intact control kidney cortex, but the tissue levels of cGMP were reported to be increased (Criss et al., 1976).

Enzymes of cyclic NMP metabolism were explored directly in human renal adenocarcinoma (Kim et al., 1977a; Hunt et al., 1978). The subcellular distribution of GnC was reversed in the human renal tumor with the highest activity of GnC in the soluble fraction, compared to the subcellular distribution of GnC in normal cortex where highest activity is in particulate fractions (Kim et al., 1977a). In human renal adenocarcinoma, cGMP-PDIE tended to be lower than in normal tissue. The abovementioned enzyme changes could favor the increased accumulation of cGMP in the tumor. In one of these studies (Kim et al., 1977), no major differences were found in the basal and nonspecifically stimulated AdC activities between normal cortex and renal adenocarcinoma.

An interesting abnormality found in AdC from renal adenocarcinoma was a complete unresponsiveness to PTH, CT, and VP (Kim et al., 1977). In "clear cell-type" tumors (which are abundant in lipids and glycogen), the response of AdC to glucagon and isoproterenol is absent; in "dark cell-type" tumors (which are rich in mitochondria and without stored lipids or glycogen), AdC had an even higher response to glucagon and isoproterenol than normal cortex. The significance of abnormalities in hormonal responsiveness for tumorogenesis is not clear at the present time, but differential sensitivity to hormones regulating lipolysis and glycolysis could perhaps account for the different metabolic behavior of these two types of renal adenocarcinoma (Kim et al., 1977). In a similar study, conducted under slightly different methodological conditions, basal AdC was found to be higher in tumors than in intact cortex; however, the hormonal responsiveness to PTH and PG was also severely diminished or abolished in tumors (Hunt et al., 1978). In the context of renal tumorogenesis, it is of interest that some carcinogens are potent stimulators of cGMP formation in renal cortex in vitro (DeRubertis and Craven, 1977). Thus, while in general, the directionality of changes seem to favor the concept of high cGMP levels are associated with accelerated growth, conclusions should be guarded at the present time and the role of cNMP in the pathogenesis of renal tumor remains to be established. In some types of experimental renal tumors in rat, high rates of urinary cGMP (but not cAMP) excretion have been observed (Criss and Murad, 1976). This may promise that the measurement of urinary N-cGMP excretion has potential use in clinical diagnosis of renal neoplasia.

Inflammatory and metabolic renal diseases

As summarized in recent reviews, cNMP may be involved in mechanisms of inflammation in several different ways (Melmon and Insel, 1977; Parker, Sullivan, and Wedner, 1974; Kaliner and Austen, 1975; Lichtenstein, 1976). cNMP may be involved in the action of local mediators of inflammation such as histamine, serotonin, PG, and bradykinin. These agents, formed and/or released locally as a result of immune injury, may modulate chemotaxis, lysosomal activity, permeability, and smooth muscle contraction (Melmon and Insel, 1977; Parker et al., 1974; Kaliner and Austen, 1975; Lichtenstein, 1976). Since glomeruli are a primary site of deleterious immunological inflammatory renal injuries, it is of interest that some mediators of inflammation affect markedly cNMP systems in glomeruli (Dousa, Shah and Abboud, 1980). Histamine causes a striking, manifold, dose-dependent increase in glomerular cAMP. This stimulation can be completely blocked by H_2-antagonists but not H_1-antihistaminics; histamine also causes, to a smaller extent, the accumulation of glomerular cGMP (Torres et al., 1978). It is of interest that glomeruli are site of active histamine formation (Abboud, Ou and Dousa, 1979). On the other hand, carbamylcholine (or acetylcholine) causes a marked increase in glomerular cGMP levels via muscarinic receptors, with little or no changes in cAMP (Torres et al., 1978b). Serotonin causes a striking increase of cAMP in glomeruli, with minimal changes in tubules (Shah et al., 1979) but does not influence cGMP. Serotonin effect on glomeruli is dose-dependent and is blocked by serotonin antagonists (Shah et al., 1979). Bradykinin had no noticeable effect of glomerular cNMP, and angiotensin II decreased cAMP but not cGMP (Torres et al., 1978b). In contrast to histamine and serotonin, dopamine and α-adrenergic agent (Abboud, Shah and Dousa, 1979a) did not influence cNMP or levels in glomeruli; β-adrenergic agent isoproterenol only slightly increased cAMP but not cGMP. From PG tested in our laboratory PGE_2, and to lesser extent $PGF_{2\alpha}$, caused a modest increase in cAMP and to a much lesser extent increase of cGMP in glomeruli. These agents had virtually no effects on cNMP in cortical tubules (Abboud, Shah and Dousa, 1979a). AdC from isolated glomeruli was reported to be stimulated by the beta-adrenergic agonist isoproterenol (Imbert et al., 1974; Schlondorff et al., 1977; Sraer et al., 1974), lipopolysaccharides from bacteria (Baud et al., 1977) and by prostaglandins PGE_2, PGE_1, and PGA (Beck and Patak, 1978; Schlondorff et al., 1977). Because the above-mentioned agents can potentially be involved in the modulation of inflammatory changes and/or because, when infused into the kidney, they cause a marked change in glomerular microcirculation (Brenner, Baylis, and Deen, 1976), cNMP-mediated effects of these compounds deserve attention as factors in the pathogenesis of glomerular inflammatory injuries.

It is of interest that the short-term treatment with glucocorticoid dexamethasone diminished significantly the elevation of cAMP in glomeruli elicited by histamine and serotonin as well as the increases in cGMP caused by histamine and carbachol. On the other hand, the response of glomerular cGMP system to non-hormonal stimulating agent sodium nitroprusside was not affected by treatment with dexamethasone (Abboud, Shah and Dousa, 1979c).

Results of the initial investigations on cAMP and cGMP in the experimental models of glomerular diseases revealed alterations of metabolism of these cNMP. In the experimental nephrotic syndrome induced by aminonucleoside of puromycin, the stimulation of cAMP by histamine and by serotonin in glomeruli was severely decreased, and also stimulatory effect of histamine and carbachol on cGMP in glomeruli was almost abolished (Dousa, Shah, and Abboud 1980, Velosa, et al., 1979). The basal levels of cAMP and cGMP in glomeruli were not different between nephrotic and control glomeruli; non-hormonal stimuli such as choleratoxin for cAMP and nitroprusside for cGMP caused elevations of cNMP to a similar extent in normal and nephrotic glomeruli. The elevation of tubular cAMP in a response to PTH did not differ between control tubules and the tubules prepared for the nephrotic kidneys (Dousa, Shah and Abboud, 1980). It is of interest in this context that in glomeruli isolated from kidney cortex of rats with streptozotocin-induced diabetes mellitus, the basal levels as well as the levels of cAMP and cGMP elevated by hormonal agents, were not significantly different from glomeruli prepared from age- and sex-matched control rats (Dousa et al., unpublished results). These observations taken together suggest that alterations in cAMP and cGMP metabolism in some glomerular diseases may play a prominent role in the pathogenesis either as causal or as contributory factors.

The role of cNMP in immune injury to tubules has been recently investigated in rats immunized with antibodies against tubular basement membrane (Loreau et al., 1977). Binding of CT and stimulation of AdC by PTH, CT and NaF, in membrane fractions from renal cortex of immunized rats was substantially diminished and likewise the phosphaturic response to PTH was reduced (Loreau et al., 1977). Although the exact mechanism of this experimental immune injury is not quite clear (in terms of whether or not antibodies are bound both on the tubular basement membrane and on plasma membrane of tubule epithelial cells), these results suggest that immune injury to tubules may be associated both with impaired cAMP systems and tubular function.

Erythropoiesis

The renal erythropoietic system seems to involve a regulatory role of cNMP (Rodgers, Fisher, and George, 1975b); factors that stimulate renal erythropoietic systems, such as lactate, PG, or cobalt, all increase renal cortical tissue cAMP and/or cGMP levels (Rodgers et al., 1975a, 1975b). Implication of such associations for pathological states, including lactic acidosis, renal cortical ischemia, or overdose of PG-synthesis inhibitors is of potential interest (Rodgers et al., 1975b).

Miscellaneous pathological disorders

Several recent reports explore the role of cNMP in renal diseases in which the pathogenesis is very complex and the contribution of various pathogenic factors is particularly difficult to evaluate. In several reports, mostly preliminary, an alteration of cAMP systems in experimental renal insufficiency has been described. According to one report, when an experimental renal insufficiency was induced in rats, the basal activity of AdC was increased and the stimulation by PTH was decreased in the cortex; inner medullary AdC was lower in uremia but stimulation by VP was normal (Weber, Schlondorff, and Trizna, 1976). In another form of uremia in rat, renal medullary AdC and its stimulation by VP were not changed, but extracts from uremic kidney homogenates depressed the response of AdC to VP (Webster and Beck, 1976). In rabbits with experimental renal insufficiency, AdC, in isolated cortical collecting tubules, was stimulated less by VP than in control tubules (Fine et al., 1978), and the hydroosmotic response to exogenous cAMP was lower. A common feature of all the abovementioned observations seems to be that hormone sensitive AdC-cAMP systems are lower in renal insufficiency, but the disparity between uremic models makes even tentative generalization very difficult.

According to a preliminary report, in unilateral kidney obstruction in rat, cortical basal AdC was higher and less stimulated by PTH and renal medullary AdC was unchanged (Weber et al., 1976). In bilateral obstruction, renal medullary AdC was unchanged , but the addition of boiled homogenate from obstructed kidneys reportedly caused decreases in AdC stimulation by VP (Webster and Beck, 1976). In another study, basal cAMP levels in cortical tubules and its increase in response to PTH was not altered in the obstructed kidney (Nito et al., 1978). Also, no abnormality was found in the urinary excretion of N-cAMP after relief of the block of previously obstructed kidney (Purkerson et al., 1974).

A few comments should be made on the extracellular cNMP dynamics in renal insufficiency. As documented in several reports, levels of extracellular cAMP and cGMP are increased in renal failure with markedly lowered GFR (Broadus, 1977; Hamet et al., 1975). Diminished renal clearance of cAMP and cGMP seems to be a major factor, but slower degradation in extrarenal tissues may also contribute. Anomalous renal handling of cNMP in renal insufficiency makes determination of renal response to hormones (in terms of measurement of urinary N-cNMP) more difficult (Broadus, 1977); whether or not the evaluated levels of circulating cNMP have a pathologic effect is unclear.

CONCLUSIONS AND PERSPECTIVES

The role of cNMP in the regulation of kidney function, and also in renal pathophysiology, has received the vigorous attention of nephrologists, and investigations on renal cNMP system seem to enter a new phase with the advance of new methodologies. As in other areas of nephrology (use of micropuncture, microperfusion), emphasis is currently more and more directed towards studies of cNMP metabolism and action in individual segments of nephrons and specific cellular and subcellular structures. Future studies call for utilization of measurements of extracellular cNMP in a more sophisticated, parametric way, as a tool to measure the renal responsiveness to hormones by noninvasive means in a variety of clinical situations. A vigorous search for animal models of human renal diseases, spontaneous or induced, is in order because human renal tissue material is available on only a few occasions for direct investigations of cNMP. Finally, every advantage should be taken from the progress in techniques in cNMP research developed in nonrenal tissues, and the most advanced methodology should be applied without delay to the renal investigations.

ACKNOWLEDGMENTS

Experimental work from this laboratory reported in this article was supported by U.S. Public Health Service grants AM-16105, AM-21114; Grant-in-Aid from the American Heart Association, contributed in part by the Minnesota Heart Association and by the Mayo Foundation. Dr. Thomas E. Northrup provided help in the editing of the manuscript.

Thomas P. Dousa, M.D., is an Established Investigator of the American Heart Association (74-147).

Mrs. Ardith Walker provided excellent secretarial assistance.

REFERENCES

Abboud, H. E., Shah, S. V. & Dousa, T. P. (1979a). Effects of biogenic amines and prostaglandins on cAMP and cGMP in isolated glomeruli. *Clinical Research*, 27:406A.

Abboud, H. E., Ou, S.-Y. L. & Dousa, T. P. (1979b). Intrarenal localization and dynamics of histamine in the rat. *Clinical Research*, 27:405A.

Abboud, H. E., Shah, S. V. & Dousa, T. P. (1979c). Effects of dexamethasone on cyclic nucleotide accumulation in glomeruli. *Journal of Laboratory and Clinical Medicine*, 94, in press.

Anderson, R. J., Berl, T., McDonald, K. M. & Schrier, R. W. (1976). Prostaglandins: Effects on blood pressure, renal blood flow, sodium and water excretion. *Kidney International*, 10, 205–215.

Ashby, J. P., MacPherson, J. N. & Strong, J. A. (1977). The relationship between thyroid function and the renal response to parathyroid hormone. *Clinical Endocrinology*, 7, 167–170.

Aurbach, G. D. & Heath, D. (1974). Parathyroid hormone and calcitonin regulation of renal function. *Kidney International*, 6, 331–345.

Aurbach, G. D., Keutmann, H. T., Niall, H. D., Tregear, G. W., O'Riordan, J. L. H., Marcus, R., Marx, S. J. & Potts, J. T., Jr. (1972). Structure, synthesis, and mechanism of action of parathyroid hormone. *Recent Progress in Hormone Research*, 28, 353–398.

Aurbach, G. D., Marcus, R., Winickoff, R. N., Epstein, E. H., Jr., & Nigra, T. P. (1970). Urinary excretion of 3',5'-AMP in syndromes considered refractory to parathyroid hormone. *Metabolism*, 19, 799–808.

Baran, D. T., Shires, R., Klahr, S., Slatopolsky, E. & Avioli, L. V. (1978). Effect of acetazolamide (AC) in type I pseudohypoparathyroidism (PHP). *Clinical Research*, 26, 410A.

Baud, L., Sraer, J., Sraer, J-D, & Ardaillou, R. (1977). Effects of *Escherichia coli* lipopolysaccharide on renal glomerular and tubular adenylate cyclase. *Nephron* 19, 342–349.

Beck, N. (1976). Effect of dietary phosphorus (P) intake on renal actions of parathyroid hormone (PTH) and cyclic AMP (cAMP). *Kidney International*, 10, 487.

Beck, N. & Davis, B. F. (1975a). Effects of lithium on vasopressin-dependent cyclic AMP in rat renal medulla. *Endocrinology*, 97, 202–227.

Beck, N. & Davis, B. B. (1975b). Impaired renal response to parathyroid hormone in potassium depletion. *American Journal of Physiology*, 228, 179–183.

Beck, N., Kim, H. P., and Kim, K. S. (1975). Effect of metabolic acidosis on renal action of parathyroid hormone. *American Journal of Physiology*, 228, 1483–1488.

Beck, N. & Patak, R. V. (1978). Effect of prostaglandin E_2 (PGE$_2$) on cyclic AMP (cAMP) generation in isolated dog glomeruli. *Clinical Research*, **26**, 540A.

Beck, N., Reed, S. W. & Davis, B. B. (1973). Inability to concentrate urine in potassium-depleted (K↓) kidney due to impaired cyclic AMP (cAMP) system in renal medulla. *Abstracts of the 6th Annual Meeting of the American Society of Nephrology*, p. 9.

Beck, N., Singh, H., Reed, S. W. & Davis, B. B. (1974). Direct inhibitory effect of hypercalcemia on renal actions of parathyroid hormone. *Journal of Clinical Investigation*, **53**, 717–725.

Beck, N. & Webster, S. K. (1976). Impaired urinary concentrating ability and cyclic AMP in K$^+$-depleted rat kidney. *American Journal of Physiology*, **231**, 1204–1208.

Bell, N. H., Avery, S., Sinha, T., Clark, C. M., Jr., Allen, D. O. & Johnston, C., Jr. (1972). Effects of dibutyryl cyclic adenosine 3′,5′-monophosphate and parathyroid extract on calcium and phosphorus metabolism in hypoparathyroidism and pseudohypoparathyroidism. *Journal of Clinical Investigation*, **51**, 816–823.

Berndt, T., Marchand, G., Sell, T., Haas, J., Dousa, T. & Knox, F. (1978). The effects of parathyroid hormone (PTH) and calcitonin (CT) on electrolyte and cyclic AMP (cAMP) excretion in the rabbit. *Federation Proceedings, Federation of American Societies for Experimental Biology*, **37**, 728.

Blonde, L., Wehmann, R. E. & Steiner, A. L. (1974). Plasma clearance rates and renal clearance of ^{3}H-labeled cyclic AMP and ^{3}H-labeled cyclic GMP in the dog. *Journal of Clinical Investigation*, **53**, 163–172.

Bonjour, J. P., Preston, C. & Fleisch, H. (1977). Effect of 1,25-dihydroxy-vitamin D_3 on the renal handling of P$_i$ in thyroparathyroidectomized rats. *Journal of Clinical Investigation*, **60**, 1419–1428.

Boumendil-Podevin, E. F. & Podevin, R. A. (1977). Transport and metabolism of adenosine 3′,5′-monophosphate and N^6-O^2-dibutyryl adenosine 3′,5′-monophosphate by isolated renal tubules. *Journal of Biological Chemistry*, **252**, 6676–6681.

Bradley, S. E., Stephan, F., Coelho, J. B. & Reville, P. (1974). The thyroid and the kidney. *Kidney International*, **6**, 346–365.

Bradshaw, R. A. & Frazier, W. A. (1977). Hormone receptors as regulators of hormone action. In *Current Topics in Cellular Regulation*, ed. Horecker, B. L. & Stadtman, E. R. Pp. 1–37. New York: Academic Press.

Brenner, B. M., Baylis, C. & Deen, W. M. (1976). Transport of molecules across renal glomerular capillaries. *Physiological Reviews*, **56**, 502–534.

Broadus, A. E. (1977). Clinical cyclic nucleotide research. *Advances in Cyclic Nucleotide Research*, **8**, 509–548.

Broadus, A. E., McCaffrey, J. E., Bartter, F. C. & Neer, R. M. (1977). Nephrogenous cyclic adenosine monophosphate as a parathyroid function test. *Journal of Clinical Investigation*, **60**, 771–783.

Broadus, A. E., Deftos, L. J. & Bartter, F. C. (1978). Effects of the intravenous administration of calcium on nephrogenous cyclic AMP: Use as a parathyroid suppression test. *Journal of Clinical Endocrinology and Metabolism*, **46**:477–487.

Brunette, M. G., Chabardes, D., Imbert-Teboul, M., Clique, A., Montegut, M. & Morel, F. (1979). Hormone sensitive adenylate cyclase activity along the nephron of genetically hypophosphatemic mice. *Kidney International*, **15**, 357–369.

Butlen, D. & Jard, S. (1972). Renal handling of 3′,5′-cyclic AMP in the rat. The possible role of luminal 3′,5′-cyclic AMP in the tubular reabsorption of phosphate. *Pflügers Archiv*, **331**, 172–190.

Carnes, D. L., Anast, C. S., and Forte, L. R. (1978). Impaired renal adenylate cyclase response to parathyroid hormone in the calcium-deficient rat. *Endocrinology*, **102**, 45–51.

Cech, S. Y. & Ignarro, L. J. (1977). Cytidine 3′,5′-monophosphate (cyclic CMP) formation in mammalian tissues. *Science*, **198**, 1063–1065.

Chase, L. R. & Slatopolsky, E. (1974). Secretion and metabolic efficacy of parathyroid hormone in patients with severe hypomagnesemia. *Journal of Clinical Endocrinology and Metabolism*, **38**, 363–371.

Chase, L. R., Melson, G. L. & Aurbach, G. D. (1969). Pseudohypoparathyroidism: Defective excretion of 3′,5′-AMP in response to parathyroid hormone. *Journal of Clinical Investigation*, **48**, 1832–1844.

Coulson, R. (1976). Metabolism and excretion of exogenous adenosine 3′,5′-monophosphate and guanosine 3′,5′-monophosphate. Studies in the isolated perfused rat kidney and in the intact rat. *Journal of Biological Chemistry*, **251**, 4958–4967.

Craven, P. A. & DeRubertis, F. R. (1976). Properties and subcellular distribution of guanylate cyclase activity in rat renal medulla: Correlation with tissue content of guanosine 3',5'-monophosphate. *Biochemistry*, **15**, 6131–6137.

Criss, W. E. & Murad, F. (1976). Urinary excretion of cyclic guanosine 3',5'-monophosphate and cyclic adenosine 3',5'-monophosphate in rats bearing transplantable liver and kidney tumors. *Cancer Research*, **36**, 1714–1716.

Criss, W. E., Murad, F. & Kimura, H. (1976). Properties of guanylate cyclase from rat kidney cortex and transplantable kidney tumors. *Journal of Cyclic Nucleotide Research*, **2**, 11–19.

Czekalski, S., Loreau, N., Paillard, F., Ardaillou, R., Fillastre, J-P., & Mallet, E. (1974). Effect of bovine parathyroid hormone 1–34 fragment on renal production and excretion of adenosine 3',5'-monophosphate in man. *European Journal of Clinical Investigation*, **4**, 85–92.

Davis, B., Zor, U., Kaneko, T., Minz, D. H. & Field, J. B. (1969). Effects of parathyroid extract (PTE), arginine vasopressin (AVP) and prostaglandin E₁ (PGE₁) on urinary and renal tissue cyclic 3',5'-adenosine monophosphate cAMP. *Clinical Research*, **17**, 458.

DeRubertis, F. R. & Craven, P. A. (1977). Activation of the renal cortical and hepatic guanylate cyclase-guanosine 3',5'-monophosphate systems by nitrosoureas. Divalent cation requirements and relationship to thiol reactivity. *Biochimica et Biophysica Acta*, **499**, 337–351.

de Troyer, A. & Demanet, J-C. (1975). Correction of antidiuresis by demeclocycline. *New England Journal of Medicine*, **293**, 915–918.

Dicker, S. E. & Greenbaum, A. L. (1977). Changes in renal cyclic nucleotide content as a possible trigger to the initiation of compensatory renal hypertrophy in rats. *Journal of Physiology*, **271**, 505–514.

Dousa, T. P. (1974a). Interactions of lithium with vasopressin-sensitive cyclic AMP system of human renal medulla. *Endocrinology*, **95**, 1359–1366.

Dousa, T. P. (1974b). Modern medical physiology. Cellular action of antidiuretic hormone in nephrogenic diabetes insipidus. *Mayo Clinic Proceedings*, **49**, 188–199.

Dousa, T. P. (1976). Drugs and other agents affecting the renal adenylate cyclase system. In *Methods in Pharmacology*, ed. Martinez-Maldonado, M. Vol. 4A, pp. 293–331. New York: Plenum Press.

Dousa, T. P. & Barnes, L. D. (1977a). Cyclic nucleotides in regulation of renal function. In *Cyclic 3',5'-nucleotides: Mechanism of Action*, ed. Cramer, H. & Schultz, J. Pp. 251–262. New York: John Wiley & Sons.

Dousa, T. P. & Barnes, L. D. (1977b). Regulation of protein kinase by vasopressin in renal medulla in situ. *American Journal of Physiology*, **232**, F50–F57.

Dousa, T. P., Barnes, L. D. & Kim, J. K. (1977a). The role of the cyclic-AMP-dependent protein phosphorylations and microtubules in the cellular action of vasopressin in mammalian kidney. In *Neurohypophysis*, ed. Moses, A. M. & Share, L. Pp. 220–235. Basel, Switzerland: S. Karger.

Dousa, T. P., Barnes, L. D., Ong, S-H. & Steiner, A. L. (1977b). Immunohistochemical localization of 3',5'-cyclic AMP and 3',5'-cyclic GMP in rat renal cortex: Effect of parathyroid hormone. *Proceedings of the National Academy of Sciences (U.S.A.)*, **74**, 3569–3573.

Dousa, T. P., Hui, Y. S. F. & Barnes, L. D. (1975). Renal medullary adenylate cyclase in rats with hypothalamic diabetes insipidus. *Endocrinology*, **97**, 802–807.

Dousa, T. P., Hui, Y. S. F. & Barnes, L. D. (1978). Microtubule assembly in renal medullary slices: effects of vasopressin, vinblastine, and lithium. *Journal of Laboratory and Clinical Medicine*, **91**, 252–264.

Dousa, T. P. & Northrup, T. E. (1978). Cellular interactions between vasopressin and prostaglandins in the mammalian kidney. In *Contributions to Nephrology*, **12**, 106–115 (Karger, Basel).

Dousa, T. P. & Rychlik, I. (1970). The metabolism of adenosine 3',5'-cyclic phosphate. II. Some properties of adenosine 3',5'-cyclic phosphate phosphodiesterase from the rat kidney. *Biochimica et Biophysica Acta*, **204**, 10–17.

Dousa, T. P., Shah, S. V. & Abboud, H. E. (1980). Potential role of cyclic nucleotides in glomerular disorders. *Advances in Cyclic Nucleotide Research*, **12**, in press.

Dousa, T. P. & Valtin, H. (1974). Cellular action of antidiuretic hormone in mice with inherited vasopressin-resistant urinary concentrating defects. *Journal of Clinical Investigation*, **54**, 753–762.

Dousa, T. P. & Valtin, H. (1976). Cellular actions of vasopressin in the mammalian kidney. *Kidney International*, **10**, 46–63.

Drezner, M. K. & Burch, W. M., Jr. (1978). Altered activity of the nucleotide regulatory site in the parathyroid hormone-sensitive adenylate cyclase from the renal cortex of a patient with pseudohypoparathyroidism. *Journal of Clinical Investigation*, **62**, 1222–1227.

Drezner, M. K. & Haussler, M. R. (1978). Normocalcemic pseudohypoparathyroidism (PsH): Association with normal vitamin D_3 metabolism. *Clinical Research*, **26**, 413A.

Drezner, M., Neelon, F. A. & Lebovitz, H. E. (1973). Pseudohypoparathyroidism type II: A possible defect in the reception of the cyclic AMP signal. *New England Journal of Medicine*, **289**, 1056–1060.

Earp, H. S. & Steiner, A. L. (1978). Compartmentalization of cyclic nucleotide-mediated hormone action. *Annual Review of Pharmacology and Toxicology*, **18**, 431–459.

Edwards, R. M., Hui, Y. S. F., Torres, V. E., Northrup, T. E. & Dousa, T. P. (1978). Adenylate cyclase in glomeruli and tubules isolated from rat kidney: Effect of parathyroid hormone (PTH). *Abstracts of the 60th Annual Meeting of the Endocrine Society* (Miami, FL), p. 481.

Edwards, R. M., Jackson, B. A. & Dousa, T. P. (1979). Protein kinase activity in microdissected medullary collecting tubule (MCT) and medullary ascending limb of Henle's loop (ALH): Effects of cyclic AMP (cAMP) and vasopressin (VP). *Clinical Research*, **27**, 496A.

Edwards, R. M., Jackson, B. A. & Dousa, T. P. (1979a). Vasopressin-sensitive adenylate cyclase in ascending limb of Henle's loop and in collecting tubules of mice with hereditary nephrogenic diabetes insipidus. *The Physiologist*, **22**, in press.

Feldman, H. A. & Singer, I. (1974). Comparative effects of tetracyclines on water flow across toad urinary bladders. *Journal of Pharmacology and Experimental Therapeutics*, **190**, 358–364.

Fine, L. G., Schlondorff, D., Trizna, W., Gilbert, R. M. & Bricker, N. S. (1978). Functional profile of the isolated uremic nephron. Impaired water permeability and adenylate cyclase responsiveness of the cortical collecting tubule to vasopressin. *Journal of Clinical Investigation*, **21**, 1519–1527.

Finn, A. L., Handler, J. S. & Orloff, J. (1966). Relation between toad bladder potassium content and permeability response to vasopressin. *American Journal of Physiology*, **210**, 1279–1284.

Forte, L. R., Nickols, G. A., and Anast, C. S. (1976). Renal adenylate cyclase and the interrelationship between parathyroid hormone and vitamin D in the regulation of urinary phosphate and adenosine cyclic 3′,5′-monophosphate excretion. *Journal of Clinical Investigation*, **57**, 559–568.

Frandsen, E. K. & Krishna, G. (1976). A simple ultrasensitive method for the assay of cyclic AMP and cyclic GMP in tissues. *Life Sciences*, **18**, 529–542.

Friedler, R. M., Descoeudres, C., Kurokawa, K., Kreusser, W. J. & Massry, S. G. (1977). Role of cyclic AMP in the natriuresis of extracellular fluid volume expansion in the dog. *Clinical Science and Molecular Medicine*, **53**, 563–571.

Friedman, D. L. (1976). Role of cyclic nucleotides in cell growth and differentiation. *Physiological Reviews*, **56**, 652–708.

Galvez, O., Roberts, B., Bay, W. & Ferris, T. (1976). Studies of mechanism of polyuria with hypokalemia. *Clinical Research*, **24**, 544A.

Gengler, W. R. & Forte, L. R. (1972). Neonatal development of rat kidney adenyl cyclase and phosphodiesterase. *Biochimica et Biophysica Acta*, **279**, 367–372.

Gilbert, P. J., Schlondorff, D., Trizna, W. & Fine, L. G. (1978). Absence of PTH-induced phosphaturia with normal adenylate cyclase in the rabbit. *Abstracts of the 7th International Congress of Nephrology*, (Montreal, Canada), p. E–11.

Glorieux, F. & Scriver, C. R. (1972). Loss of a parathyroid hormone-sensitive component of phosphate transport in X-linked hypophosphatemia. *Science*, **175**, 997–1000.

Goldberg, N. D. & Haddox, M. K. (1977). Cyclic GMP metabolism and involvement in biological regulation. *Annual Review of Biochemistry*, **46**, 823–896.

Goldberg, N. D., Haddox, M. K., Nicol, S. E., Acott, T. S., Glass, D. B. & Zeilig, C. E. (1976). Cyclic GMP and cyclic AMP in biological regulation. In *Control Mechanisms in Cancer*, ed. Criss, W. E., Ono, T. & Sabine, J. R. Pp. 99–108. New York: Raven Press.

Goldring, S. R., Dayer, J.-M., Ausiello, D. A. & Krane, S. M. (1978). A cell strain cultured from porcine kidney increases cyclic AMP content upon exposure to calcitonin or vasopressin. *Biochemical and Biophysical Research Communications*, **83**, 434–440.

Grantham, J. J. & Orloff, J. (1968). Effect of prostaglandin E$_1$ on the permeability response of the isolated collecting tubule to vasopressin, adenosine 3',5'-monophosphate and theophylline. *Journal of Clinical Investigation,* **47,** 1154–1161.

Hahn, T. J., Chase, L. R. & Avioli, L. V. (1972). Effect of magnesium depletion on responsiveness to parathyroid hormone in parathyroidectomized rats. *Journal of Clinical Investigation,* **51,** 886–891.

Hall, D. A., (1979). Possible role of vasopressin in regulating solute transport in mouse medullary thick ascending limb of Henle's loop. *Clinical Research,* **27,** 416A.

Hall, D. A., Barnes, L. D. & Dousa, T. P. (1977). Cyclic AMP in action of antidiuretic hormone: Effects of exogenous cyclic AMP and its new analogue. *American Journal of Physiology,* **232,** F368–F376.

Hamet, P., Stouder, D. A., Ginn, H. E., Hardman, J. G. & Liddle, G. W. (1975). Studies of the elevated extracellular concentration of cyclic AMP in uremic man. *Journal of Clinical Investigation,* **56,** 339–345.

Handler, J. S. & Orloff, J. (1973). The mechanism of action of antidiuretic hormone. In *Handbook of Physiology,* ed. Orloff, J. & Berliner, R. W. Section 8, Renal Physiology, p. 791. Washington, D.C.: American Physiology Society.

Harkcom, T. M., Kim, J. K., Palumbo, P. J., Hui, Y. S. F. & Dousa, T. P. (1978). Modulatory effect of thyroid function on enzymes of vasopressin-sensitive cyclic AMP system in renal medulla. *Endocrinology,* **102,** 1475–1484.

Harper, J. F. & Brooker, G. (1975). Femtomole sensitive radioimmunoassay for cyclic AMP and cyclic GMP after 2'0 acetylation by acetic anhydride in aqueous solution. *Journal of Nucleotide Research,* **1,** 207–218.

Helwig, J-J., Bollack, C., Mandel, P. & Goridis, C. (1975). Renal cortex guanylate cyclase preferential enrichment in glomerular membranes. *Biochimica et Biophysica Acta,* **377,** 463–472.

Horiuchi, N., Suda, T., Takahashi, H., Shimazwa, E. & Ogta, E. (1977). In vivo evidence for the intermediary role of 3',5'-cyclic AMP in parathyroid hormone-induced stimulation of 1α,25-dihydroxyvitamin D$_3$ synthesis in rats. *Endocrinology,* **101,** 969–974.

Humes, H. D., Ichikawa, I., Troy, J. L. & Brenner, B. M. (1978). Evidence for a parathyroid hormone-dependent influence of calcium on the glomerular ultrafiltration coefficient. *Journal of Clinical Investigation,* **61,** 32–40.

Humes, H. D., Simmons, C. F., Jr., & Brenner, B. M. (1978). The effect of ADH on renal phosphate excretion: Evidence that ADH influences parathormone release. *Clinical Research,* **26,** 565A.

Hunt, N. H., Shortland, J. R., Michelangeli, V. P., Hammonds, J. C., Atkins, D. & Martin, T. J. (1978). Adenylate cyclase activity of renal cortical carcinoma and its relation to histology and ultrastructure. *Cancer Research,* **38,** 23–31.

Ichikawa, I., Humes, H. D., Dousa, T. P. & Brenner, B. M. (1978). Influence of parathyroid hormone on glomerular ultrafiltration in the rat. *American Journal of Physiology,* **234,** F393–F401; or *American Journal of Physiology; Renal Fluid Electrolyte Physiology,* **3,** F393–F401.

Imbert, M., Chabardes, D., Montegut, M., Clique, A. & Morel, F. (1975). Vasopressin-dependent adenylate cyclase in single segments of rabbit kidney tubule. *Pflügers Archiv,* **357,** 173–186.

Imbert, M., Chabardes, D. & Morel, F. (1974). Hormone sensitive adenylate cyclase in isolated rabbit glomeruli. *Molecular and Cellular Endocrinology,* **1,** 295–304.

Imbert-Teboul, M., Chabardes, D., Montegut, M., Clique, A. & Morel, F. (1978a). Vasopressin-dependent adenylate cyclase activities in the rat kidney medulla: Evidence for two separate sites of action. *Endocrinology,* **102,** 1254–1261.

Imbert-Teboul, M., Chabardes, D., Montegut, M., Cique, A., & Morel, F. (1978b). Impaired response to vasopressin of adenylate cyclase of the thick ascending limb of Henle's loop in Brattleboro rats with diabetes insipidus. *Renal Physiolopy,* Basel **1,** 3–10.

Ishizuka, I., Tadano, K., Nagata, N., Nümura, Y. & Nagai, Y. (1978). Hormone-specific responses and biosynthesis of sulfolipids in cell lines derived from mammalian kidney. *Biochimica et Biophysica Acta,* **541,** 467–482.

Jackson, B. A., Northrup, T. E. & Dousa, T. P. (1978a). Differential response of adenylate cyclase (AC) to vasopressin (VP), parathyroid hormone (PTH) and calcitonin (CT) in rat, rabbit and dog kidney. *The Physiologist,* **21,** 58.

Jackson, B. A., Edwards, R. M. & Dousa, T. P. (1978). Cyclic AMP phosphodiesterase in microdissected medullary ascending limb of Henle's loop (ALH) and medullary collecting tubule (MCT). *Clinical Research*, **26**, 780A.

Jackson, B. A., Hui, Y. S. F., Northrup, T. E. & Dousa, T. P. (1979a). Differential responsiveness of adenylate cylase from rat, dog and rabbit kidney to parathyroid hormone, vasopressin and calcitonin. *Mineral Electrolyte Metabolism*, in press.

Jackson, B. A., Edwards, R. M., Heublein, D. M. & Dousa, T. P. (1979b). Effects of adrenalectomy (AdX) and dexamethasone on cAMP phosphodiesterase (PDE) in microdissected medullary ascending limb (ALH) and medullary collecting tubule (MCT). *Clinical Research*, **27**, 418A.

Jackson, B. A., Edwards, R. M. & Dousa, T. P. (1979c). Differential effect of Ibuprofen on vasopressin-sensitive adenylate cyclase in medullary collecting tubule (MCT) and in medullary thick ascending limb of Henle's loop (ALH). *The Physiologist*, **22**, in press.

Kahn, C. R. (1976). Membrane receptors for hormones and neurotransmitters. *Journal of Cellular Biology*, **70**, 261–286.

Kakuta, S., Sato, C., Suda, T., Kimura, N., Araki, N., Ono, Y. & Nagata, N. (1978). Relationship between parathyroid hormone and adenosine 3′,5′-monophosphate metabolism in the kidney of vitamin D-deficient rats. *Biochimica et Biophysica Acta*, **539**, 173–180.

Kaliner, M. & Austen, K. F. (1975). Immunologic release of chemical mediators from human tissues. *Annual Review of Pharmacology*, **15**, 117–189.

Kim, J. K., Frohnert, P. P., Hui, Y. S. F., Barnes, L. D., Farrow, G. M. & Dousa, T. P. (1977a). Enzymes of cyclic 3′,5′-nucleotide metabolism in human renal cortex and renal adenocarcinoma. *Kidney International*, **12**, 172–183.

Kim, J. K., Hui, Y. S. F., Northrup, T. E., Valtin, H. & Dousa, T. P. (1977b). Activation of protein kinase (PK) by [8-Arg]-vasopressin (AVP) in renal medulla (RM) slices from mice with nephrogenic diabetes insipidus (NDI). *Federation Proceedings, Federation of American Societies for Experimental Biology*, **36**, 592.

Kimura, H. & Murad, F. (1975). Subcellular localization of guanylate cyclase. *Life Sciences*, **17**, 837–843.

Knox, F. G., Hoppe, A., Kempson, S. A., Shah, S. V. & Dousa, T. P. (1979). Cellualr mechanisms of phosphate transport. In *Renal Handling of Phosphate*, ed. Massry, S. G. New York, Plenum Press. (in press).

Knox, F. G., Preiss, J., Kim, J. K. & Dousa, T. P. (1977). Mechanism of resistance to the phosphaturic effect of the parathyroid hormone in the hamster. *Journal of Clinical Investigation*, **59**, 675–683.

Kuo, F. J. & Greengard, P. (1969). Cyclic nucleotide-dependent protein kinases. IV. Widespread occurrence of adenosine 3′,5′-dependent protein kinase in various tissues and phyla of the animal kingdom. *Proceedings of the National Academy of Sciences (U.S.A.)*, **64**, 1349–1355.

Kuo, J. F., Brackett, N. L., Shoji, M. & Tse, J. (1978). Cytidine 3′,5′-monophosphate phosphodiesterase in mammalian tissues. Occurrence and biological involvement. *Journal of Biological Chemistry*, **253**, 2518–2521.

Kuo, J. F., Malveaux, E. J., Patrick, J. G., Davis, C. W., Kuo, W-N. & Puritt, A. W. (1977). Cyclic GMP-dependent and cyclic AMP-dependent protein kinases, protein kinase modulators and phosphodiesterases in arteries and veins of dogs. Distribution and effects of arteriovenous fistula and arterial occlusion. *Biochimica et Biophysica Acta*, **497**, 785–796.

Kurokawa, K., Aznar, E., Descoeudres, C., Zulueta, A. & Massry, S. G. (1978). Effects of glucocorticoid deficiency on renal medullary cyclic adenosine monophosphate of rats. *Clinical Science and Molecular Medicine*, **54**, 573–577.

Kurokawa, K., Kreusser, W. J., Aznar, E. & Massry, S. G. (1977). In vivo renal cyclic AMP levels and cyclic AMP dependent protein kinase (PK) activity in phosphate depletion (PD). *Clinical Research*, **24**, 439A.

Lang, M. A. & Edelman, I. S. (1972). Effects of aldosterone and vasopressin on adenylate cyclase activity of rat kidney. *American Journal of Physiology*, **272**, 21–24.

Lichtenstein, L. M. (1976). Hormone receptor modulation of cAMP in the control of allergic and inflammatory responses. In *The Role of Immunological Factors in Infections, Allergic and Anti-immune Processes*, ed. Beers, R. F., Jr. & Bassett, E. G. Ch. 30, pp. 339–354. New York: Raven Press.

Lincoln, T. M. & Corbin, J. D. (1978). On the role of the cAMP and cGMP-dependent protein kinases in cell function. *Journal in Cyclic Nucleotide Research*, **4**, 3–14.

Lincoln, T. M., Hall, C. L., Park, C. R. & Corbin, J. C. (1976). Guanosine 3′,5′-cyclic monophosphate binding proteins in rat tissues. *Proceedings of the National Academy of Sciences (U.S.A.)*, **73**, 2559–2563.

Loreau, N., Cosyns, J. P., Lepreux, C., Verroust, P. & Ardaillou, R. (1977). Renal calcitonin receptors and adenylate cyclase in rats immunized against tubular basement membrane. *Kidney International*, **12**, 184–192.

Marcus, R., Wilber, J. F. & Aurbach, G. D. (1971). Parathyroid hormone-sensitive adenyl cyclase from the renal cortex of a patient with pseudohypoparathyroidism. *Journal of Clinical Endocrinology*, **33**, 537–541.

Melmon, K. L. & Insel, P. A. (1977). Inflammatory and immune responses: Cell individuality amidst ubiquitous hormonal signals. *Johns Hopkins Medical Journal*, **141**, 15–22.

Metz, S. A., Baylink, D. J., Huighes, M. R., Haussler, M. R. & Robertson, R. P. (1977). Selective deficiency of 1,25-dihydroxycholecalciferol. A cause of isolated skeletal resistance to parathyroid hormone. *New England Journal of Medicine*, **297**, 1084–1090.

Michael, U. F., Kelley, J., Alpert, H. & Vaamonde, C. A. (1976). Role of distal delivery of filtrate in impaired renal dilution of the hypothyroid rat. *American Journal of Physiology*, **230**, 699–705.

Mittal, K-C. & Murad, F. (1977). Properties and oxidative regulation of guanylate cyclase. *Journal in Cyclic Nucleotide Research*, **3**, 381–391.

Morel, F., Chabardes, D. & Imbert, M. (1975). Target sites of antidiuretic hormone (ADH) and parathyroid hormone (PTH) along the segments of the nephron. In *Advances in Nephrology*, ed. Hamburger, J., Crosiner, J. & Maxwell, M. H. Vol. 5, pp. 283–300. Chicago: Yearbook Medical.

Morel, F., Chabardes, D. & Imbert-Teboul, M. (1978a). Heterogeneity of hormonal control in the distal nephron. In *Proc. 7th International Congress of Nephrology*, eds. Barcelo, R., Bergeron, M., Carriere, S., Dirks, J. H., Drummond, K., Guttmann, R. D., Lemieux, G., Mongeau, J-G. & Seely, J. F. Pp. 209–216. Basel: S. Karger.

Morel, F., Chabardes, D. & Imbert-Teboul, M. (1978b). Methodology for enzymatic studies of isolated tubular segments: Adenylate cyclase. In *Methods in Pharmacology*, ed. Martinex-Maldonado, M. Vol. 4B, pp. 297–323. New York: Plenum.

Morel, F., Imbert, M. & Chabardes, D. (1976). Measurement of hormone dependent adenylate cyclase activity in single pieces of rabbit kidney tubules. In *Renal Metabolism in Relation to Renal Function* (Current Problems in Clinical Biochemistry, No. 6), eds. Schmidt, U. & Dubach, U.C. Pp. 214–222. Bern: Hans Huber.

Murad, F. (1973). Clinical studies and applications of cyclic nucleotides. *Advances in Cyclic Nucleotide Research*, **3**, 355–383.

Nakajima, T., Naitoh, F. & Kuruma, I. (1977). Elevation of adenosine 3′,5′-monophosphate in the perfusate of rat kidney after addition of dopamine. *European Journal of Pharmacology*, **45**, 195–197.

Nimmo, H. G. & Cohen, P. (1977). Hormonal control of protein phosphorylation. *Advances in Cyclic Nucleotide Research*, **8**, 145–266.

Nito, H., Descoeudres, C., Kurokawa, K. & Massry, S. G. (1978). Effect of unilateral ureteral obstruction on renal cell metabolism and function. *Journal of Laboratory and Clinical Medicine*, **91**, 60–71.

Parker, C. W., Sulivan, T. J. & Wedner, H. J. (1974). Cyclic AMP and the immune response. *Advances in Cyclic Nucleotide Research*, **4**, 1–79.

Pawlson, L. G., Taylor, A., Mintz, D. H., Field, J. B. & Davis, B. B. (1970). Effect of vasopressin on renal cyclic AMP generation in potassium deficiency and patients with sickle hemoglobin. *Metabolism*, **19**, 694–700.

Purkerson, M. L., Rolf, D. B., Chase, L. R., Slatopolsky, E. & Klahr, S. (1974). Tubular reabsorption of phosphate after release of complete ureteral obstruction in the rat. *Kidney International*, **5**, 326–336.

Raisz, L. G., Mundy, G. R., Dietrich, J. W. & Canalis, E. M. (1977). Hormonal regulation of mineral metabolism. In *Endocrine Physiology II*, ed. McCann, S. M. Vol. 16, Ch. 6. Baltimore: University Park Press.

Rajerison, R. M., Butlen, D. & Jard, S. (1976). Ontogenic development of antidiuretic hormone receptors in rat kidney: Comparison of hormonal binding and adenylate cyclase activation. *Molecular and Cellular Endocrinology* (Amsterdam), **4**, 271–285.

Rajerison, R. M., Butlen, D. & Jard, S. (1977). Effects of in vivo treatment with vasopressin and analogues on renal adenylate cyclase responsiveness to vasopressin stimulation in vitro. *Endocrinology*, **101**, 1–12.

Rajerison, R., Marchetti, J., Roy, C., Bockaert, J. & Jard, S. (1974). The vasopressin-sensitive adenylate cyclase of the rat kidney: Effect of adrenalectomy and corticosteroids on hormonal receptor-enzyme coupling. *Journal of Biological Chemistry*, **249**, 6390–6400.

Robison, G. A., Butcher, R. W. & Sutherland, E. W. (1971). *Cyclic AMP*. New York: Academic Press.

Rodgers, G. M., Fisher, J. W. & George, W. J. (1975a). Renal cyclic AMP accumulation and adenylate cyclase stimulation by erythropoietic agents. *American Journal of Physiology*, **229**, 1387–1392.

Rodgers, G. M., Fisher, J. W. & George, W. J. (1975b). The role of renal adenosine 3′,5′-monophosphate in the control of erythropoietin production. *American Journal of Medicine*, **58**, 31–38.

Rodriguez, H. J., Villarreal, H., Jr., Klahr, S. & Slatopolsky, E. (1974). Pseudohypoparathyroidism type II: Restoration of normal renal responsiveness to parathyroid hormone by calcium administration. *Journal of Endocrinology and Metabolism*, **39**, 693–701.

Rubin, C. S. & Rosen, O. M. (1975). Protein phosphorylation. *Annual Review of Biochemistry*, **44**, 83–161.

Rutecki, G. W., Nally, J. V., Bay, W. H. & Ferris, T. F. (1977). The acute effects of lithium (Li) on renal function. *Kidney International*, **12**, 571.

Schlondorff, D. & Weber, H. (1976). Cyclic nucleotide metabolism in compensatory renal hypertrophy and neonatal kidney growth. *Proceedings of the National Academy of the Sciences (U.S.A.)*, **73**, 524–528.

Schlondorff, D., Weber, H., Trizna, W. & Fine, L. G. (1978). Vasopressin responsiveness of renal adenylate cyclase in newborn rats and rabbits. *American Journal of Physiology*, **234**, F16–F21.

Schlondorff, D., Yoo, P. & Alpert, B. E. (1978). Stimulation of adenylate cyclase in isolated rat glomeruli by prostaglandins. *American Journal of Physiology*, **235**, F458–F468.

Seif, S. M., Zenser, T. V., Huellmantel, A. B. & Davis, B. B. (1977). Elevated plasma vasopressin and impaired renal cyclic nucleotide generation in myxedematous rats. *Abstracts of the 59th Annual Meeting of Endocrine Society*, (Abstr. #374) p. 243, Chicago, IL.

Shah, S. V., Northrup, T. E., Hui, Y. S. F. & Dousa, T. P. (1979). Action of serotonin (5-hydroxytryptamine) on cyclic nucleotides in glomeruli of rat renal cortex. *Kidney International*, **15**, 463–472.

Shaw, J. W., Oldham, S. B., Rosoff, L., Bethune, J. E. & Fichman, M. P. (1977). Urinary cyclic AMP analyzed as a function of the serum calcium and parathyroid hormone in the differential diagnosis of hypercalcemia. *Journal of Clinical Investigation*, **59**, 14–21.

Shoji, M. & Kuo, W-N. (1978). Molecular and pathophysiologic aspects of mammalian cyclic GMP-dependent protein kinase. *American Review of Pharmacology and Toxicology*, **18**, 341–355.

Singer, I. & Forrest, J. N., Jr., (1976). Drug-induced states of nephrogenic diabetes insipidus. *Kidney International*, **10**, 82–95.

Sinha, T. K., DeLuca, H. F. & Bell, N. H. (1977). Evidence for a defect in the formation of 1α-25-dihydroxyvitamin D in pseudohypoparathyroidism. *Metabolism*, **26**, 731–738.

Slatopolsky, E., Mercado, A., Morrison, A., Yates, T. & Klahr, S. (1976). Inhibitory effects of hypomagnesemia on the renal action of parathyroid hormone. *Journal of Clinical Investigation*, **58**, 1273–1279.

Sovik, O. & Apold, J. (1976). Urinary cyclic AMP: High concentrations in vitamin D-deficient and -dependent rickets. *Journal of Pediatrics*, **89**, 946–949.

Sraer, J., Ardaillou, R. & Couette, S. (1974a). Increased binding of calcitonin to renal receptors in parathyroidectomized rats. *Endocrinology*, **95**, 632–637.

Sraer, J., Ardaillou, R., Loreau, N. & Sraer, J. D. (1974b). Evidence for parathyroid hormone sensitive adenylate cyclase in rat glomeruli. *Molecular and Cellular Endocrinology*, **1**, 285–294.

Stadel, J. M. & Goodman, D. B. P. (1978). 8-p-chrophenylthio-cyclic AMP: a potent partial simulator of antidiuretic hormone action. *Journal of Cyclic Nucleotide Research*, **4**, 35–43.

Steele, T. H. (1976). Renal resistance ot parathyroid hormone during phosphorus deprivation. *Journal of Clinical Investigation*, **58**, 1461–1464.

Steiner, A. L., Parker, C. W. & Kipnis, D. M. (1972). Radioimmunoassay for cyclic nucleotides. I. Preparation of antibodies and iodinated cyclic nucleotides. *Journal of Biological Chemistry*, **247**, 1106–1113.

Steiner, A. L., Ong, S-H. & Wedner, H. J. (1976). Cyclic nucleotide immunocytochemistry. *Advances in Cyclic Nucleotide Research*, **7**, 115–155.

Stoff, J. S., Handler, J. S. & Orloff, J. (1972). The effect of aldosterone on the accumulation of adenosine 3′,5′-cyclic monophosphate in toad bladder epithelial cells in response to vasopressin and theophylline. *Proceedings of the National Academy of Sciences (U.S.A.)*, **69**, 805–808.

Stoff, J. S., Silva, P., Rosa, R. & Epstein, F. H. (1978). Effect of indomethacin on water excretion in diabetes insipidus: Possible action of prostaglandins independent of antidiuretic hormone. *Clinical Research*, **26**, 477A.

Strada, S. J. & Thompson, W. J. (1978). Multiple forms of cyclic nucleotide phosphodiesterases: anomalies or biologic regulators? *Advances in Cyclic Nucleotide Research*, **9**, 265–283.

Strewler, G. J., Manganiello, V. C. & Vanghan, M. (1978). Phosphodiesterase activator from rat kidney cortex. *Journal of Biological Chemistry*, **253**, 390–393.

Strewler, G. J. & Orloff, J. (1977). Role of cyclic nucleotides in the transport of water and electrolytes. *Advances in Cyclic Nucleotide Research*, **8**, 311–361.

Tomlinson, S., Hendy, G. W., Pemberton, D. M. & O'Riordan, J. L. H. (1976). Reversible resistance to renal action of parathyroid hormone in rat. *Clinical Science and Molecular Medicine*, **51**, 59–69.

Torres, V. E., Hui, Y. S. F., Shah, S. V., Northrup, T. E. & Dousa, T. P. (1978a). Cyclic nucleotide phosphodiesterases in glomeruli of rat renal cortex. *Kidney International*, **14**, 444–451.

Torres, V. E., Northrup, T. E., Edwards, R. M., Shah, S. V. & Dousa, T. P. (1978b). Modulation of cyclic nucleotides in isolated glomeruli: role of histamine, carbamylcholine, parathyroid hormone and angiotensin II. *Journal of Clinical Investigation*, **62**, 1334–1343.

Ueland, P. M. & Doskeland, S. O. (1977). An adenosine 3′,5′-monophosphate-adenosine binding protein from mouse liver. *Journal of Biological Chemistry*, **252**, 677–686.

Vainsel, M., Manderlier, T. & Otten, J. (1976). Urinary excretion of adenosine 3′,5′-monophosphate in vitamin D deficiency. *European Journal of Clinical Investigation*, **6**, 127–130.

Valtin, H., Sokoi, H. W. & Sunde, D. (1975). Genetic approaches to the study of the regulation and actions of vasopressin. *Recent Progress in Hormone Research*, **31**, 447–486.

Van Inwegan, R. G., Swafford, R. L., Strada, S. J. & Thompson, W. J. (1977). Characterization of particulate cyclic nucleotide phosphodiesterases of rat kidney. *Archives of Biochemistry and Biophysics*, **178**, 58–68.

Velosa, J. A., Shah, S. V., Abboud, H. E. & Dousa, T. P. (1980). Impaired accumulation of glomerular cAMP in response to histamine (Hi) and serotonin (SE) in experimental nephrosis. *Advances in Cyclic Nucleotide Research*, **12**, in press.

Wald, H., Gutman, Y. & Czaczkes, W. (1977). Effect of salt loading in the rat on adenylate cyclase and phosphodiesterase activity in kidney cortex, medulla and papilla. *Enzyme*, **22**, 336–340.

Wallin, J. D. & Kaplan, R. A. (1977). Effect of sodium fluoride on concentrating and diluting ability in the rat. *American Journal of Physiology*, **232**, F355–F340.

Wallin, J. D., Kaplan, R. A., Clifton, G. & Leichter, S. B. (1978). Biochemical basis for the fluoride-induced urinary concentrating defect in the rat. *Clinical Research*, **26**, 478A.

Weber, H., Schlondorff, D. & Trizna, W. (1976). Renal adenylate cyclase (AC) in experimental kidney disease. *Clinical Research*, **24**, 415A.

Webster, S. K. & Beck, N. (1976). Impairment of vasopressin (VP)-dependent cyclic AMP (cAMP) and urinary concentrating ability in uremia. *Clinical Research*, **24**, 415A.

Wells, J. N. & Hardman, J. G. (1977). Cyclic nucleotide phosphodiesterases. *Advances in Cyclic Nucleotide Research*, **8**, 119–143.

Zenser, T. V., Robinson, A. G., Seif, S. M. & Davis, B. B. (1978). Impaired inner medullary production of prostaglandin E_2 in the kidney of myxedematous rat. *Endocrinology*, **102**, 884–888.

Zusman, R. M. & Keiser, H. R. (1977). Prostaglandin biosynthesis by rabbit renomedullary interstitial cells in tissue culture. Stimulation by angiotensin II, bradykinin, and arginine vasopressin. *Journal of Clinical Investigation*, **60**, 215–223.

Zusman, R. M., Keiser, H. R. & Handler, J. S. (1977a). Inhibition of vasopressin-stimulated prostaglandin E biosynthesis by chlorpropamide in the toad urinary bladder. Mechansim of enhancement of vasopressin-stimulated water flow. *Journal of Clinical Investigation*, **60**, 1348–1353.

Zusman, R. M., Keiser, H. R. & Handler, J. S. (1977b). Vasopressin-stimulated prostaglandin E biosynthesis in the toad urinary bladder. Effect on water flow. *Journal of Clinical Investigation*, **60**, 1339–1347.

Zusman, R. M., Keiser, H. R. & Handler, J. S. (1978). Effect of adrenal steroids on vasopressin-stimulated PGE synthesis and water flow. *American Journal of Physiology*, **234**, F532–F540.

Index

Page numbers in *italics* represent illustrations;
page numbers followed by (t) represent tables.